D1740559

THYROID FUNCTION TESTING

6 WEEK LOAN

040112

ENDOCRINE UPDATES
Shlomo Melmed, M.D., Series Editor

For further volumes:
http://www.springer.com/series/5917

THYROID FUNCTION TESTING

Edited by

Gregory A. Brent
Professor of Medicine and Physiology
David Geffen School of Medicine at UCLA
Los Angeles, CA, USA

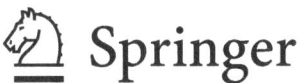 Springer

Editor
Gregory A. Brent
Departments of Medicine and Physiology
David Geffen School of Medicine at UCLA
Los Angeles, CA, USA
gbrent@ucla.edu

ISSN 1566-0729
ISBN 978-1-4614-2575-5   e-ISBN 978-1-4419-1485-9
DOI 10.1007/978-1-4419-1485-9
Springer New York Dordrecht Heidelberg London

Preface

Thyroid function tests are utilized by essentially all medical practitioners, across every clinical setting, in patients from newborns to the elderly. They are the most frequently measured endocrine tests. The sensitive thyrotropin (TSH) assay reflects thyroid hormone feedback to the pituitary, and is diagnostic of both thyroid hormone excess as well as deficiency. The log–linear relationship between serum TSH and thyroxine concentrations means that small changes in serum thyroxine are amplified by changes in serum TSH. The availability of the sensitive TSH assay in essentially all clinical laboratories has improved and simplified the assessment of thyroid function for the diagnosis of thyroid disease and to monitor treatment. Serum free thyroxine and thyrotropin concentrations, as well as other thyroid tests, can be measured utilizing an automated immunoassay platform that provides rapid and accurate results. This simplified approach to thyroid assessment, often requiring only a serum TSH measurement, and rapid availability of the thyroid function tests results, has expanded the scope of thyroid testing and clinicians ordering and interpreting thyroid tests.

There remain, however, many challenges in selecting the appropriate thyroid function test to order, the correct interpretation of results, and applying these results to the diagnosis and management of thyroid diseases. It is especially important to be aware of limitations of thyroid function tests, as well as special clinical circumstances that can influence thyroid function measurements. The serum TSH concentration, for example, may not accurately reflect thyroid status in many situations including after prolonged hyperthyroidism when serum TSH remains suppressed for months, in the presence of hypothalamic or pituitary disease, or due to a number of interfering medications. The serum free thyroxine, measured by the analog method, is not accurate with high or low serum binding proteins and during pregnancy. Hospitalized patients often have thyroid function test abnormalities that are transient and return to normal after recovery from the acute illness. Iodine excess and deficiency can dramatically influence thyroid function tests.

Significant insights have been gained into the regulation of thyroid hormone synthesis and especially the role of thyroid hormone metabolism in supplying tissues locally with an adequate supply of thyroid hormone. In a number of instances, these factors influence the selection and interpretation of thyroid function tests. Polymorphisms, common sequence variations, in genes of components that regulate thyroid function and thyroid hormone action may also contribute to variability in thyroid function tests in a population.

This volume draws on an outstanding international panel of experts in thyroid function tests and thyroid function assessment. They represent clinicians, clinical researchers, and basic science researchers, all with a focus on some aspect of the assessment of thyroid function. The chapters all provide a clinical perspective, but are informed by the most recent scientific advancements.

The first section of the book (Chaps. 1–3) presents the most recent advances in thyroid physiology, a review of genetic influences on thyroid function tests, and a discussion on the influence of iodine on thyroid function. In Chap. 1, Drs. Huang and de Castro Neves describe thyroid hormone metabolism, emphasizing the key role of thyroid hormone activation and inactivation in thyroid hormone action. Dr. Visser is a world leader in studies of thyroid metabolism and genetic influences on thyroid function. In Chap. 2, Dr. Visser and his colleagues, Drs. van der Deure, Medici, and Peeters, provide a clear view of this important and rapidly expanding field. The population variation in the TSH "set point" (relationship between serum TSH and thyroxine in an individual), for example, is thought to be genetically determined, and influences the evaluation of thyroid function and thyroid function targets for treatment of thyroid disease. Dr. Zimmerman, an internationally recognized expert in iodine, and his colleague, Dr. Andersson, provide in Chap. 3 an in-depth treatment of the most significant influence on thyroid function throughout the world—iodine intake. The influence of iodine deficiency and excess on individual thyroid function is discussed, as well as the population effects on thyroid diseases and especially fetal and neonatal development.

The basics of thyroid function measurements, approaches, limitations, and clinical applications are described for the major categories of thyroid function tests (Chaps. 4–7). The authors of these chapters are innovators in the field, strongly identified with the origination or significant refinement of the core tests utilized in thyroid assessment. In Chap. 4, Dr. Hershman describes the measurement of TSH, the clinical application and utilization. This remains the cornerstone of thyroid testing, but must be interpreted with an understanding of the dynamics of thyroid regulation. An active controversy in thyroid measurement involves the appropriate use of serum thyroxine measurements and especially the value of the analog free thyroxine measurement, the most commonly used thyroxine assay. In Chap. 5, Dr. Stockigt provides a detailed assessment of thyroxine and triiodothyronine measurements and a clear message for their use and limitations. The most common etiology of thyroid disease is autoimmune, and the appropriate use of thyroid autoantibody measurements remains confusing to many clinicians. In Chap. 6, Dr. Weetman and his colleague, Dr. Ajjan, clearly describe the range of thyroid autoantibody tests and how they should be utilized clinically. Thyroglobulin measurement is the key tumor marker to follow thyroid cancer patients and Dr. Spencer and her colleague, Ivana Petrovic, describe the essential features of this measurement in Chap. 7. It is essential that clinicians using thyroglobulin measurements to monitor thyroid cancer are aware of the performance of the assay being used and the factors that can interfere with the measurement.

Application of thyroid function testing to the key clinical settings is discussed by expert clinicians and clinical researchers in Chaps. 8–13. The appropriate selection of thyroid function tests in the diagnosis and monitoring of thyroid disease in the ambulatory setting is discussed by Drs. Farwell and Leung in Chap. 8. This is the most common setting for thyroid function test measurement and a rational approach is described. Specific issues of thyroid function in infants and children are discussed in Chap. 9 by Drs. LaFranchi and Balogh. Screening for thyroid disease among newborns has been a highly effective approach to prevent mental retardation. The assessment of thyroid function in newborns, especially premature infants, is challenging as are the interpretation of thyroid function tests in infancy through childhood. Illness has a significant impact on thyroid function tests and assessment in this group is described by Drs. LoPresti and Patil in Chap. 10. A logical approach to these patients is provided as are ways to identify those patients with thyroid disease that need to be treated. Assessment of thyroid function in pregnancy is challenging and is being increasing recognized as a crucial time to normalize maternal thyroid status. Adverse outcome for mother and her child can result from thyroid hormone deficiency or excess. In Chap. 11, Drs. Lazarus, Soldin, and Evans carefully describe the use and limitations of thyroid tests in pregnancy and provide an approach to testing and monitoring thyroid function. The incidence of autoimmune thyroid disease increases significantly with age and in Chap. 12 Dr. Samuels provides a clear approach to the assessment of thyroid status in the elderly and interpretation of thyroid studies. The influence of drugs on thyroid function testing remains a major clinical issue with recognition of an ever increasing list of medications that influence thyroid function and thyroid testing. In Chap. 13, Drs. Pearce and Ananthakrishnan comprehensively describe these medications with a special emphasis on their mechanism of action and on iodine-containing medications.

I am most grateful to my colleagues for their enthusiasm and willingness to provide such outstanding contributions to this book. The editorial team at Springer is excellent and has been highly supportive and effective. My special thanks to Editor Laura Walsh, Associate Editor Dianne Wuori, Editorial Assistant Stacy Lazar, Senior Production Editor Jenny Wolkowicki and Crest Premedia Solutions for final production.

Los Angeles, CA   Gregory A. Brent

Contents

Contributors

1. R. A. Ajjan
   Leeds General Infirmary, Department of Diabetes and Endocrinology, Great George Street, Leeds, UK, r.ajjan@leeds.ac.uk
2. Sonia Ananthakrishnan
   Assistant Professor of Medicine, Department of Medicine/Section of Endocrinology, Diabetes and Nutrition, Boston University School of Medicine, Boston, MA, USA, soniaa@bu.edu
3. Maria Andersson
   Swiss Federal Institute of Technology Zurich (ETH Zurich), Human Nutrition Laboratory, Institute of Food, Nutrition and Health, Zurich, Switzerland, maria.andersson@ilw.agrl.ethz.ch
4. Luciana Audi de Castro Neves
   Research Fellow, Children's Hospital Boston, Division of Endocrinology, Boston, MA, USA, luciana.neves@childrens.harvard.edu
5. Carol Evans
   University Hospital of Wales, Cardiff School of Medicine, Department of Medical Biochemistry and Immunology, Cardiff, Wales, UK, carol.evans@cardiffandvale.wales.nhs.uk
6. Alan P. Farwell
   Associate Professor of Medicine, Boston University School of Medicine, Division of Endocrinology, Diabetes and Nutrition, Boston Medical Center, Boston, MA, USA, alan.farwell@bmc.org
7. Jerome M. Hershman
   Distinguished Professor of Medicine, David Geffen School of Medicine at UCLA, West Los Angeles VA Medical Center, Division of Endocrinology and Diabetes, Los Angeles, CA, USA, jhershmn@ucla.edu
8. Stephen Albert Huang
   Assistant Professor of Pediatrics, Thyroid Program, Children's Hospital Boston, Harvard Medical School, Division of Endocrinology, Boston, MA, USA, stephen.huang@childrens.harvard.edu
9. Stephen H. LaFranchi
   Professor of Pediatrics, Oregon Health & Science University, Department of Pediatrics, Division of Endocrinology, Portland, OR, USA, lafrancs@ohsu.edu

10. John H. Lazarus
    Professor of Clinical Endocrinology, University Hospital of Wales, Centre for Endocrine and Diabetes Sciences, Cardiff, Wales, UK, lazarus@cardiff.ac.uk

11. Angela M. Leung
    Division of Endocrinology, Diabetes and Nutrition, Boston University School of Medicine, Boston Medical Center, Boston, MA, USA, angela.leung@bmc.org

12. Jonathan S. LoPresti
    Associate Professor of Clinical Medicine, University of Southern California, Keck School of Medicine, LAC-USC Medical Center, Department of Internal Medicine, Division of Endocrinology, Los Angeles, CA, USA, jlopresti@socal.rr.com

13. Alicia G. Marks
    Fellow, Pediatric Endocrinology, Oregon Health & Science University, Department of Pediatrics, Division of Endocrinology, Portland, OR, USA, balogha@ohsu.edu

14. Marco Medici
    Erasmus University Medical Center, Department of Internal Medicine, Rotterdam, The Netherlands, m.medici@erasmusmc.nl

15. Komal S. Patil
    Fellow in Endocrinology, Los Angeles County Hospital, University of Southern California, Los Angeles, CA, USA, komal.patil.md@gmail.com

16. Elizabeth N. Pearce
    Associate Professor of Medicine, Department of Medicine/Section of Endocrinology, Diabetes and Nutrition, Boston University School of Medicine, Boston, MA, USA, elizabeth.pearce@bmc.org

17. Robin P. Peeters
    Erasmus University Medical Center, Department of Internal Medicine, Rotterdam, The Netherlands, r.peeters@erasmusmc.nl

18. Ivana Petrovic
    Research Lab Specialist, University of Southern California, Keck School of Medicine, USC Endocrine Laboratories, Los Angeles, CA, USA, ivapet70@hotmail.com

19. Mary H. Samuels
    Professor of Medicine, Oregon Health & Science University, Division of Endocrinology, Diabetes, and Clinical Nutrition, Portland, OR, USA, samuelsm@ohsu.edu

20. Offie P. Soldin
    Associate Professor of Oncology, Division of Endocrinology and Metabolism and Department of Oncology, Division of Cancer Genetics and Epidemiology, Lombardi Comprehensive Cancer Center, Georgetown University Medical Center, Washington D.C., USA, os35@georgetown.edu

21. Carole Spencer
    Professor of Medicine, University of Southern California, Keck School of Medicine, Los Angeles, CA, USA, cspencer@usc.edu

22. Jim R. Stockigt
Professor of Medicine, Epworth and Alfred Hospitals, Monash University, Melbourne, Victoria, Australia, jrs@netspace.net.au

23. Wendy M. van der Deure
Erasmus University Medical Center, Department of Internal Medicine, Rotterdam, The Netherlands, w.vanderdeure@erasmusmc.nl

24. Theo J. Visser
Professor of Medicine, Erasmus University Medical Center, Department of Internal Medicine, Rotterdam, The Netherlands, t.j.visser@erasmusmc.nl

25. A. P. Weetman
Professor of Medicine, University of Sheffield, Sheffield Teaching Hospital, Beech Hill Road, Sheffield, UK, a.p.weetman@sheffield.ac.uk

26. Michael B. Zimmermann
Professor, Swiss Federal Institute of Technology Zurich (ETH Zurich), Human Nutrition Laboratory, Institute of Food, Nutrition and Health, Zurich, Switzerland, michael.zimmermann@ilw.agrl.ethz.ch

Chapter 1
Thyroid Hormone Metabolism

Stephen A. Huang and Luciana A. de Castro Neves

1.1 Introduction

Thyroid hormone is a potent regulator of cellular proliferation and metabolic rate and must be maintained within an optimal range for normal development and health. The severe growth and neurologic injuries observed in children with untreated congenital hypothyroidism illustrate this. Thyroid hormone metabolism, which describes the biochemical activation and inactivation of thyroid hormones, is a powerful mechanism regulating thyroid hormone action. In this chapter, we will review the glandular synthesis of thyroid hormone and then discuss the metabolic pathways responsible for its activation and inactivation in peripheral tissues, focusing on deiodination as the dominant pathway in postnatal vertebrates and the most clinically relevant for thyroid function testing in patients. Subsequent chapters will discuss other sites of regulation, including the genes regulating thyroid hormone production and action (Chap. 2), availability of iodine (Chap. 3), and thyrotropin regulation of the thyroid gland (Chap. 4).

While most treatable thyroid diseases are due to abnormal glandular secretion rather than deranged hormone metabolism, an understanding of the major metabolic pathways is invaluable in the interpretation of thyroid function tests, allowing the clinician to avoid the misdiagnosis of thyroid dysfunction in euthyroid individuals with altered metabolism and conversely to recognize the rare diseases that are caused by primary defects in metabolism.

S. A. Huang (✉)

Division of Endocrinology, Children's Hospital Boston, Harvard Medical School, Boston, MA 02115, USA

e-mail: stephen.huang@childrens.harvard.edu

G. A. Brent (ed.), *Thyroid Function Testing,*
DOI 10.1007/978-1-4419-1485-9_1, © Springer Science+Business Media, LLC 2010

1.2 Thyroid Hormone Synthesis and Plasma Transport

Thyroid hormone secretion is regulated by the hypothalamic-pituitary-thyroid axis and this system is discussed in depth in Chap. 4. In brief (Fig. 1.1), the hypothalamus produces thyrotropin releasing hormone (TRH), which stimulates the pituitary to secrete thyrotropin. Thyrotropin, also called thyroid stimulating hormone (TSH), stimulates thyroid hormone synthesis and glandular secretion. Both active thyroid hormones, thyroxine (T4) and triiodothyronine (T3), exert negative feedback upon the hypothalamus and the pituitary. Assays to measure serum TSH, T4, and T3 are all routinely available in clinical laboratories and are adequate to diagnosis primary and central thyroid dysfunction.

Thyroid hormones are composed mostly of iodine (65% of T4's weight; 58% of T3's weight) which is primarily derived from the diet. In nonpregnant adults, a daily dietary iodine intake of 100–150 μg is sufficient to meet the synthetic requirements of the normal thyroid [1]. Ingested iodine is rapidly absorbed from the stomach and intestine and, once in the circulation, it becomes available for uptake into the thyroid gland. Thyroid follicular cells are uniquely adapted to concentrate iodine and to incorporate it into thyroid hormone (Fig. 1.2). The sodium/iodide symporter (NIS) is a membrane protein on the basolateral surface of thyroid follicular cells that actively transports circulating iodide into the thyrocyte. This property of NIS is exploited in clinical practice to perform diagnostic thyroid imaging (scintigraphy) with tracer amounts of I-123 and also to deliver ablative therapies with I-131.

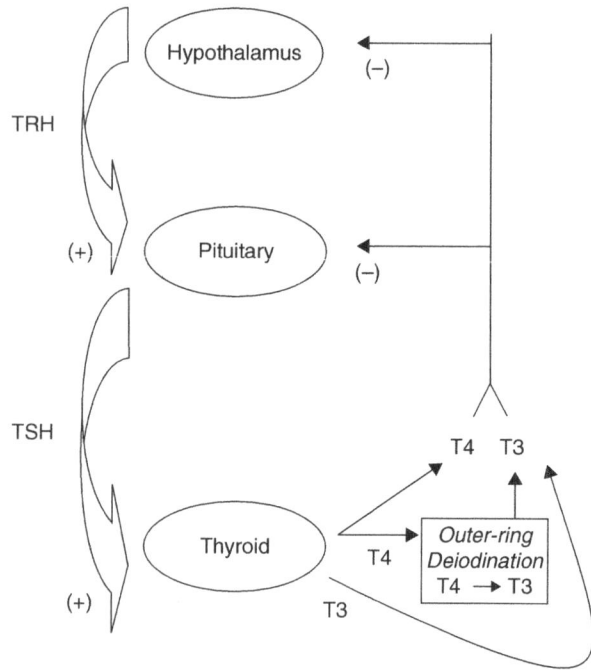

Fig. 1.1 Hypothalamic-pituitary-thyroid axis. The hypothalamus and pituitary stimulate thyroid secretion, primarily in the form of the prohormone T4 which is then converted into T3 by outer-ring deiodination in peripheral tissues. Both T4 and T3 feedback negatively on the hypothalamus and pituitary

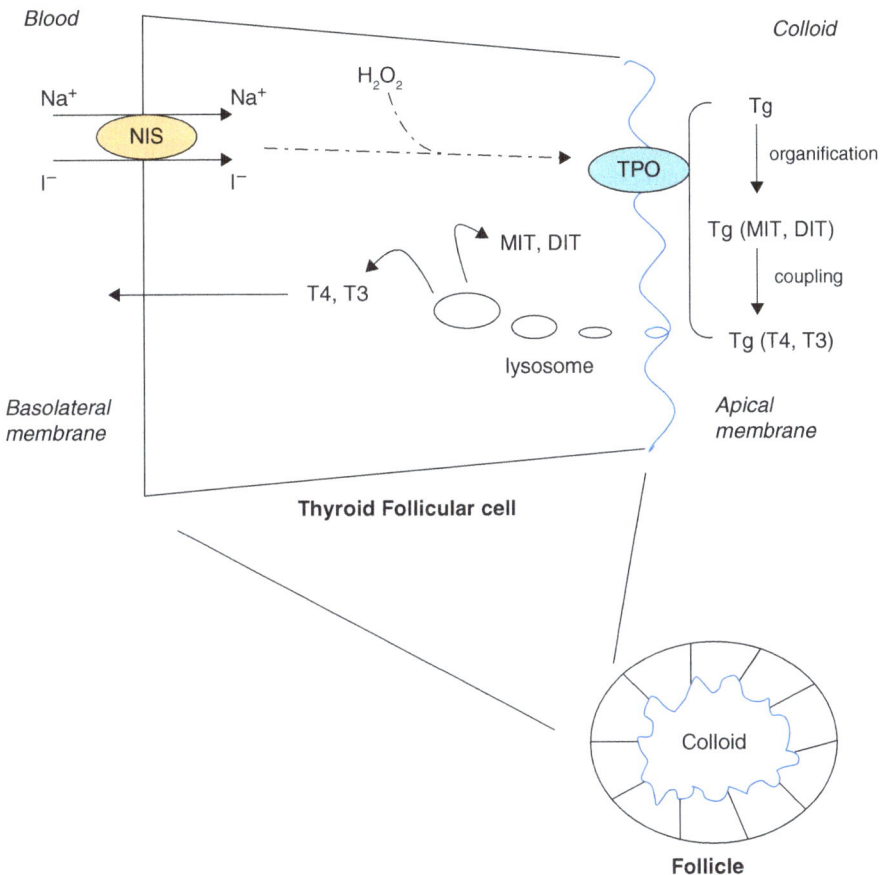

Fig. 1.2 Thyroid hormone synthesis. Circulating iodide (I^-) is transported into the thyroid follicle by the sodium/iodide symporter (*NIS*). Thyroperoxidase (*TPO*) catalyzes the oxidation and organification of intracellular iodine onto tyrosine residues of thyroglobulin (*Tg*), forming monoiodotyrosine (*MIT*) and diiodotyrosine (*DIT*). Iodinated tyrosine residues couple to form T4 and T3. Thyroglobulin is endocytosed, undergoes proteolysis in lysosomes, and T4 and T3 are released into the bloodstream

Intracellular iodide is then oxidized and conjugated onto tyrosine residues of the large glycoprotein thyroglobulin via a process called "organification". This tyrosine iodination reaction can add either one iodine atom (resulting in monoiodotyrosine or MIT) or two (resulting in diiodotyrosine or DIT), and the subsequent "coupling" of two iodinated tyrosines produces both T4 (formed by the coupling of two DIT molecules) and T3 (formed by the coupling of one DIT molecule and one MIT molecule). Mature thyroglobulin thus contains both T4 and T3, present in a ratio of about 15:1 [2].

Thyroglobulin is stored within the center of thyroid follicles in a matrix called colloid and this constitutes a large reservoir of preformed hormone, equivalent to several weeks of normal secretion. This storage property is unique to the endocrine glands and permits continued thyroid hormone availability during transient iodine deficiency and other environmental goitrogen exposures which might otherwise temporarily impair thyroid hormone synthesis. Thyroid hormone secretion begins with the endocytosis of colloid from the apical membrane of thyroid follicular cells. Thyroglobulin then undergoes lysosomal proteolysis to release T4 and T3, which subsequently enter the circulation at a ratio of about 11:1 [3]. The difference between this secreted T4 to T3 ratio and the 15:1 T4 to T3 ratio in thyroglobulin can be explained by the intrathyroidal conversion of T4 to T3 as discussed below in the section on deiodination. Thyroglobulin proteolysis also releases uncoupled iodinated tyrosine residues which are metabolized by iodotyrosine deiodinases to release free iodide which in turn is recycled for organification.

Many of the biochemical reactions required for thyroid hormone synthesis are catalyzed by the thyroperoxidase enzyme. In addition, several other thyroid-specific proteins such as NIS, the thyroid oxidases which generate H_2O_2 for iodine oxidation [4], and the iodotyrosine deiodinases responsible for iodine recycling [5] are also required for normal thyroid hormone synthesis. These thyroid-specific proteins have been investigated in animal models, and also in humans through the clinical study of patients with germline mutations that present as congenital hypothyroidism or euthyroid goiter [6].

Thyroid hormones have poor aqueous solubility and most T4 and T3 in the circulation are bound to plasma proteins. The major binding protein in humans is thyroxine-binding globulin, which binds about 68% of circulating T4 and 80% of circulating T3, followed by albumin and transthyretin (previously termed thyroxine binding prealbumin) [7]. Only about 0.02% of serum T4 and 0.3% of serum T3 is normally free (unbound) and available to enter cells and signal thyroid hormone action. An understanding of this "free hormone concept" is important in clinical practice, as several inherited and acquired conditions can alter the amount of these serum binding proteins and/or their affinity for thyroid hormones. While free thyroid hormone concentrations are normal in such individuals, these binding abnormalities can mimic the laboratory findings of central thyroid disease and care must be taken to avoid misdiagnosis. For example, congenital thyroxine-binding globulin deficiency presents with a low serum total T4 and normal serum TSH (mimicking central hypothyroidism) and familial dysalbuminemic hyperthyroxinemia (caused by a mutant albumin protein with abnormally high T4 avidity) presents with a high serum total T4 and a normal serum TSH (mimicking syndromes of inappropriate TSH secretion). In addition, as discussed in Chap. 13, many common medications can induce binding abnormalities and abnormal serum thyroid function tests by increasing (estrogen) [7] or decreasing (L-asparaginase) [8] serum thyroxine-binding globulin or by decreasing T4 binding affinity (salicylates, phenytoin) [9]. Diagnostic considerations in the measurement of free versus total thyroid hormone in such patients are discussed in depth in Chap. 5.

Serum thyroid hormone binding proteins serve two important physiologic functions. The first is to prolong the serum half-life of thyroid hormones by reducing their renal clearance. The second is to promote a homogenous level of T4 and T3 in the circulation. This latter allows local thyroid status to be governed by tissue specific factors that regulate intracellular T3 availability, such as thyroid hormone transporters (Chap. 2) and the metabolic pathways (conjugation, deiodination) described in the following sections.

1.3 Thyroid Hormone Action

In brief, thyroid hormone signaling begins with the binding of either T4 or T3 to nuclear thyroid hormone receptors (discussed in Chap. 2). Upon ligand binding, these receptors complex with other transcriptional cofactors and then interact with regulatory sequences of thyroid hormone responsive genes to increase or decrease transcription. While both T4 and T3 can mediate thyroid hormone responses, T3 is more potent and binds the thyroid hormone receptor with 15-fold greater affinity than T4 [7]. Because of this, T3 is often referred to as the "active" ligand and T4 as the "prohormone".

1.4 Thyroid Hormone Metabolism

The majority of thyroid hormone secreted by the gland is in the form of the prohormone T4, which is later converted to T3 by deiodination in peripheral tissues. This activation pathway is responsible for the majority (80%) of T3 in the circulation, illustrating the importance of thyroid hormone metabolism in normal physiology. The term thyroid hormone metabolism refers to the activation of T4 into T3 and also the various inactivating pathways for T4 and T3. In this section, we will first review nondeiodinative "alternate" pathways of thyroid hormone metabolism and then focus on deiodination, which is the dominant pathway in humans and the most clinically relevant for thyroid function testing in patients.

1.5 Alternative Pathways of Thyroid Hormone Metabolism

This section will briefly review the two major nondeiodinative "alternate" pathways of thyroid hormone metabolism, conjugation and side-chain modification (Fig. 1.3).

1.5.1 Conjugation

The phenolic hydroxyl group of thyroid hormone can be conjugated by sulfotransferases or glucuronidases [10, 11].

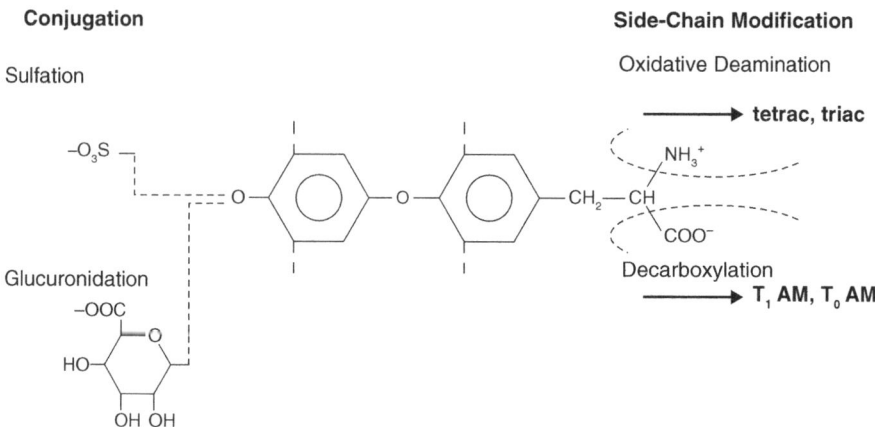

Fig. 1.3 Alternative pathways of thyroid hormone metabolism. Conjugation and side-chain modification are illustrated

The sulfation of T4 and T3 promotes their subsequent inactivation by type 1 deiodinase (D1). Because sulfotransferases are minimally expressed in postnatal tissues, this is a minor pathway in patients. However, during fetal development when there is combined high expression of sulfotransferases and D1, sulfation is a potent inactivating pathway. Interestingly, sulfation is a reversible modification and so sulfatases may "rescue" sulfated T4 and T3 from inactivation. During fetal development, it is speculated that these enzymes work in concert to generate a large reservoir of sulfated thyroid hormone that is rapidly inactivated in tissues that express D1 and reactivated in other tissues that express sulfatase activity, thus modulating thyroid hormone availability in a tissue-specific fashion.

Glucuronide conjugation also promotes the inactivation of thyroid hormone by increasing its biliary excretion. Because glucuronidase expression is normally minimal, this is a minor pathway in most patients. However, inactivation can become significant in individuals taking anticonvulsants or other medications that stimulate glucuronidation. Hypothyroid individuals taking such medications may require higher doses of levothyroxine to maintain euthyroidism.

1.5.2 Alanine Side-Chain Modification

The alanine side chain of thyroid hormone can be modified by oxidative deamination or decarboxylation [10, 11].

Oxidative deamination converts T4 and T3 into tetrac and triac, respectively. Both tetrac and triac have been identified in the serum of healthy individuals and thus occur endogenously. Both these acetic acid analogs can bind nuclear thyroid hormone receptors and possess thyromimetic activity. Of note, triac has much higher affinity for TRβ1 over TRα1. Because of this unique selectivity, triac has been explored as a therapy for TRβ specific pathologies, such as the syndrome of resistance to thyroid hormone (Chap. 2) [10].

Decarboxylation of the thyroid hormone alanine side chain produces the thyronamine derivatives of 3-T$_1$AM and T$_0$AM. These derivatives are present endogenously and, in experimental systems, mediate potent effects on cardiac function (negative inotropy and chronotropy) and body temperature (hypothermia) [12]. Early studies indicate that these actions are independent of the thyroid hormone receptor and signal instead through the G protein-coupled trace amine receptor TAAR1 [13, 14].

1.6 Thyroid Hormone Deiodination

Monodeiodination is the major pathway of thyroid hormone metabolism in humans. As illustrated in Fig. 1.4, the sequential removal of iodine atoms can lead to either substrate activation or inactivation. The prohormone T4 contains four iodine atoms, two on its "outer" phenolic ring and two on its "inner" tyrosyl ring. Removal of a

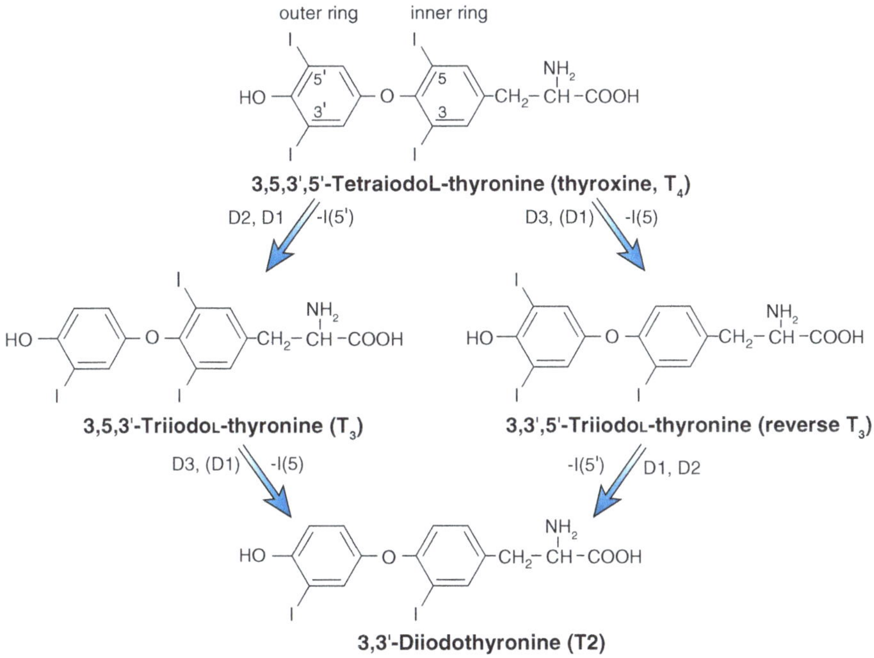

Fig. 1.4 Thyroid hormone deiodination. Outer-ring deiodination, catalyzed by D1 and D2, activates the T4 prohormone into T3. Inner-ring deiodination, catalyzed primarily by D3, inactivates T4 and T3

single iodine atom from thyroxine's outer ring converts it into the more biologically potent T3. This reaction is catalyzed by type 1 (D1) and 2 (D2) deiodinase. Conversely, inner-ring deiodination converts both T4 and T3 into inactive metabolites, rT3 and T2 respectively. While both type 1 (D1) and 3 (D3) deiodinase are capable of inner-ring deiodination, outside of embryonic development (where thyroid hormone sulfation facilitates D1-mediated inner-ring deiodination), D3 is the major inactivating enzyme.

Outer-ring deiodination is responsible for the majority of T3 production in euthyroid individuals, explaining the observation that adequate levothyroxine (T4) monotherapy produces normal serum T3 concentrations in hypothyroid patients. While a small amount of T4 activation occurs in the thyroid gland itself, the vast majority of T4 to T3 conversion occurs in peripheral tissues and is catalyzed by both D1 and D2. In the euthyroid state, D3-mediated inner-ring deiodination is responsible for inactivating 80% of daily thyroid hormone production [15].

1.7   The Iodothyronine Deiodinase Enzyme Family

Each of the three deiodinase enzymes (D1, D2, and D3) is encoded by a distinct gene (*DIO1* on human chromosome 1p32–p33; *DIO2* on human chromosome 14q24.3; *DIO3* on human chromosome 14q32). While all three deiodinases share significant sequence homology and the rare amino acid selenocysteine in their active centers, each has a unique anatomic and developmental pattern of distribution as well as distinct enzymatic properties (Table 1.1). Working in concert, these features allow the deiodinases to modulate thyroid hormone signaling in a temporally and

Table 1.1 Human iodothyronine deiodinases

	D1	D2	D3
Enzyme activity	Outer-ring deiodination *and* inner-ring deiodination	Outer-ring deiodination	Inner-ring deiodination
Tissue expression	Liver Kidney Thyroid	Central nervous system Pituitary Brown fat Cardiac and skeletal muscle	Uterus Placenta Central nervous system Skin
Substrates	rT3, T4, T3S, T4S	T4, rT3	T3, T4
Positive regulators	Thyroid hormone	Cold exposure Bile acids Cyclic AMP Deubiquitination	Thyroid hormone Angiogenic factors TGF-β family Hypoxia Hedgehog family
Negative regulators	Cytokines Illness/fasting	Thyroid hormone Sonic hedgehog	Glucocorticoids

anatomically specific manner by altering both systemic and local T3 availability. This ability of deiodination to alter local thyroid status is important for the regulation of thyroid hormone action during development and was first characterized in amphibians, where rapid peaks and D2 and D3 activity are required for normal metamorphosis [16]. More recent studies indicate that the local modulation of thyroid status by deiodination is similarly important for the development of mammalian species [17, 18], as well as for cellular proliferation and metabolism in injured tissues such the ischemic myocardium [19] and certain cancers [20]. The molecular features of the deiodinases and their impact on local thyroid status is beyond the scope of this chapter, so the reader is directed to a number of excellent reviews listed in the references [21–23]. This section will focus specifically on the impact of deiodination on systemic thyroid status as these manifest as changes in serum thyroid function tests.

1.7.1   Type 1 Deiodinase (D1)

D1 is unique amongst the deiodinases in its ability to catalyze both outer-ring and inner-ring deiodination. D1 is also the only deiodinase with high sensitivity to inhibition by propylthiouracil, a feature that is exploited clinically in the treatment of thyrotoxicosis and also experimentally in enzymatic studies of deiodination. While D1 is capable of both T4 activation and inactivation, it has much higher affinity for the activating pathway and its contribution to thyroid hormone inactivation is normally minimal. A single exception to this occurs during embryonic development, when fetal sulfotransferases are highly expressed and conjugate large amounts of T4 and T3 into sulfated forms which are excellent substrates for D1-mediated inner-ring deiodination. D1 is also the major clearance pathway for the inactive metabolite rT3, via outer-ring deiodination.

In postnatal humans, high D1 activity has been documented in the liver and kidney, with lower expression in the thyroid and pituitary. Together with D2, D1 catalyzes the outer-ring deiodination of T4 in peripheral tissues, which is the major source of T3 in the circulation. Clinical studies of hypothyroid adults performed in the presence or absence of propylthiouracil (which inhibits D1, but not D2), indicate that D1 is likely the minor source of serum T3 in the euthyroid state [24, 25]. However, in the setting of thyrotoxicosis, D1's contribution increases and about half of serum T3 production is attributed to D1 [26]. Because of this, propylthiouracil is often used in the therapy of severely hyperthyroid adults as it not only decreases glandular secretion but also rapidly inhibits D1-catalyzed T4 to T3 conversion.

1.7.2   Type 2 Deiodinase (D2)

D2 catalyzes the outer-ring deiodination of T4 into T3, and is the major source of serum T3 production in the euthyroid state. In comparison to D1 (the other activating deiodinase), D2 has a much higher affinity for T4 (with a low nanomolar Michaelis constant), and its enzymatic activity is insensitive to inhibition by propylthiouracil.

In humans, D2 is expressed in the central nervous system, thyroid, placenta, and cardiac and skeletal myocytes. In addition to its major role in the provision of circulating T3, D2 is a potent mechanism to increase local T3 concentrations in critical structures such as the pituitary (where D2-generated T3 is required for feedback regulation of TSH secretion) [27] and brown fat (where D2-generated T3 is required to promote uncoupling and adaptive thermogenesis) [28, 29]. This theme has been recapitulated more recently in other settings, including the developing growth plate of embryonic bones [17].

1.7.3   Type 3 Deiodinase (D3)

D3 is the physiologic inactivator of thyroid hormones, catalyzing the inner-ring deiodination of both T4 and T3 into rT3 and T2, respectively. During pregnancy, D3 is highly expressed in the uteroplacental unit [30, 31] and also in the tissues of the developing fetus itself [32]. This activity limits the transfer of maternal thyroid hormone to the fetus, thus explaining the high maternal-to-fetal gradients of serum thyroid hormone that are characteristic of normal gestation. While D3 expression falls precipitously at birth, becoming undetectable in most tissues other than the central nervous system and skin, it remains the major path of thyroid hormone degradation, inactivating 80% of daily thyroid hormone production in adults [15].

1.8   Thyroid Hormone Metabolism and T3 Homeostasis

Thyroid hormone metabolism is a powerful homeostatic mechanism that reacts dynamically during iodine deficiency and the derangement of glandular secretion to maintain normal concentrations of the active thyroid hormone T3 (discussed in depth in Chap. 3).

1.8.1   Iodine Deficiency

Iodine is the major component of thyroid hormone, and when dietary iodine intake falls below 100 μg/day, thyroid hormone synthesis is compromised. Clinical manifestations of iodine deficiency include goiter and, in the young, growth failure and a form of mental retardation called cretinism. Recent estimates indicate that 2 billion individuals, including one third of the world's pediatric population, have insufficient iodine intake and are at risk for iodine-deficiency disorders [33]. Cretinism thus remains the most common preventable cause of mental retardation worldwide and the elimination of iodine deficiency is an ongoing international health effort [1]. Of note, all negative sequelae of iodine deficiency can be prevented (but not reversed) by increasing dietary intake, either through supplementation or food fortification.

A number of compensatory mechanisms work in concert during iodine deficiency to preserve T3 availability. Within the thyroid gland itself, tyrosine iodination shifts to favor monoiodination over diiodination. This increases the MIT to DIT ratio in thyroglobulin and, consequently, the T3 to T4 ratio of secreted thyroid hormones. Iodine deficiency also increases the fractional conversion of T4 to T3 in peripheral tissues. This outer-ring deiodinase activity is largely PTU-insensitive, indicating catalysis by D2 [21]. The net effect of these changes is a decrease in the serum T4 to T3 ratio, which is characteristic of both iodine deficiency and early hypothyroidism. This explains the observation that serum T3 concentrations are often normal in early iodine deficiency, even in individuals with hyperthyrotropinemia and marked hypothyroxinemia. While these compensatory mechanisms cannot prevent the pathology of severe iodine deficiency, they are protective when deficiency is transient or mild.

1.8.2 Hypothyroidism

Thyroid hormone deiodination is altered in the hypothyroid state. As with iodine deficiency, the fractional conversion of T4 to T3 by D2 in peripheral tissues is increased, leading to a decrease in the serum T4 to T3 ratio. This explains why serum T3 is typically normal in mild or early hypothyroidism, even after hyperthyrotropinemia and hypothyroxinemia develop. The serum T4 to T3 ratio may be depressed even further in those patients who have autoimmune thyroiditis as the cause of their hypothyroidism, due to impaired thyroperoxidase activity and inefficient organification.

In addition, tracer kinetic experiments and clinical studies of serum thyroid function tests obtained during levothyroxine therapy indicate that thyroid hormone clearance is decreased in hypothyroid patients [34, 35]. This is the rationale for the clinical recommendation to reassess thyroid function 6 months after the restoration of euthyroidism, after thyroid hormone clearance has normalized [36]. Recent animal studies have provided an explanation for this reduced clearance by documenting decreased expression of D3, the thyroid hormone-inactivating enzyme, in the setting of hypothyroidism [37].

The net effect of these two changes, increased T4 to T3 conversion and decreased thyroid hormone turnover, is to maintain normal serum T3 concentrations in the setting of early thyroid insufficiency. Because of this, the measurement of serum T3 is not helpful in the diagnosis of hypothyroidism.

1.8.3 Hyperthyroidism

Tracer kinetic studies in adults indicate that the plasma turnover of thyroid hormones is increased during hyperthyroidism [34], and rodent studies support that this is due to increased expression of the thyroid hormone-inactivating deiodinase D3 [37]. This accelerated clearance of circulating thyroid hormones can be viewed as a general adaption to reduce the severity of biochemical thyrotoxicosis, and the induction of high focal D3-expression reported in certain structures like the brain [37] suggests that critical tissues such as the central nervous system may be afforded even greater protection by local T3 inactivation.

While TSH suppression is the most sensitive single indicator of primary hyperthyroidism, serum T4 and T3 measurements are also helpful to assess the severity of biochemical derangement and to gauge the response to therapy. This is especially true early in treatment as TSH secretion may take many months to recover. Discordance between serum T4 and serum T3 is, not infrequently, a source of confusion in the treatment of hyperthyroid patients and this is usually characterized by a disproportionately high T3 (a low serum T4 to T3 ratio). While in rare cases this is due to thyrotoxicosis facticia from exogenous liothyronine (T3), it is most often due to changes in thyroid hormone synthesis and metabolism.

Graves' disease is the most common cause of hyperthyroidism and it is often associated with T3 predominance (a low T4 to T3 ratio). Intrathyroidal changes are a major contributor to this, as both the T3 to T4 ratio in thyroglobulin and glandular D2 activity (which promotes intrathyroidal conversion of T4 into T3) are increased in Graves' disease. These effects are compounded by the administration of thionamide medications, which antagonize tyrosine iodination and further raise both the MIT to DIT ratio and the T3 to T4 ratio in thyroglobulin. All these effects contribute to a higher T3 to T4 ratio in secreted thyroid hormones. In addition, the peripheral conversion of T4 into T3 is increased in hyperthyroidism by the induction of hepatic D1, which is paradoxically stimulated by high levels of thyroid hormone. This deiodinase activity is specifically targeted in thyroid storm by high dose propylthiouracil therapy which, in addition to its primary antithyroid action, inhibits D1 activity.

All the above factors decrease the serum T4 to T3 ratio in hyperthyroid patients, and an awareness of this is helpful in the management of patients who have low serum TSH, low free T4, but a high serum free T3. While these results are sometimes mistaken for central hypothyroidism or overtreatment with antithyroid medication, the hypertriiodothyronemia usually signifies persistent hyperthyroidism and antithyroid therapy should be increased accordingly.

1.9 Altered Thyroid Hormone Metabolism as a Cause of Abnormal Thyroid Function Testing

The preceding section describes the homeostatic role of thyroid hormone metabolism in the maintenance of T3 availability during iodine deficiency and thyroid dysfunction. In contrast, this section describes primary changes in thyroid hormone metabolism which cause secondary changes in thyroid status. Because such changes commonly occur in response to illness and the administration of certain medications, an understanding of these effects is important for the interpretation of serum thyroid function tests (discussed in detail in Chap. 10). Finally, we will review two rare conditions where tumoral deiodinase expression causes clinically significant derangement of systemic thyroid status.

1.9.1 Low-T3 Syndrome

Critical illness is commonly associated with the derangement of serum thyroid function tests. These changes are variable [38], but almost always include a fall in serum T3 and a rise in serum rT3. For this reason, they are referred to as the "low-T3 syndrome", and the terms "nonthyroidal illness" and "euthyroid sick syndrome" are synonyms. While the low-T3 syndrome is common, affecting up to 75% of hospitalized patients [39], its etiology is incompletely understood and there is controversy regarding the role of thyroid hormone supplementation in affected patients [39–41].

The physiology of the low-T3 syndrome is multifactorial and complex. Because it is discussed in depth in Chap. 10, this section will only focus on specific changes in thyroid hormone metabolism. T3 production is decreased in the low-T3 syndrome, due both to the suppression of the hypothalamic-pituitary-thyroid axis and to a decrease in peripheral T4 to T3 conversion [39]. Animal and patient studies indicate that a fall in D1 [42–45], rather than D2 [46], accounts for the latter. Of note, while this decrease in D1 contributes to both the high serum T4 to T3 ratio (from decreased T4 outer-ring deiodination) and the high serum rT3 (from decreased rT3 clearance) that are characteristic of the low-T3 syndrome, D1 deficiency alone cannot explain the primary finding of hypotriiodothyronemia, illustrated by the fact that mice with genetic D1 deficiency have normal serum T3 concentrations [47–49].

In addition to the above changes, recent postmortem studies also implicate D3 reactivation as a contributor to the low-T3 syndrome [50]. While high D3 expression is normally restricted to embryonic development, the reactivation of high D3 activity in the liver and skeletal muscle has been documented in critically ill patients [44, 51]. The specific D3 activity in these tissues correlates with the serum rT3 to T4 ratio, indicating that this inner-ring deiodinase activity contributes to the derangement of serum thyroid function tests. In certain patients, the accelerated inactivation of circulating thyroid hormone may be facilitated by an increase in the free hormone fraction due to a decrease in the quantity [52, 53] and/or binding affinity [54, 55] of thyroxine binding globulin.

The net effect of this decrease in D1 and increase in D3 is a shift from T4 activation to T4 inactivation. Combined with a D3-mediated increase in thyroid hormone clearance, this shift in the pattern of thyroid hormone deiodination can explain many of the changes observed in the low-T3 syndrome, especially in those patients where serum T3 falls rapidly. From the standpoint of clinical practice, an appreciation of the low-T3 syndrome's high incidence is helpful to avoid misdiagnosing central hypothyroidism in critically ill patients who have low circulating thyroid hormone concentrations and simultaneously normal serum TSH concentrations. Serial monitoring of thyroid function tests in such patients will often reveal that endogenous thyroid function is normal on recovery.

1.9.2 Medications that Alter Thyroid Hormone Metabolism

Medications are a common cause of abnormal thyroid function tests (discussed in detail in Chap. 13). This section focuses specifically upon those medications which alter thyroid hormone metabolism via either deiodinative or nondeiodinative pathways.

Certain medications decrease T4 to T3 conversion and thus raise the serum T4 to T3 ratio (Table 1.2). As described above, propylthiouracil is a specific inhibitor of D1 activity and this feature is exploited in the treatment of thyroid storm. A number of other medications with unrelated indications also share the property of inhibiting T4 outer-ring deiodination, including propranolol, amiodarone [56], and iopanoic acid [57]. In certain euthyroid individuals who chronically take propranolol or amiodarone, compensatory mild hyperthyroxinemia may develop [58], similar to the pattern observed in mice with genetic D1 deficiency [47, 48, 59]. Such individuals generally have normal serum TSH concentrations and a careful medication history is helpful to distinguish this medication effect from the rare syndrome of inappropriate TSH secretion. The initiation of high glucocorticoid doses is also associated with an acute increase in the serum T4 to T3 ratio. This effect is usually transient and resolves spontaneously during chronic glucocorticoid administration [57].

In contrast, other medications accelerate the metabolism of circulating thyroid hormone via a nondeiodinative hepatic pathway that likely involves the glucoronidation and subsequent biliary excretion of thyroid hormones [7]. This group of drugs includes rifampin, phenobarbitol, and the anticonvulsants phenytoin and carbamazepine. In general, these medications preferentially promote the clearance of T4 over T3. In patients with preexisting hypothyroidism, this acceleration in thyroid hormone clearance can increase requirements for exogenous levothyroxine, and

Table 1.2 Changes in thyroid hormone metabolism can alter the serum T4 to T3 ratio

Serum T4 to T3 ratio	Potential causes
Decreased	Iodine deficiency
	Mild hypothyroidism
	Hyperthyroidism
	T4 to T3 hyperconversion in D2-expressing follicular thyroid cancer
	Medications: thionamides, anticonvulsants
Increased	Selenium deficiency
	SBP2 deficiency
	Illness, the "low-T3 syndrome"
	Medications: amiodarone, propranolol

biochemical monitoring is recommended after the initiation of these medications. In contrast, in the absence of coexisting thyroid disease, glandular secretion compensates for increased inactivation and, as a rule, euthyroidism is maintained with normal serum thyroid function tests. However, there are rare reports of children on chronic anticonvulsant therapy who manifest the combination of mild hypothyroxinemia with simultaneously normal TSH and T3 concentrations (Table 1.2) [60]. An awareness of medication effects is important to avoid the misdiagnosis of central hypothyroidism in such patients.

1.9.3 Tumoral D3 and Consumptive Hypothyroidism

D3 activity has been documented in several human tumors, including glioblastoma multiforme, astrocytomas, and TSH-secreting pituitary adenomas [61, 62]. In rare patients who have the combination of both high specific D3 activity and large tumor burden, the amount of circulating thyroid hormone inactivated by inner-ring deiodination can exceed the synthetic capacity of even the normal hypothalamic-pituitary-thyroid axis. This condition is termed consumptive hypothyroidism and it has been reported in children with large infantile hemangiomas [63] as well in adults with massive vascular [64] or fibrous [65] tumors.

Like primary hypothyroidism, affected individuals present with hyperthyrotropinemia +/− low serum concentration of T4 and T3. In addition, serum concentrations of rT3, the byproduct of T4 inactivation, are markedly elevated. Unlike other forms of hypothyroidism, serum T3 often falls to a greater degree than T4 in individuals with consumptive hypothyroidism.

Because the clearance of circulating T4 and T3 is accelerated, frequent laboratory monitoring is indicated and supernormal doses of thyroid hormone may be required to restore euthyroidism. Since consumptive hypothyroidism is due to tumoral enzyme activity rather than thyroid deficiency, hypothyroidism resolves spontaneously with tumor involution or resection [15, 66].

1.9.4 Tumoral D2 in Metastatic Follicular Thyroid Carcinoma

While most patients with thyroid cancer have normal thyroid function tests upon presentation, a low serum T4 to T3 ratio has been observed in certain individuals with follicular thyroid carcinoma and large tumor burden. This phenomenon is distinct from the general thyrotoxicosis described in other patients with functional metastases of follicular thyroid cancer. A recent clinical study revealed that this depressed T4 to T3 ratio is due to T4 to T3 hyperconversion from tumoral D2 expression, with specific D2 activity manyfold higher than in normal thyroid tissue [67]. Affected individuals can have persistent hypothyroxinemia despite levothyroxine doses sufficient to cause TSH suppression and hypertriiodothyronemia [68].

Consistent with the above pathophysiology, this unusual thyroid function test pattern resolves with tumor resection.

1.9.5 Selenium Deficiency and Inborn Errors in Selenoprotein Synthesis

Because the iodothyronine deiodinases are selenoproteins, dietary selenium deficiency and defective selenoproteins synthesis can both impact thyroid hormone metabolism. While mild selenium deficiency typically has no impact on thyroid status, a high serum T4 to T3 ratio has been reported in children with severe deficiency [21, 69]. This is hypothesized to be due to decreased T4 to T3 conversion and, consistent with this, hepatic D1 activity is decreased in rodent models of selenium deficiency [70].

Of note, certain populations have coexisting iodine deficiency and selenium deficiency. In this scenario, the supplementation of selenium without iodine can precipitate a rapid fall in circulating thyroid hormones, presumably due to the restoration of normal inactivating pathways that require selenium-containing deiodinases. Because this can cause severe hypothyroidism in such at-risk individuals, iodine supplementation should begin before or simultaneously with selenium supplementation [71].

The synthesis of eukaryotic selenoproteins, including the deiodinases, requires specialized trans-acting factors including selenocysteine insertion sequence (SECIS) binding protein 2 (SBP2) and the elongation factor EF-sec. Recently, human mutations in SBP2 have been reported [72, 73]. These mutations are associated with decreased deiodinase activity (D2) and affected individuals have abnormal serum thyroid function tests characterized by high serum T4, low serum T3, and mild hyperthyrotropinemia. This pattern can be explained by impaired outer-ring deiodination and it is reminiscent of the phenotype observed in mice with genetic deficiencies of D2 [29, 74] +/− D1 [47, 59]. While the prevalence of this or similar defects are unknown, these families represent the first and novel demonstration of altered deiodination from a human germline mutation and suggest the possibility that genetic abnormalities in selenoprotein function may impact thyroid status in other clinical settings.

References

1. Delange F, Burgi H, Chen ZP, Dunn JT. World status of monitoring iodine deficiency disorders control programs. *Thyroid.* 2002;12:915-924.
2. Izumi M, Larsen PR. Triiodothyronine, thyroxine, and iodine in purified thyroglobulin from patients with Graves' disease. *J Clin Invest.* 1977;59:1105-1112.

3. Larsen PR. Thyroidal triiodothyronine and thyroxine in Graves' disease: correlation with pre-surgical treatment, thyroid status, and iodine content. *J Clin Endocrinol Metab.* 1975;41:1098-1104.

4. Moreno JC, Bikker H, Kempers MJ, et al. Inactivating mutations in the gene for thyroid oxidase 2 (THOX2) and congenital hypothyroidism. *N Engl J Med.* 2002;347:95-102.

5. Moreno JC, Klootwijk W, van Toor H, et al. Mutations in the iodotyrosine deiodinase gene and hypothyroidism. *N Engl J Med.* 2008;358:1811-1818.

6. Kopp P. Perspective: genetic defects in the etiology of congenital hypothyroidism. *Endocrinology.* 2002;143:2019-2024.

7. Larsen PR, Davies TF. Thyroid physiology and diagnostic evaluation of patients with thyroid disorders. In: Kronenberg HM, Melmed S, Polonsky KS, Larsen PR, eds. *Williams Textbook of Endocrinology.* 11th ed. Philadelphia, PA: Saunders Elsevier; 2008:299-332.

8. Garnick MB, Larsen PR. Acute deficiency of thyroxine-binding globulin during L-asparaginase therapy. *N Engl J Med.* 1979;301:252-253.

9. Larsen PR. Salicylate-induced increases in free triiodothyronine in human serum. Evidence of inhibition of triiodothyronine binding to thyroxine-binding globulin and thyroxine-binding prealbumin. *J Clin Invest.* 1972;51:1125-1134.

10. Wu SY, Green WL, Huang WS, Hays MT, Chopra IJ. Alternate pathways of thyroid hormone metabolism. *Thyroid.* 2005;15:943-958.

11. Vissor TJ. Hormone Metabolism. Thyroid Disease Manager. http://www.thyroidmanager.org/Chapter3/3c/3c-frame.htm. Updated May 20, 2008.

12. Moreno M, de Lange P, Lombardi A, Silvestri E, Lanni A, Goglia F. Metabolic effects of thyroid hormone derivatives. *Thyroid.* 2008;18:239-253.

13. Scanlan TS, Suchland KL, Hart ME, et al. 3-Iodothyronamine is an endogenous and rapid-acting derivative of thyroid hormone. *Nat Med.* 2004;10:638-642.

14. Chiellini G, Frascarelli S, Ghelardoni S, et al. Cardiac effects of 3-iodothyronamine: a new aminergic system modulating cardiac function. *FASEB J.* 2007;21:1597-1608.

15. Huang SA. Physiology and pathophysiology of type 3 deiodinase in humans. *Thyroid.* 2005;15:875-881.

16. Brown DD. The role of deiodinases in amphibian metamorphosis. *Thyroid.* 2005;15:815-821.

17. Dentice M, Bandyopadhyay A, Gereben B, et al. The Hedgehog-inducible ubiquitin ligase subunit WSB-1 modulates thyroid hormone activation and PTHrP secretion in the developing growth plate. *Nat Cell Biol.* 2005;7:698-705.

18. Hernandez A, Martinez ME, Fiering S, Galton VA, St Germain D. Type 3 deiodinase is critical for the maturation and function of the thyroid axis. *J Clin Invest.* 2006;116:476-484.

19. Simonides WS, Mulcahey MA, Redout EM, et al. Hypoxia-inducible factor induces local thyroid hormone inactivation during hypoxic-ischemic disease in rats. *J Clin Invest.* 2008;118:975-983.

20. Dentice M, Luongo C, Huang S, et al. Sonic hedgehog-induced type 3 deiodinase blocks thyroid hormone action enhancing proliferation of normal and malignant keratinocytes. *Proc Natl Acad Sci U S A.* 2007;104:14466-14471.

21. Bianco AC, Salvatore D, Gereben B, Berry MJ, Larsen PR. Biochemistry, cellular and molecular biology, and physiological roles of the iodothyronine selenodeiodinases. *Endocr Rev.* 2002;23:38-89.

22. Gereben B, Zavacki AM, Ribich S, et al. Cellular and molecular basis of deiodinase-regulated thyroid hormone signaling. *Endocr Rev.* 2008;29:898-938.

23. Bianco AC, Kim BW. Deiodinases: implications of the local control of thyroid hormone action. *J Clin Invest.* 2006;116:2571-2579.

24. Saberi M, Sterling FH, Utiger RD. Reduction in extrathyroidal triiodothyronine production by propylthiouracil in man. *J Clin Invest.* 1975;55:218-223.

25. Geffner DL, Azukizawa M, Hershman JM. Propylthiouracil blocks extrathyroidal conversion of thyroxine to triiodothyronine and augments thyrotropin secretion in man. *J Clin Invest.* 1975;55:224-229.

26. Abuid J, Larsen PR. Triiodothyronine and thyroxine in hyperthyroidism. Comparison of the acute changes during therapy with antithyroid agents. *J Clin Invest*. 1974;54:201-208.
27. Silva JE, Larsen PR. Pituitary nuclear 3,5,3'-triiodothyronine and thyrotropin secretion: an explanation for the effect of thyroxine. *Science*. 1977;198:617-620.
28. Bianco AC, Silva JE. Cold exposure rapidly induces virtual saturation of brown adipose tissue nuclear T3 receptors. *Am J Physiol*. 1988;255:E496-E503.
29. de Jesus LA, Carvalho SD, Ribeiro MO, et al. The type 2 iodothyronine deiodinase is essential for adaptive thermogenesis in brown adipose tissue. *J Clin Invest*. 2001;108:1379-1385.
30. Roti E, Fang SL, Green K, Emerson CH, Braverman LE. Human placenta is an active site of thyroxine and 3,3',5-triiodothyronine tyrosyl ring deiodination. *J Clin Endocrinol Metab*. 1981;53:498-501.
31. Mortimer RH, Galligan JP, Cannell GR, Addison RS, Roberts MS. Maternal to fetal thyroxine transmission in the human term placenta is limited by inner ring deiodination. *J Clin Endocrinol Metab*. 1996;81:2247-2249.
32. Huang SA, Dorfman DM, Genest DR, Salvatore D, Larsen PR. Type 3 iodothyronine deiodinase is highly expressed in the human uteroplacental unit and in fetal epithelium. *J Clin Endocrinol Metab*. 2003;88:1384-1388.
33. Zimmermann MB, Jooste PL, Pandav CS. Iodine-deficiency disorders. *Lancet*. 2008;372:1251-1262.
34. Bianchi R, Zucchelli GC, Giannessi D, et al. Evaluation of triiodothyronine (T3) kinetics in normal subjects, in hypothyroid, and hyperthyroid patients using specific antiserum for the determination of labeled T3 in plasma. *J Clin Endocrinol Metab*. 1978;46:203-214.
35. Brown ME, Refetoff S. Transient elevation of serum thyroid hormone concentration after initiation of replacement therapy in myxedema. *Ann Intern Med*. 1980;92:491-495.
36. Mandel SJ, Brent GA, Larsen PR. Levothyroxine therapy in patients with thyroid disease. *Ann Intern Med*. 1993;119:492-502.
37. Tu HM, Legradi G, Bartha T, Salvatore D, Lechan RM, Larsen PR. Regional expression of the type 3 iodothyronine deiodinase messenger ribonucleic acid in the rat central nervous system and its regulation by thyroid hormone. *Endocrinology*. 1999;140:784-790.
38. Kaplan MM, Larsen PR, Crantz FR, Dzau VJ, Rossing TH, Haddow JE. Prevalence of abnormal thyroid function test results in patients with acute medical illnesses. *Am J Med*. 1982;72:9-16.
39. Adler SM, Wartofsky L. The nonthyroidal illness syndrome. *Endocrinol Metab Clin North Am*. 2007;36:657-672, vi.
40. De Groot LJ. Dangerous dogmas in medicine: the nonthyroidal illness syndrome. *J Clin Endocrinol Metab*. 1999;84:151-164.
41. Brent GA, Hershman JM. Thyroxine therapy in patients with severe nonthyroidal illnesses and low serum thyroxine concentration. *J Clin Endocrinol Metab*. 1986;63:1-8.
42. Yu J, Koenig RJ. Regulation of hepatocyte thyroxine 5'-deiodinase by T3 and nuclear receptor coactivators as a model of the sick euthyroid syndrome. *J Biol Chem*. 2000;275:38296-38301.
43. Yu J, Koenig RJ. Induction of type 1 iodothyronine deiodinase to prevent the nonthyroidal illness syndrome in mice. *Endocrinology*. 2006;147:3580-3585.
44. Peeters RP, Wouters PJ, Kaptein E, van Toor H, Visser TJ, Van Den Berghe G. Reduced activation and increased inactivation of thyroid hormone in tissues of critically ill patients. *J Clin Endocrinol Metab*. 2003;88:3202-3211.
45. Koenig RJ. Regulation of type 1 iodothyronine deiodinase in health and disease. *Thyroid*. 2005;15:835-840.
46. Mebis L, Langouche L, Visser TJ, Van Den Berghe G. The type II iodothyronine deiodinase is up-regulated in skeletal muscle during prolonged critical illness. *J Clin Endocrinol Metab*. 2007;92:3330-3333.
47. Berry MJ, Grieco D, Taylor BA, et al. Physiological and genetic analyses of inbred mouse strains with a type I iodothyronine 5' deiodinase deficiency. *J Clin Invest*. 1993;92:1517-1528.

48. St Germain DL, Hernandez A, Schneider MJ, Galton VA. Insights into the role of deiodinases from studies of genetically modified animals. *Thyroid.* 2005;15:905-916.

49. Christoffolete MA, Arrojo e Drigo R, Gazoni F, et al. Mice with impaired extrathyroidal thyroxine to 3,5,3′-triiodothyronine conversion maintain normal serum 3,5,3′-triiodothyronine concentrations. *Endocrinology.* 2007;148:954-960.

50. Huang SA, Bianco AC. Reawakened interest in type III iodothyronine deiodinase in critical illness and injury. *Nat Clin Pract.* 2008;4:148-155.

51. Peeters RP, Wouters PJ, van Toor H, Kaptein E, Visser TJ, Van Den Berghe G. Serum 3,3′,5′-triiodothyronine (rT3) and 3,5,3′-triiodothyronine/rT3 are prognostic markers in critically ill patients and are associated with postmortem tissue deiodinase activities. *J Clin Endocrinol Metab.* 2005;90:4559-4565.

52. Janssen OE, Golcher HM, Grasberger H, Saller B, Mann K, Refetoff S. Characterization of T(4)-binding globulin cleaved by human leukocyte elastase. *J Clin Endocrinol Metab.* 2002;87:1217-1222.

53. Jirasakuldech B, Schussler GC, Yap MG, Drew H, Josephson A, Michl J. A characteristic serpin cleavage product of thyroxine-binding globulin appears in sepsis sera. *J Clin Endocrinol Metab.* 2000;85:3996-3999.

54. Chopra IJ, Teco GN, Nguyen AH, Solomon DH. In search of an inhibitor of thyroid hormone binding to serum proteins in nonthyroid illnesses. *J Clin Endocrinol Metab.* 1979;49:63-69.

55. den Brinker M, Joosten KF, Visser TJ, et al. Euthyroid sick syndrome in meningococcal sepsis: the impact of peripheral thyroid hormone metabolism and binding proteins. *J Clin Endocrinol Metab.* 2005;90:5613-5620.

56. Iervasi G, Clerico A, Bonini R, et al. Acute effects of amiodarone administration on thyroid function in patients with cardiac arrhythmia. *J Clin Endocrinol Metab.* 1997;82:275-280.

57. Surks MI, Sievert R. Drugs and thyroid function. *N Engl J Med.* 1995;333:1688-1694.

58. Cooper DS, Daniels GH, Ladenson PW, Ridgway EC. Hyperthyroxinemia in patients treated with high-dose propranolol. *Am J Med.* 1982;73:867-871.

59. Schneider MJ, Fiering SN, Thai B, et al. Targeted disruption of the type 1 selenodeiodinase gene (Dio1) results in marked changes in thyroid hormone economy in mice. *Endocrinology.* 2006;147:580-589.

60. Vainionpaa LK, Mikkonen K, Rattya J, et al. Thyroid function in girls with epilepsy with carbamazepine, oxcarbazepine, or valproate monotherapy and after withdrawal of medication. *Epilepsia.* 2004;45:197-203.

61. Mori K, Yoshida K, Kayama T, et al. Thyroxine 5-deiodinase in human brain tumors. *J Clin Endocrinol Metab.* 1993;77:1198-1202.

62. Tannahill LA, Visser TJ, McCabe CJ, et al. Dysregulation of iodothyronine deiodinase enzyme expression and function in human pituitary tumours. *Clin Endocrinol.* 2002;56:735-743.

63. Huang SA, Tu HM, Harney JW, et al. Severe hypothyroidism caused by type 3 iodothyronine deiodinase in infantile hemangiomas. *N Engl J Med.* 2000;343:185-189.

64. Huang SA, Fish SA, Dorfman DM, et al. A 21-year-old woman with consumptive hypothyroidism due to a vascular tumor expressing type 3 iodothyronine deiodinase. *J Clin Endocrinol Metab.* 2002;87:4457-4461.

65. Ruppe MD, Huang SA, Jan de Beur SM. Consumptive hypothyroidism caused by paraneoplastic production of type 3 iodothyronine deiodinase. *Thyroid.* 2005;15:1369-1372.

66. Balazs AE, Athanassaki I, Gunn SK, et al. Rapid resolution of consumptive hypothyroidism in a child with hepatic hemangioendothelioma following liver transplantation. *Ann Clin Lab Sci.* 2007;37:280-284.

67. Kim BW, Daniels GH, Harrison BJ, et al. Overexpression of type 2 iodothyronine deiodinase in follicular carcinoma as a cause of low circulating free thyroxine levels. *J Clin Endocrinol Metab.* 2003;88:594-598.

68. Miyauchi A, Takamura Y, Ito Y, et al. 3,5,3′-Triiodothyronine thyrotoxicosis due to increased conversion of administered levothyroxine in patients with massive metastatic follicular thyroid carcinoma. *J Clin Endocrinol Metab.* 2008;93:2239-2242.

69. Jochum F, Terwolbeck K, Meinhold H, Behne D, Menzel H, Lombeck I. Effects of a low selenium state in patients with phenylketonuria. *Acta Paediatr.* 1997;86:775-777.
70. DePalo D, Kinlaw WB, Zhao C, Engelberg-Kulka H, St Germain DL. Effect of selenium deficiency on type I 5′-deiodinase. *J Biol Chem.* 1994;269:16223-16228.
71. Vanderpas JB, Contempre B, Duale NL, et al. Selenium deficiency mitigates hypothyroxine-mia in iodine-deficient subjects. *Am J Clin Nutr.* 1993;57:271S-275S.
72. Dumitrescu AM, Liao XH, Abdullah MS, et al. Mutations in SECISBP2 result in abnormal thyroid hormone metabolism. *Nat Genet.* 2005;37:1247-1252.
73. Schomburg L, Dumitrescu AM, Liao XH, et al. Selenium supplementation fails to correct the selenoprotein synthesis defect in subjects with sequence binding protein 2 gene mutations. *Thyroid.* 2009;19:277-281.
74. Schneider MJ, Fiering SN, Pallud SE, Parlow AF, St Germain DL, Galton VA. Targeted disruption of the type 2 selenodeiodinase gene (DIO2) results in a phenotype of pituitary resistance to T4. *Mol Endocrinol.* 2001;15:2137-2148.

Chapter 2
Genetic Influences on Thyroid Function Tests[*]

Wendy M. van der Deure, Marco Medici, Robin P. Peeters and Theo J. Visser

In this review we will discuss the possible effects of polymorphic variation in the genes important for thyroid hormone synthesis, metabolism, and action, on the interindividual variation in thyroid functions tests. The genes involved are summarized in the following outline of thyroid hormone production and action, but their role is discussed in detail in other sections (Chaps. 1 and 4). In addition to these genes, we will also briefly discuss the possible contribution of genetic variation in the thyroid-specific transcription factors which are known to be important for thyroid development and regulation: TTF1, TTF2, and Pax8.

2.1 The Hypothalamus-Pituitary-Thyroid Axis

The production of thyroid hormone occurs in the follicular cells of the thyroid and involves the following steps (Fig. 2.1) [1]:

1. Cellular uptake of iodide by the Na/I symporter (NIS) located in the basolateral membrane.
2. Release of iodide through the apical membrane into the follicular lumen via pendrin and/or other transporters.
3. Generation of H_2O_2 by the enzyme dual oxidase 2 (DUOX2) located in the apical membrane.
4. Iodination of tyrosine residues in thyroglobulin (Tg) with generation of mono- and diiodotyrosine (MIT, DIT); generation of thyroxine (T4) by coupling of two

T. J. Visser (✉)
Department of Internal Medicine, Erasmus MC, Room Ee502,
Erasmus University Medical School, Dr. Molewaterplein 50,
3015 GE Rotterdam, The Netherlands
e-mail: t.j.visser@erasmusmc.nl

[*] **Disclosure statement:** *The authors have nothing to disclose.*

G. A. Brent (ed.), *Thyroid Function Testing,*
DOI 10.1007/978-1-4419-1485-9_2, © Springer Science+Business Media, LLC 2010

Follicular lumen

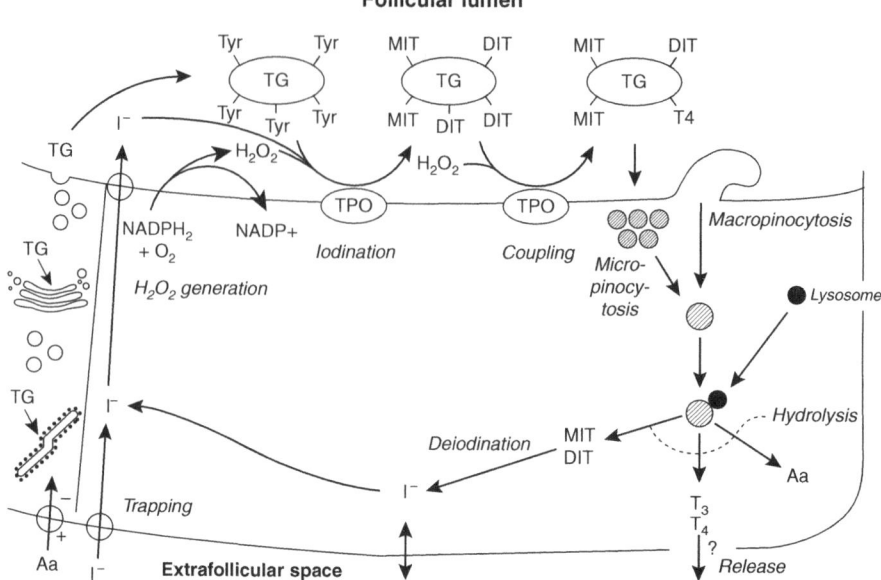

Fig. 2.1 Overview of thyroid hormone synthesis

DITs and of triiodothyronine (T3) by coupling of MIT and DIT. Both iodination and coupling are catalyzed by thyroid peroxidase (TPO) and require H_2O_2.

5. Endocytosis of Tg and hydrolysis by lysosomal enzymes, resulting in the liberation of MIT, DIT, T4, and T3.
6. Deiodination of excess MIT and DIT residues by iodotyrosine dehalogenase (DEHAL), and reutilization of the iodide liberated for thyroid hormone synthesis.
7. Secretion of T4 and T3 at the apical membrane by an as yet unknown mechanism.

Under normal conditions the thyroid predominantly secretes the prohormone T4 and only a small amount of the active hormone T3. Most T3 is generated by enzymatic outer-ring deiodination of T4 in peripheral tissues. Alternative inner-ring deiodination of T4 results in the generation of the inactive metabolite rT3. Inner-ring deiodination is also an important route for the degradation of T3. Three deiodinases (D1-3) are involved in these reactions; D1 and D2 are capable of activating T4 to T3, whereas D3 is responsible for inactivation of T4 to rT3 and of T3 to 3,3′-T2. These deiodinases are expressed in various tissues, including liver, kidney, brain, pituitary, thyroid, and skeletal muscle.

The production of thyroid hormone by the thyroid gland is regulated by the hypothalamus-pituitary-thyroid (HPT) axis (Fig. 2.2) [2]. Thyroid hormone is secreted in response to thyroid-stimulating hormone (TSH), which is synthesized in and released from the pituitary. TSH consists of a (common) α subunit and a TSH-specific β subunit, and exerts its effect via binding to the TSH receptor (TSHR) on the thyroid follicular cells. In turn, TSH production is stimulated by hypothalamic thyrotropin-releasing hormone (TRH). The production of TRH and

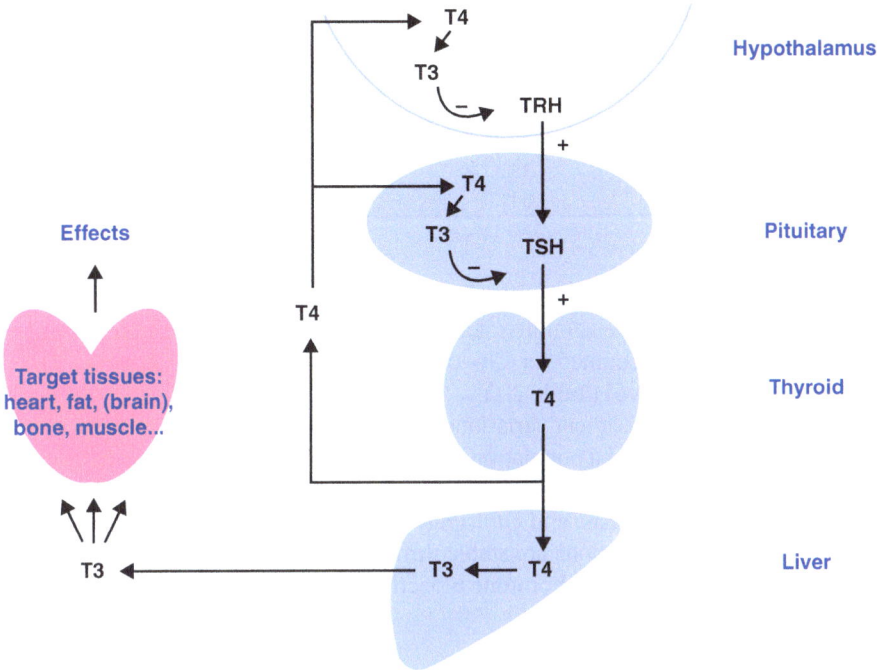

Fig. 2.2 Overview of hypothalamus-pituitary-thyroid-peripheral tissues axis

TSH is down-regulated by thyroid hormones, a process known as negative feedback regulation. Also, other hypothalamic hormones and drugs, such as somatostatin, cortisol, and bromocriptine lower TSH production. Besides the regulation by TSH, thyroid hormone synthesis is also dependent on the availability of iodine.

Thyroid hormone is transported in the circulation tightly bound to different proteins, largely, thyroxine-binding globulin (TBG), transthyretin (TTR), and albumin. However, it is the free fraction of T4 and T3 which is available for metabolism and action in the tissues. The above mentioned deiodinases have their active sites located in the cytoplasm, and most thyroid hormone actions are initiated by binding of T3 to its nuclear receptors (TRs). Cellular uptake of thyroid hormone does not occur by passive diffusion, but is mediated by specific transporters. These include different members of the monocarboxylate transporter (MCT) and organic anion transporting polypeptide (OATP) families. TRs are encoded by two genes: THRA which codes for different TRα isoforms and THRB which codes for different TRβ isoforms.

2.2   Influence of Genetic Variation on Thyroid Function Tests

In healthy subjects, serum thyroid parameters show substantial interindividual variability, whereas the intraindividual variability is within a narrow range [3]. Together with environmental factors such as diet and smoking, genetic factors contribute

Table 2.1 Estimates of the genetic contribution to the variation in serum thyroid hormone levels from different studies

	Proportion of variance in serum thyroid hormone levels attributable to genetic effects		
	Hansen et al. [4]	Samollow et al. [5]	Panicker et al. [6]
TSH	64%	37%	65%
FT4	65%	35%	39%
FT3	64%	64%	23%

significantly to this interindividual variability, resulting in a thyroid function set-point that is different for each individual. This is demonstrated by different studies in which heritability accounted for ~30–65% of the overall variation in serum TSH, FT4, and FT3 levels [4–6] (Table 2.1).

Polymorphisms are frequent variations in the nucleotide sequence of the genome that occur in at least 1% of a population, whereas mutations have a lower frequency. These variations seem to play an important role in the interindividual variation in serum thyroid function tests, and contribute to each individual's unique HPT axis setpoint. Since these variations are stable throughout life, they may not only affect serum levels, but also thyroid hormone bioactivity throughout life.

Table 2.2 Genetic defects associated with abnormal thyroid function tests

Phenotype	Gene	Inheritance	Chromosome
Central hypothyroidism	TRHR	AR	8p23
	TSHβ	AR	1p13
Resistance to TSH, thyroid hypoplasia, and hypothyroidism	TSHR	AR	14q13
Hyperthyroidism and goiter	TSHR	AD	14q13
Thyroid dysgenesis and hypothyroidism	PAX8	AR	2q12–q14
	TTF1	AD	14q13.3
	TTF2	AD	22q33
Thyroid dyshormonogenesis, hypothyroidism, and goiter	NIS	AR	19p13.2–p12
	Tg	AR	8q24.2–q24.3
	DUOX2	AR	15q15
	TPO	AR	2p25
	DEHAL1	AR	6q24q25
Hypothyroidism, goiter, and deafness	Pendrin	AR	7q31
High total T4/T3, normal FT4/FT3	TBG	X-linked	Xq22
	TTR	AD	18q11
	ALB	AD	4q11
Low total T4/T3, normal FT4/FT3	TBG	X-linked	Xq22
Mental retardation, high serum T3	MCT8	X-linked	Xq13
High TSH/FT4/rT3, low T3	SBP2	AR	9q22

TRHR thyrotropin releasing hormone receptor, *TSHβ* thyroid stimulating hormone β subunit, *TSHR* TSH receptor, *PAX8/TTF1/TTF2* thyroid transcription factors, *NIS* sodium iodide symporter, *Tg* thyroglobulin, *DUOX2* dual oxidase 2, *TPO* thyroid peroxidase, *DEHAL1* iodotyrosine dehalogenase 1, *TBG* thyroid binding globulin, *TTR* transthyretin, *ALB* albumin, *MCT8* monocarboxylate transporter 8, *SBP2* selenocysteine *cis* element binding protein 2, *AR* autosomal recessive, *AD* autosomal dominant

Many studies, in which the effects of certain polymorphisms on serum thyroid hormone levels are studied, have been published in the last few years. These studies usually involve comparisons of many polymorphisms with several clinical endpoints, resulting in a high risk of type I statistical errors. For this reason, replication of data in independent cohorts is essential before any conclusions can be drawn. In this chapter we review the different studies that have been published on this subject, and discuss the consequences of polymorphisms and mutations in different thyroid hormone pathway genes on serum thyroid function tests. An overview of the genetic defects associated with abnormal thyroid function tests can be found in Table 2.2.

2.3   Genetic Variation in Thyroid-Regulating Genes: TRH, TRHR, TSH, TSHR

Central hypothyroidism is a rare disorder with an estimated frequency of 0.005% in the general population [7]. It is characterized by insufficient TSH secretion resulting in low levels of thyroid hormones, caused by either pituitary or hypothalamic defects. Theoretically, it could result from mutations in the TRH, TRHR, and TSHβ genes. Several clinical reports have suggested isolated TRH deficiency as a cause of central hypothyroidism [8, 9]. However, to date, no patients with mutations in the TRH gene have been described. Collu et al. described the first patient with a mutation in the TRHR causing central hypothyroidism. A 9-year-old boy was found to have compound heterozygous mutations in the 5'-part of the gene [10]. Recently, a family has been described with complete resistance to TRH due to a homozygous nonsense mutation in the TRH receptor [11].

Central hypothyroidism due to a mutation in the TSHβ gene was first described in 1990 [12]. In these patients, TSH is undetectable or very low, and the administration of TRH does not result in a rise in serum TSH. Among the currently known mutations, most are located in the coding region of the gene [12, 13]. However, a mutation that led to TSH deficiency caused by exon skipping has also been described [14]. All affected patients were homozygous. No data regarding the influence of polymorphisms in TRH, TRHR, and TSHβ genes on thyroid function tests are available.

Many mutations in TSHR have been described which can be divided into germline or acquired mutations. Acquired gain-of-function mutations result in a phenotype of toxic adenoma or toxic multinodular goiter [15]. Germline gain-of-function TSHR mutations were first identified in two French families in 1992 [16]. It causes autonomous thyroid growth and function, resulting in a phenotype of hyperthyroidism and goiter. On the other hand, germline loss-of-function TSHR mutations are associated with TSH resistance and congenital hypothyroidism [17]. In a subset of these patients, the mutations in the TSHR are partially inactivating [18]. In partial resistance TSH is elevated, but the peripheral hormone levels are normal: a condition known as euthyroid hyperthyrotropinemia [18]. In these patients, the size of the thyroid is normal or enlarged.

Polymorphisms in TSHR have been extensively studied in the context of the development of autoimmune thyroid disease. Although early studies investigating TSHR polymorphisms in Graves' disease proved inconclusive, more recent studies have provided convincing evidence for association of the TSHR region with Graves' disease. Strongest associations were obtained for two SNPs (single nucleotide polymorphisms) (rs179247 and rs12101255), both located in intron 1 of the TSHR. [19–21]. Data on the influence of TSH polymorphisms on thyroid function tests, on the other hand, are sparse: so far only one polymorphism has been shown to influence serum thyroid hormone levels. In several Caucasian populations, the TSHR-Asp727Glu polymorphism is associated with lower levels of plasma TSH, but not with FT4 [22–24]. This could point toward a higher sensitivity of the variant versus the wild-type TSHR, since less TSH is needed to produce normal FT4 levels. Although there is one *in vitro* study showing that the TSHR-Glu^{727} variant results in an increased cAMP response of the receptor to TSH [25], others have not been able to replicate this [26, 27]. A different explanation would be that the Asp727Glu polymorphism is linked to another polymorphism elsewhere in the gene. The TSHR-Asp727Glu polymorphism is found to be within a linkage disequilibrium block starting at intron 8 and extending about 10 kb beyond the 3′-UTR of the TSHR gene [28].

2.4 Genetic Variation in Thyroid Transcription Factors: PAX8, TTF1, TTF2

The paired-box gene PAX8 is important for the development of the thyroid gland and for the regulation thyroid-specific gene expression, including NIS, Tg, and TPO [29]. The PAX8 gene is located on human chromosome 2q12–q14. Homozygous inactivation of the *Pax8* gene in mice results in a complete lack of the development of thyroid follicles [30]. Most animals die within the first 3 weeks of life unless they are treated with thyroid hormone. The first patient with thyroid dysgenesis resulting from a heterozygous nonsense mutation in PAX8 was reported in 1998 by the group of Di Lauro [31]. Since then several other patients with congenital hypothyroidism have been identified with heterozygous mutations in the paired-box domain of the PAX8 protein.

No associations have been reported between polymorphisms in PAX8 and thyroid function tests. A nonsynonymous Phe329Leu SNP has been identified, but it lies outside the paired-box domain and probably has little effect on PAX8 function [32]. In addition to the thyroid, PAX8 is also expressed in the central nervous system and the kidneys.

TTF1 is a homeobox-containing protein belonging to the NKX2 family of transcription factors and is also referred to as NKX2.1. TTF1 is expressed predominantly in the thyroid, lung, and brain, in particular the basal ganglia. Homozygous *Ttf1* knockout mice are born without thyroid gland and also lack lung parenchyma [33]. In patients, different mutations in TTF1 result in varying dysfunction of the organs where TTF1 is expressed, including congenital hypothyroidism, respiratory distress, and choreoathetosis [34–36]. In the deCODE population study in Iceland, polymorphisms in the region of the TTF1 gene on chromosome 14q13.3 have recently been associated with an increased risk of thyroid cancer as well as with lower serum TSH levels [37].

TTF2 is a forkhead gene which is now also termed FOXE1. Like PAX8 and TTF1, TTF2 is an essential transcription factor for the development of the thyroid gland, but it is not involved in the regulation of thyroid function. Mice with homozygous inactivation of the *Foxe1* gene exhibit an ectopic or absent thyroid gland and a cleft palate [38]. Heterozygous missense mutations have been identified in patients with thyroid dysgenesis, cleft palate, choanal atresia and spiky hair [39, 40]. After the first report, this is also referred to as the Bamforth–Lazarus syndrome.

In the deCODE study, polymorphisms in the FOXE1 locus on human chromosome 22q33 have been associated with an increased risk for thyroid cancer as well as with lower serum TSH and T4 levels and higher serum T3 levels [37]. Contradictory reports have appeared on the possible association of the poly-Ala stretch (14 or 16 residues) in TTF2 with thyroid dysgenesis [41, 42]. Furthermore, an SNP in the 5′-UTR of FOXE1 has been associated with cleft palate [43].

2.5   Genetic Variation in Thyroid Hormone Synthesis Genes: NIS, Pendrin, Tg, TPO, DUOX2, DEHAL

The cloning and characterization of NIS was reported in 1996 by the group of Carrasco [44, 45]. It mediates the electrogenic thyroidal uptake of I^- together with Na^+ in a stoichiometry of 1:2. NIS is also involved in iodide transport in other tissues such as the breast and intestine [46, 47]. The NIS gene is located on chromosome 19p13.2–p12 and consists of 15 exons. Different homozygous and compound heterozygous NIS mutations have been reported in patients with congenital hypothyroidism because of a thyroid hormone synthesis defect [48]. To our knowledge, no studies have been reported regarding the possible effects of polymorphisms in the NIS gene.

The precise role of pendrin in the transport of iodide in the thyroid follicle is still subject to debate [48, 49]. Pendrin earned its name because mutations in this gene have been identified in patients with Pendred syndrome, which is a recessive disorder characterized by sensorineural deafness and hypothyroidism resulting from a thyroid hormone synthesis defect (dyshormonogenesis) [48, 49]. However, pendrin mutations may also result in a selective hearing defect without thyroid dysfunction [50]. The hearing impairment is the result of a malformation of the cochlea, where pendrin plays an important role in the secretion of bicarbonate into the endolymph [51]. As far as we know, there have been no reports of an association of polymorphisms in the pendrin gene with thyroid function.

Human Tg is a large 660 kDa protein consisting of two identical subunits consisting of 2,748 amino acids. The gene covers ~300 kb on chromosome 8q24.2–q24.3

and contains 37 exons; the mature mRNA is ~8.7 kb in size [52, 53]. Tg provides the substrate for the synthesis of thyroid hormone and is the most abundant protein in the follicular lumen. It is not surprising, therefore, that Tg is a major antigen against which antibodies are produced in patients with autoimmune thyroid disorders.

Many mutations in Tg have been identified in patients with congenital hypothyroidism due to dyshormonogenesis. The interested reader is referred to the OMIM section of the NCBI website (http://www.ncbi.nlm.nih.gov/omim). Also, the *cog/cog* mouse has severe hypothyroidism because of a homozygous missense mutation in Tg [54]. Polymorphisms in the *Tg* gene have been associated with a risk for autoimmune thyroid disease [53, 55, 56], but to our knowledge no evidence has been reported for the association of Tg polymorphisms with thyroid function tests.

Human DUOX2 is a large and complex protein containing 1,548 amino acids, the sequence of which indicates the presence of 7 transmembrane domains, an NADPH-binding domain, an FAD-binding domain, a heme-binding domain, two calcium-binding EF hands, and a peroxidase domain. It catalyzes the oxidation of NADPH from the cytoplasm and delivers its product (H_2O_2) to the luminal surface of the apical membrane where it is utilized as a substrate for TPO [57]. Proper expression of DUOX2 requires the presence of the maturation factor DUOXA2, a protein consisting of 320 amino acids and five transmembrane domains [58]. They are encoded by genes located in a cluster on human chromosome 15q15 which also contains the homologous DUOX1 and DUOXA1 genes [58].

A variety of mutations have been identified in DUOX2 [59, 60] and recently also in DUOXA2 [60, 61] in patients with thyroid dyshormonogenesis. However, associations of polymorphisms in these genes with thyroid function tests have so far not been reported.

TPO is a glycoprotein consisting of 933 amino acids and containing a single transmembrane domain. A short C-terminal domain is located in the cytoplasm, but most of the protein is exposed on the luminal surface of the apical membrane which also contains a heme-binding domain, the active center of the enzyme [62]. TPO is encoded by a gene which covers about 150 kb on chromosome 2p25, distributed over 17 exons. In addition to full-length TPO-1, different splice variants have been characterized, including the TPO-2 variant which is generated by skipping of exon 10, resulting in the loss of 57 amino acids in the middle of the protein [62]. TPO-2 has no enzyme activity and its function is unknown.

Many TPO mutations have been identified in patients with thyroid dyshormonogenesis, see for instance [63, 64]. To our knowledge association have not been reported so far of polymorphisms in TPO with thyroid function tests.

DEHAL1 is a 289-amino acid protein containing an N-terminal membrane anchor and a conserved nitroreductase domain with an FMN-binding site [65–67]. Functional DEHAL1 probably exists as a homodimer. The DEHAL1 gene is located on chromosome 6q24–q25 and consists of 5 exons. DEHAL1, also termed IYD, catalyzes the reductive deiodination of MIT and DIT by NADH. Since DEHAL1 lacks an NADH-binding sequence, iodotyrosine deiodinase activity requires the involvement of a reductase, which has not yet been identified.

Recently, homozygous missense mutations in DEHAL1 have been identified in patients with hereditary hypothyroidism [68, 69]. Remarkably, patients are not always identified at neonatal screening, and hypothyroidism develops later in life, probably depending on the iodine intake. Since this may occur in the first year(s) and is not immediately recognized, it may result in mental retardation. So far, associations of polymorphisms in DEHAL1 with thyroid function tests have not been reported.

2.6   Genetic Variation in Thyroid Hormone Receptor Genes: TRα, TRβ

Thyroid hormone action is initiated by binding of T3 to its receptor (TR), which is located in the nucleus. TRs are associated with T3 response elements of target genes, and binding of T3 to the TR leads to stimulation or suppression of gene transcription. TRs are encoded by the THRA gene located on chromosome 17q11.2 and the THRB gene located on chromosome 3p24.3. THRA encodes five proteins, of which only TRα1 has intact DNA and T3 binding domains. THRB encodes three proteins that can bind DNA and T3. TRα is the predominant TR in brain, heart, and bone, whereas TRβ is the predominant TR in the liver, kidney, thyroid, and pituitary [70, 71].

Mutations in TRβ can lead to thyroid hormone resistance syndrome. Over 100 different heterozygous TRβ mutations have been identified, almost all located in the ligand-binding domain. The estimated frequency is 1/50,000 [72, 73]. As TRβ is the predominant TR in the negative feedback regulation of the HPT axis, increased serum thyroid hormones and nonsuppressed TSH are the hallmarks of the diagnosis. Amongst others, clinical features include goiter, short stature, decreased weight, tachycardia, cardiomyopathy, hearing loss, attention deficit hyperactivity disorder, decreased IQ, and dyslexia. These are due to a relative hypothyroid state in TRβ-expressing tissues and a relative hyperthyroid state in TRα-expressing tissues [74].

A limited number of studies have been published about the association of genetic variation in TRβ and serum thyroid parameters [23, 75]. Sørensen et al. found the THRB-intron9-G>A polymorphism to be associated with higher serum TSH in a Danish twin population. Although replication in a Caucasian population showed a similar trend, it did not reach statistical significance [75].

No patients with mutations in TRα have been identified yet. Various mouse models with knock-in mutations in TRα have been generated [76–79]. In all models, TSH was (moderately) elevated. Depending on the mutation, T3 and T4 levels ranged from slightly decreased to slightly increased. In general, these mice showed a higher mortality, delayed growth, reduced fertility, delayed bone development and signs of impaired cardiac function and neuropsychiatric abnormalities (e.g., ataxia and anxiety-related behavior).

Sørensen et al. studied the possible relationship of two polymorphisms in THRA (i.e., THRA-A2390G, rs12939700) with serum thyroid parameters in a large population of Danish twins and found no significant associations [75]. Furthermore, no studies have been published on the association of genetic variation in TRα and serum thyroid parameters.

2.7 Genetic Variation in Serum TH Transport Proteins: TBG, TTR, and Albumin

Thyroid hormones circulate in serum bound to the carrier proteins TBG, TTR (formerly known as thyroxine-binding prealbumin or TBPA) and albumin. These proteins provide a large and stable pool of circulating thyroid hormone, distributing the water-insoluble hormone to all tissues. In humans TBG, TTR, and albumin carry about 75%, 15%, and 10%, respectively, of T4 and T3 [80–82].

The TBG gene is located on the long arm of the X chromosome (Xq22.2) and is composed of five exons [83]. Mutations in the TBG gene can lead to three different phenotypes according to serum TBG concentrations in affected hemizygous males: complete TBG deficiency, partial TBG deficiency, and TBG excess [84]. TBG deficiency is associated with very low levels of total T4 and T3. Since unbound hormone levels are normal, patients are euthyroid and TSH levels are normal. TBG excess gives rise to increased levels of total T4 and T3, again with normal levels of FT4 and FT3. To date, approximately 30 variants have been associated with TBG defects [83]. These are either nonsense or missense mutations, randomly distributed throughout the TBG gene. Gene duplications or triplications have been shown to be the cause of TBG excess [85].

The TTR gene is located on chromosome 18q11.2–q12.1. Circulating TTR is a tetramer of identical 127-amino acid subunits. More than 80 different mutations in this gene have been reported. Most mutations are related to amyloid deposition, affecting predominantly peripheral nerves and/or the heart. These mutations can lead to diseases such as amyloidotic polyneuropathy, amyloidotic vitreous opacities, cardiomyopathy, oculoleptomeningeal amyloidosis, meningocerebrovascular amyloidosis, and carpal tunnel syndrome [86]. Interestingly, only a small portion of the gene mutations is nonamyloidogenic. Some mutations increase the affinity of T4, leading to a state called euthyroid hyperthyroxinemia: increased total T4 and T3 levels, with normal levels of FT4, FT3, and TSH. This has been shown for the Ala109Thr, Ala109Val and Thr119Met mutations [87, 88]. A decreased concentration or affinity of TTR is not associated with variations in serum concentrations of thyroid hormones [89].

Familial dysalbuminemic hyperthyroxinemia (FDH) was first identified in 1979 by Hennemann et al. [90]. Like other conditions associated with euthyroid hyperthyroxinemia, it is characterized by increased levels of total T4, but normal levels of FT4 and TSH. It is caused by mutations in the albumin gene. The most common mutation in this respect is Arg218His: it produces an albumin molecule with 10- to 15-fold higher affinity for T4 than wild-type albumin, and a fivefold increase in affinity for T3 [91]. Two other mutations have been identified, i.e., Arg218Pro and Leu66Pro [91]. The latter induces a selective increase in affinity for T3.

Although polymorphisms have been identified in the TBG, TTR, and albumin genes, none has been linked to alterations in serum thyroid hormone levels.

2.8   Genetic Variation in TH Transporters: MCT8, MCT10, OATPs

Both TRs and deiodinases are located intracellularly. Therefore, transport of thyroid hormone across the cell membrane is required for hormone action and metabolism. Based on the lipophilic structure of thyroid hormones, it was assumed that they enter cells through passive diffusion. However, it has become increasingly clear that there are specific thyroid hormone transporters, and that the activity of these transporters in part determines the intracellular thyroid hormone concentration [92].

2.8.1   MCT8 and MCT10

Monocarboxylate transporter 8 (MCT8) has been characterized as an active and specific thyroid hormone transporter [93]. The MCT8 gene is located on the X chromosome (Xq13.2) and contains six exons. Mutations in the MCT8 gene cause a syndrome of severe psychomotor retardation and high serum T3 levels in affected male patients, known as the Allan–Herndon–Dudley syndrome [94, 95]. The neurological deficits are probably explained by an impeded uptake of T3 in MCT8-expressing central neurons and, hence, an impaired brain development. This has been reviewed in detail elsewhere [94, 95].

Since mutations in the MCT8 gene have such profound effects, the question arises whether small changes in the MCT8 gene may affect transport activity as well. Only two studies exist on the relationship between MCT8 polymorphic variants and serum thyroid hormone levels [96–98] (Table 2.3). Dominguez-Gerpe and colleagues studied the Ser107Pro polymorphism (rs6647476), which is the only established nonsynonymous polymorphism in MCT8 [98]. In their study, 276 healthy Spanish men were genotyped for this polymorphism. They found no association with serum thyroid hormone levels or with mRNA levels coding for MCT8 or thyroid hormone-responsive genes in white blood cells or in T3-stimulated

Table 2.3 Effect of common variation in MCT8 and MCT10 on thyroid function tests

Gene	Polymorphism	Location	Change	Effect on serum thyroid hormone levels	*In vitro* effect
MCT8	–	Exon	Ser33Pro	No effect observed	Not determined
	rs6647476	Exon	Ser107Pro	No effect observed	No effect observed
	rs5937843	Intron	G > T	Not consistent	Not determined
MCT10	rs14399	3'-UTR	C > A	No effect observed	Not determined

fibroblasts. We also genotyped this polymorphism in a population of 156 healthy men and women and found no association between this variant and serum thyroid parameters. Hemizygous carriers of a different polymorphism, i.e., rs5937843, located in intron 5 of the MCT8 gene, had lower FT4 levels compared to wild-type male subjects. However, we failed to replicate these findings in the homozygous female carriers in the same population.

MCT10 has been characterized by Kim et al. in 2002 [99] as a T-type amino acid transporter, facilitating the cellular uptake and efflux of aromatic amino acids. Although this was not immediately clear, we have later shown that MCT10 is an active iodothyronine transporter [100]. The MCT10 gene is located on chromosome 6q21–q22 and has the same gene structure as MCT8. The MCT10 protein also has ~50% amino acid identity with the MCT8 protein.

To date, only one study has been published regarding the possible association of genetic variation in the MCT10 gene with serum thyroid parameters. We showed that a common polymorphism (rs14399) in the 3'-UTR region of the MCT10 gene is not associated with serum thyroid hormone levels [97]. The only established nonsynonymous polymorphism identified in human MCT10 is Lys508Gln (rs17072442), with a minor allele frequency of ~2%. Considering the type of amino acid change, it would be interesting to investigate the association of this polymorphism with serum thyroid parameters and other thyroid-related endpoints.

So far, patients with mutations in MCT10 have not been identified. Considering the wide tissue distribution of MCT10 expression and its swift T3 transport, it is quite likely that MCT10 mutations are associated with significant alterations in tissue and/or serum thyroid hormone concentration. As is the case with MCT8, mutations in MCT10 may well result in a significant impairment of tissue T3 uptake and, thus, in manifestations of thyroid hormone resistance. To predict the phenotype of patients with MCT10 mutations, it would be highly interesting to study MCT10 knockout mice, although it should be realized that MCT8 knockout mice do not show any neurological abnormality in sharp contrast with the clinical condition of patients with MCT8 mutations [101–103].

2.8.2   OATP1A2, 1B1, 1B3, and 1C1

The organic anion transporting polypeptides (OATPs) are a large family of transporters responsible for Na^+-independent transmembrane transport of amphipathic organic compounds, including bile salts, bromosulfophthalein, steroid hormones and numerous drugs [104]. Among the many ligands transported by OATPs, several members of this large family also facilitate uptake of thyroid hormone. These include members of the OATP1 subfamily: 1A2 [105, 106], 1B1 [105, 107], 1B3 [105], and 1C1 [108]; a member of the OATP2 subfamily: 2B1 [105]; and members of the OATP4 subfamily: 4A1 [106] and 4C1 [109]. The focus in this review will be on OATP1A2, 1B1, 1B3, and 1C1, since data regarding the effect of genetic variants on serum thyroid hormone levels is available for only these four genes. These transporters show high sequence homology and are encoded by a gene cluster located on chromosome 12p12.

OATP1A2 has been shown to transport T3 and T4 with K_m values of 7 μM and 8 μM, respectively [106]. In addition, it was demonstrated that OATP1A2 facilitates not only transport of T4, T3, and rT3, but also of their sulfates T4S, T3S, and rT3S in transfected cells [110]. We analyzed the OATP1A2-Ile13Thr and -Glu-172Asp polymorphisms for association with serum thyroid hormone levels. For the Ile13Thr polymorphism, no consistent associations with serum thyroid hormone levels were found. In addition, no differences in thyroid hormone transport were observed between this variant and wild-type OATP1A2 *in vitro*. However, cells transfected with the Glu172Asp variant showed decreased transport compared to cells transfected with wild-type OATP1A2. This variant was, however, not associated with serum thyroid parameters in two populations of Caucasians. It could, therefore, be concluded that this polymorphism might affect tissue thyroid hormone concentrations independent of serum levels. Alternatively, OATP1A2 might not play an important role in thyroid hormone transport in a physiological situation.

OATP1B1 and OATP1B3 are exclusively expressed in the liver and share approximately 80% amino acid identity with each other [107, 111]. Recent studies have shown that OATP1B1 markedly stimulates uptake of the iodothyronine sulfates T4S, T3S, and rT3S but has little activity toward nonsulfated T4, T3, and rT3 [112]. Like OATP1B1, OATP1B3 preferentially transports the sulfated iodothyronines as well as rT3 [110]. Polymorphisms in the OATP1B1 and OATP1B3 genes have been extensively studied as they impact on the interindividual variability of drug disposition and drug response [113]. To date, only one study has focused on associations between a polymorphism in the OATP1B1 gene, Val174Ala, and serum thyroid hormone levels. This polymorphism has been studied extensively: Niemi and colleagues have shown that the Val174Ala polymorphism leads to decreased function of OATP1B1 and thereby increases the systemic bioavailability of lipid-lowering drugs [114].

As we saw that OATP1B1 preferentially transports sulfated hormones, i.e., T4S, T3S, rT3S, and E1S [112], we expected that the Val174Ala polymorphism would be associated with serum levels of iodothyronine sulfates and E1S. Indeed, this polymorphism was associated with higher serum T4S levels in 155 blood donors, while in a larger cohort of elderly Caucasians this same polymorphism was associated with 40% higher serum E1S levels. *In vitro*, OATP1B1-Ala[174] showed a 40% lower induction of transport and metabolism of these substrates than OATP1B1-Val[174] [112]. Decreased hepatic uptake of T4S and E1S by OATP1B1-Ala[174] compared with OATP-Val[174] *in vivo* thus gives rise to higher T4S and E1S levels.

To date, no associations have been found between genetic variation in the OATP1B3 gene and serum thyroid hormone levels [110]: the OATP1B3-Ser112Ala and Met233Ile polymorphisms showed no association with serum thyroid parameters in a population of Caucasian blood donors. OATP1C1 shows a high preference for

T4 and rT3 [108]. In addition, T4S uptake is also facilitated by OATP1C1, although less effectively than T4 [115]. Together with the almost exclusive expression at the blood–brain barrier, this suggests that OATP1C1 is critical for T4 uptake into the brain. This important role is substantiated by Sugiyama and colleagues who showed that expression levels of Oatp1c1 in isolated rat brain capillaries are regulated by thyroid hormone concentrations [116]. Oatp1c1 is up-regulated in hypothyroid rats and down-regulated in hyperthyroid rats [116]. Considering the presumed function of T4 transport across the blood–brain barrier, mutations in OATP1C1 are expected to have a significant impact on brain development and function. Loss of OATP1C1 function may well lead to neuronal deficits similar to that seen in subjects with untreated congenital hypothyroidism or in patients with MCT8 mutations [116]. It seems worthwhile to study this in *Oatp1c1* knockout mice.

OATP1C1 is capable of T4, T4S, and rT3 transport, but polymorphisms in the OATP1C1 gene are not consistently associated with serum thyroid hormone levels [115]. Although, the OATP1C1-Pro143Thr and C3035T polymorphisms were associated with serum thyroid parameters in 156 blood donors, we could not replicate these findings in a much larger cohort of Danish twins. Nor did we observe any differences in uptake and metabolism of T4 and rT3 between these variants and wild-type OATP1C1. In addition, no associations were found between the OATP1C1-intron3C>T polymorphism and serum thyroid hormone levels [115]. However, both intron3C>T and C3035T polymorphisms, but not Pro143Thr, were associated with symptoms of fatigue and depression in a population of adequately treated hypothyroid patients [117]. This is of interest as recently a number of papers have reported on effects of polymorphisms in thyroid hormone pathway genes, independent of an effect on serum thyroid hormone levels [118, 119]. Many associations between polymorphisms in thyroid hormone pathway genes and different clinical endpoints are independent of serum thyroid hormone levels, highlighting the importance of local regulation of thyroid hormones in tissues [120].

Table 2.4 presents a summary of the studies discussed above regarding the possible effects of polymorphisms in the different OATP1 transporters on serum thyroid hormone levels *in vivo* and on the rate of iodothyronine transport *in vitro*.

Table 2.4 Effect of common variation in OATP1A2, OATP1B1, OATP1B3, and OATP1C1 on thyroid function tests

Gene	Polymorphism	Location	Change	Serum thyroid hormone levels	*In vitro* transport
OATP1A2	rs57921276	Exon	Ile13Thr	No effect	No effect
	rs57550534	Exon	Glu172Asp	No effect	↓
OATP1B1	rs4149056		Val174Ala	T4S↑, E1S↓ T3/rT3↓	↓
OATP1B3	rs4149117	Exon	Ser112Ala	No effect	ND
	rs7311358	Exon	Met233Ile	No effect	ND
OATP1C1	rs10770704	Intron	C/T	No effect	ND
	rs36010656	Exon	Pro143Thr	rT3↑ (not consistent)	No effect
	rs10444412	3′-UTR	C3035T	FT4↑, rT3↑ (not consistent)	No effect

2.9   Genetic Variation in Deiodinases: D1, D2, D3

All the three deiodinases have a different physiological role [121]. D1 is present in liver, kidney, and thyroid, and plays a key-role in the production of the active hormone T3 from T4 and in the clearance of the metabolite rT3. D2 is present in brain, pituitary, brown adipose tissue, thyroid, skeletal muscle, aortic smooth muscle cells, and osteoblasts; D2 mRNA has also been detected in the human heart. In tissues such as the brain, D2 is important for local production of T3, whereas D2 in skeletal muscle may also contribute to plasma T3 production. D3 is present in brain, skin, placenta, pregnant uterus, and various fetal tissues, and is induced in critical illness. D3 is the major T3 and T4 inactivating enzyme and contributes to thyroid hormone homeostasis by protecting tissues from excess thyroid hormone.

The DIO1 gene has four exons and is located on human chromosome 1p33–p32, the DIO2 gene has two exons and is located on chromosome 14q24.3, and the DIO3 gene consists of a single exon and is located on chromosome 14q32. No patients with inactivating mutations in any of the iodothyronine deiodinases have yet been described. Whether this means that these mutations are not compatible with life, that they have little or no consequences, or that they result in unexpected phenotypes is still unclear. Based on the phenotypes of mice with targeted deletions of *Dio1*, *Dio2*, or *Dio3*, the most severe effects would be expected of mutations in DIO3 [122–125]. All three deiodinases are selenoproteins, and contain a selenocysteine residue in the catalytic center, which is crucial for enzymatic activity. Interestingly, mutations that result in an incomplete loss of function of SECISBP2, which is essential for the incorporation of selenocysteine, lead to a thyroid phenotype [126]. TSH, FT4, and rT3 are high in these patients, whereas T3 levels are low. Similar thyroid function tests are observed in *Dio1xDio2* knockout mice, although these mice are still able to maintain normal levels of serum T3 [127].

In the last few years, several studies on polymorphisms in deiodinases and their association with thyroid function tests have been published (see [128] and [120] for reviews). Polymorphisms in DIO1 (rs11206244, rs12095080, rs2235544) have consistently been associated with altered thyroid hormone levels (especially T3 and rT3 levels) in different populations, without an effect on serum TSH [23, 120, 128–130]. The associations are similar in hypothyroid patients who receive levothyroxine treatment and those who are euthyroid without medication. Interestingly, a randomized placebo controlled study investigating the effect of T3 addition in the treatment of depression, showed an enhanced response to T3 in depressed patients which was associated with the rs11206244 and rs2235544 polymorphisms [131]. In other words, depressed patients who have a genetically determined lower T4 to T3 conversion may be more likely to benefit from T3 supplementation. However, these findings need replication in an independent study cohort.

On the other hand, polymorphisms in DIO2 and DIO3 show no associations with serum thyroid hormone levels [23, 120, 128, 129], expect for one study of DIO2 in younger subjects (rs12885300), the results of which have not been replicated [132]. A different polymorphism in DIO2 (rs225014) has been associated with different clinical endpoints independent of serum thyroid hormone levels, such as osteoarthritis, mental retardation in iodine deficient areas, and insulin resistance [120, 128]. This suggests that an altered D2 activity may lead to certain clinical phenotypes, without affecting serum thyroid hormone levels.

2.10   Genome-Wide Association (GWA) Studies

Besides the classical candidate gene approach, an increasing number of studies use a hypothesis-free approach by performing a genome-wide association (GWA) analysis. In such a GWA study the genome of each individual in the population is typed for more than 500,000 polymorphisms to search for variants that are associated with the phenotype of interest. GWA analysis will be very useful to identify novel loci involved in the regulation of thyroid hormone levels. Although such a study is complicated, as it requires large sample sizes, replication, and reliable geno- and phenotyping, it will unravel previously unknown pathways involved in thyroid hormone metabolism. Panicker et al. identified several loci associated with serum FT4 and TSH by a genome-wide linkage scan with 737 microsatellite markers [133], but as expected from an underpowered linkage scan in related subjects, they did not identify the actual genes explaining the variation in serum thyroid hormone levels. Arnaud-Lopez and colleagues recently demonstrated that polymorphisms in the Phosphodiesterase 8B gene are associated with serum TSH levels and thyroid function [134]. Probably, GWA studies will provide more candidate genes involved in thyroid function.

2.11   Concluding Remarks

Genetic variation has an important contribution to the overall variation in thyroid function tests, with estimates varying from 30 to 65%. Although many studies have been published in which the effects of polymorphisms on serum thyroid hormone levels have been demonstrated, only a minor fraction of the overall genetic variation is yet explained. This is clearly illustrated by two studies, in which the contribution of two polymorphisms (rs11206244 in DIO1 and rs1991517 in TSHR) to the overall genetic variation was calculated [24, 135]. Although both polymorphisms show a very significant association with serum thyroid function tests in different independent populations, the proportion of genetic influence explained by these particular polymorphisms is very small (~1%). Genome wide association strategies (and in the near future probably whole genome sequencing), made possible due to the rapid technical progress and the advancement of new techniques, will undoubtedly unravel previously unknown pathways involved in thyroid hormone metabolism, and provide new insights about their physiological function. Whether these techniques will enable us to better estimate an individual's HPT setpoint, remains to be elucidated.

References

1. Björkman U, Elkholm R. Biochemistry of thyroid hormone formation and secretion. In: Greer MA, ed. *The Thyroid Gland.* New York, NY: Raven Press; 1990:83-126.
2. Larsen PR, Davies TE, Hay ID. The thyroid gland. In: Wilson JD, Foster DW, Kronenberg HM, Larsen RR, eds. *Williams Textbook of Endocrinology.* 9th ed. Philadelphia, PA: WB Saunders; 1998:389-515.
3. Andersen S, Pedersen KM, Bruun NH, Laurberg P. Narrow individual variations in serum T(4) and T(3) in normal subjects: a clue to the understanding of subclinical thyroid disease. *J Clin Endocrinol Metab.* 2002;87:1068-1072.
4. Hansen PS, Brix TH, Sorensen TI, Kyvik KO, Hegedus L. Major genetic influence on the regulation of the pituitary-thyroid axis: a study of healthy Danish twins. *J Clin Endocrinol Metab.* 2004;89:1181-1187.
5. Samollow PB, Perez G, Kammerer CM, et al. Genetic and environmental influences on thyroid hormone variation in Mexican Americans. *J Clin Endocrinol Metab.* 2004;89:3276-3284.
6. Panicker V, Wilson SG, Spector TD, et al. Heritability of serum TSH, free T4 and free T3 concentrations: a study of a large UK twin cohort. *Clin Endocrinol (Oxford).* 2008;68:652-659.
7. Hanna CE, Krainz PL, Skeels MR, Miyahira RS, Sesser DE, LaFranchi SH. Detection of congenital hypopituitary hypothyroidism: ten-year experience in the Northwest Regional Screening Program. *J Pediatr.* 1986;109:959-964.
8. Katakami H, Kato Y, Inada M, Imura H. Hypothalamic hypothyroidism due to isolated thyrotropin-releasing hormone (TRH) deficiency. *J Endocrinol Invest.* 1984;7:231-233.
9. Niimi H, Inomata H, Sasaki N, Nakajima H. Congenital isolated thyrotrophin releasing hormone deficiency. *Arch Dis Child.* 1982;57:877-878.
10. Collu R, Tang J, Castagne J, et al. A novel mechanism for isolated central hypothyroidism: inactivating mutations in the thyrotropin-releasing hormone receptor gene. *J Clin Endocrinol Metab.* 1997;82:1561-1565.
11. Bonomi M, Busnelli M, Beck-Peccoz P, et al. A family with complete resistance to thyrotropin-releasing hormone. *N Engl J Med.* 2009;360:731-734.
12. Hayashizaki Y, Hiraoka Y, Tatsumi K, et al. Deoxyribonucleic acid analyses of five families with familial inherited thyroid stimulating hormone deficiency. *J Clin Endocrinol Metab.* 1990;71:792-796.
13. Biebermann H, Liesenkotter KP, Emeis M, Oblanden M, Gruters A. Severe congenital hypothyroidism due to a homozygous mutation of the betaTSH gene. *Pediatr Res.* 1999;46:170-173.
14. Pohlenz J, Dumitrescu A, Aumann U, et al. Congenital secondary hypothyroidism caused by exon skipping due to a homozygous donor splice site mutation in the TSHbeta-subunit gene. *J Clin Endocrinol Metab.* 2002;87:336-339.
15. Krohn K, Paschke R. Somatic mutations in thyroid nodular disease. *Mol Genet Metab.* 2002;75:202-208.
16. Duprez L, Parma J, Van Sande J, et al. Germline mutations in the thyrotropin receptor gene cause non-autoimmune autosomal dominant hyperthyroidism. *Nat Genet.* 1994;7:396-401.
17. Abramowicz MJ, Duprez L, Parma J, Vassart G, Heinrichs C. Familial congenital hypothyroidism due to inactivating mutation of the thyrotropin receptor causing profound hypoplasia of the thyroid gland. *J Clin Invest.* 1997;99:3018-3024.
18. Sunthornthepvarakui T, Gottschalk ME, Hayashi Y, Refetoff S. Brief report: resistance to thyrotropin caused by mutations in the thyrotropin-receptor gene. *N Engl J Med.* 1995;332:155-160.
19. Dechairo BM, Zabaneh D, Collins J, et al. Association of the TSHR gene with Graves' disease: the first disease specific locus. *Eur J Hum Genet.* 2005;13:1223-1230.
20. Brand OJ, Barrett JC, Simmonds MJ, et al. Association of the thyroid stimulating hormone receptor gene (TSHR) with Graves' disease. *Hum Mol Genet.* 2009;18:1704-1713.

21. Tomer Y, Barbesino G, Keddache M, Greenberg DA, Davies TF. Mapping of a major susceptibility locus for Graves' disease (GD-1) to chromosome 14q31. *J Clin Endocrinol Metab.* 1997;82:1645-1648.

22. van der Deure WM, Uitterlinden AG, Hofman A, et al. Effects of serum TSH and FT4 levels and the TSHR-Asp727Glu polymorphism on bone: the Rotterdam study. *Clin Endocrinol (Oxford).* 2008;68:175-181.

23. Peeters RP, van Toor H, Klootwijk W, et al. Polymorphisms in thyroid hormone pathway genes are associated with plasma TSH and iodothyronine levels in healthy subjects. *J Clin Endocrinol Metab.* 2003;88:2880-2888.

24. Hansen PS, van der Deure WM, Peeters RP, et al. The impact of a TSH receptor gene polymorphism on thyroid-related phenotypes in a healthy Danish twin population. *Clin Endocrinol (Oxford).* 2007;66:827-832.

25. Gabriel EM, Bergert ER, Grant CS, van Heerden JA, Thompson GB, Morris JC. Germline polymorphism of codon 727 of human thyroid-stimulating hormone receptor is associated with toxic multinodular goiter. *J Clin Endocrinol Metab.* 1999;84:3328-3335.

26. Nogueira CR, Kopp P, Arseven OK, Santos CL, Jameson JL, Medeiros-Neto G. Thyrotropin receptor mutations in hyperfunctioning thyroid adenomas from Brazil. *Thyroid.* 1999;9:1063-1068.

27. Sykiotis GP, Neumann S, Georgopoulos NA, et al. Functional significance of the thyrotropin receptor germline polymorphism D727E. *Biochem Biophys Res Commun.* 2003;301:1051-1056.

28. Dechairo BM, Zabaneh D, Collins J, et al. Association of the TSHR gene with Graves' disease: the first disease specific locus. *Eur J Hum Genet.* 2005;13(11):1223-1230.

29. Pasca di Magliano M, Di Lauro R, Zannini M. Pax8 has a key role in thyroid cell differentiation. *Proc Natl Acad Sci U S A.* 2000;97:13144-13149.

30. Mansouri A, Chowdhury K, Gruss P. Follicular cells of the thyroid gland require Pax8 gene function. *Nat Genet.* 1998;19:87-90.

31. Macchia PE, Lapi P, Krude H, et al. PAX8 mutations associated with congenital hypothyroidism caused by thyroid dysgenesis. *Nat Genet.* 1998;19:83-86.

32. Torban E, Pelletier J, Goodyer P. F329L polymorphism in the human PAX8 gene. *Am J Med Genet.* 1997;72:186-187.

33. Kimura S, Hara Y, Pineau T, et al. The T/ebp null mouse: thyroid-specific enhancer-binding protein is essential for the organogenesis of the thyroid, lung, ventral forebrain, and pituitary. *Genes Dev.* 1996;10:60-69.

34. Breedveld GJ, van Dongen JW, Danesino C, et al. Mutations in TITF-1 are associated with benign hereditary chorea. *Hum Mol Genet.* 2002;11:971-979.

35. Krude H, Schutz B, Biebermann H, et al. Choreoathetosis, hypothyroidism, and pulmonary alterations due to human NKX2-1 haploinsufficiency. *J Clin Invest.* 2002;109:475-480.

36. Pohlenz J, Dumitrescu A, Zundel D, et al. Partial deficiency of thyroid transcription factor 1 produces predominantly neurological defects in humans and mice. *J Clin Invest.* 2002;109:469-473.

37. Gudmundsson J, Sulem P, Gudbjartsson DF, et al. Common variants on 9q22.33 and 14q13.3 predispose to thyroid cancer in European populations. *Nat Genet.* 2009;41:460-464.

38. De Felice M, Ovitt C, Biffali E, et al. A mouse model for hereditary thyroid dysgenesis and cleft palate. *Nat Genet.* 1998;19:395-398.

39. Bamforth JS, Hughes IA, Lazarus JH, Weaver CM, Harper PS. Congenital hypothyroidism, spiky hair, and cleft palate. *J Med Genet.* 1989;26:49-51.

40. Clifton-Bligh RJ, Wentworth JM, Heinz P, et al. Mutation of the gene encoding human TTF-2 associated with thyroid agenesis, cleft palate and choanal atresia. *Nat Genet.* 1998;19:399-401.

41. Carre A, Castanet M, Sura-Trueba S, et al. Polymorphic length of FOXE1 alanine stretch: evidence for genetic susceptibility to thyroid dysgenesis. *Hum Genet.* 2007;122:467-476.

42. Tonacchera M, Banco M, Lapi P, et al. Genetic analysis of TTF-2 gene in children with congenital hypothyroidism and cleft palate, congenital hypothyroidism, or isolated cleft palate. *Thyroid.* 2004;14:584-588.

43. Venza M, Visalli M, Venza I, et al. Altered binding of MYF-5 to FOXE1 promoter in non-syndromic and CHARGE-associated cleft palate. *J Oral Pathol Med.* 2009;38:18-23.
44. Dai G, Levy O, Carrasco N. Cloning and characterization of the thyroid iodide transporter. *Nature.* 1996;379:458-460.
45. Eskandari S, Loo DD, Dai G, Levy O, Wright EM, Carrasco N. Thyroid Na^+/I^- symporter. Mechanism, stoichiometry, and specificity. *J Bioll Chem.* 1997;272:27230-27238.
46. Nicola JP, Basquin C, Portulano C, Reyna-Neyra A, Paroder M, Carrasco N. The Na^+/I^- symporter mediates active iodide uptake in the intestine. *Am J Physiol.* 2009;296:C654-C662.
47. Wapnir IL, Goris M, Yudd A, et al. The Na^+/I^- symporter mediates iodide uptake in breast cancer metastases and can be selectively down-regulated in the thyroid. *Clin Cancer Res.* 2004;10:4294-4302.
48. Bizhanova A, Kopp P. Minireview: the sodium-iodide symporter NIS and pendrin in iodide homeostasis of the thyroid. *Endocrinology.* 2009;150:1084-1090.
49. Kopp P, Pesce L, Solis SJ. Pendred syndrome and iodide transport in the thyroid. *Trends Endocrinol Metab.* 2008;19:260-268.
50. Azaiez H, Yang T, Prasad S, et al. Genotype-phenotype correlations for SLC26A4-related deafness. *Hum Genet.* 2007;122:451-457.
51. Wangemann P, Nakaya K, Wu T, et al. Loss of cochlear HCO_3^- secretion causes deafness via endolymphatic acidification and inhibition of Ca^{2+} reabsorption in a Pendred syndrome mouse model. *Am J Physiol Renal Physiol.* 2007;292:F1345-F1353.
52. van de Graaf SA, Ris-Stalpers C, Pauws E, Mendive FM, Targovnik HM, de Vijlder JJ. Up to date with human thyroglobulin. *J Endocrinol.* 2001;170:307-321.
53. Rivolta CM, Targovnik HM. Molecular advances in thyroglobulin disorders. *Clin Chim Acta.* 2006;374:8-24.
54. Kim PS, Hossain SA, Park YN, Lee I, Yoo SE, Arvan P. A single amino acid change in the acetylcholinesterase-like domain of thyroglobulin causes congenital goiter with hypothyroidism in the cog/cog mouse: a model of human endoplasmic reticulum storage diseases. *Proc Natl Acad Sci U S A.* 1998;95:9909-9913.
55. Gough S. The thyroglobulin gene: the third locus for autoimmune thyroid disease or a false dawn? *Trends Mol Med.* 2004;10:302-305.
56. Tomer Y, Huber A. The etiology of autoimmune thyroid disease: a story of genes and environment. *J Autoimmun.* 2009;32:231-239.
57. De Deken X, Wang D, Many MC, et al. Cloning of two human thyroid cDNAs encoding new members of the NADPH oxidase family. *J Biol Chem.* 2000;275:23227-23233.
58. Grasberger H, Refetoff S. Identification of the maturation factor for dual oxidase. Evolution of an eukaryotic operon equivalent. *J Biol Chem.* 2006;281:18269-18272.
59. Moreno JC, Bikker H, Kempers MJ, et al. Inactivating mutations in the gene for thyroid oxidase 2 (THOX2) and congenital hypothyroidism. *N Engl J Med.* 2002;347:95-102.
60. Moreno JC, Visser TJ. New phenotypes in thyroid dyshormonogenesis: hypothyroidism due to DUOX2 mutations. *Endocr Dev.* 2007;10:99-117.
61. Zamproni I, Grasberger H, Cortinovis F, et al. Biallelic inactivation of the dual oxidase maturation factor 2 (DUOXA2) gene as a novel cause of congenital hypothyroidism. *J Clin Endocrinol Metab.* 2008;93:605-610.
62. Taurog A. Molecular evolution of thyroid peroxidase. *Biochimie.* 1999;81:557-562.
63. Bakker B, Bikker H, Vulsma T, de Randamie JS, Wiedijk BM, De Vijlder JJ. Two decades of screening for congenital hypothyroidism in The Netherlands: TPO gene mutations in total iodide organification defects (an update). *J Clin Endocrinol Metab.* 2000;85:3708-3712.
64. Bikker H, Baas F, De Vijlder JJ. Molecular analysis of mutated thyroid peroxidase detected in patients with total iodide organification defects. *J Clin Endocrinol Metab.* 1997;82:649-653.
65. Gnidehou S, Caillou B, Talbot M, et al. Iodotyrosine dehalogenase 1 (DEHAL1) is a transmembrane protein involved in the recycling of iodide close to the thyroglobulin iodination site. *FASEB J.* 2004;18:1574-1576.
66. Moreno JC. Identification of novel genes involved in congenital hypothyroidism using serial analysis of gene expression. *Horm Res.* 2003;60(suppl 3):96-102.

67. Friedman JE, Watson JA Jr, Lam DW, Rokita SE. Iodotyrosine deiodinase is the first mammalian member of the NADH oxidase/flavin reductase superfamily. *J Biol Chem.* 2006;281:2812-2819.

68. Moreno JC, Klootwijk W, van Toor H, et al. Mutations in the iodotyrosine deiodinase gene and hypothyroidism. *N Engl J Med.* 2006;358:1811-1818.

69. Afink G, Kulik W, Overmars H, et al. Molecular characterization of iodotyrosine dehalogenase deficiency in patients with hypothyroidism. *J Clin Endocrinol Metab.* 2006;93:4894-4901.

70. Cheng SY. Multiple mechanisms for regulation of the transcriptional activity of thyroid hormone receptors. *Rev Endocr Metab Disord.* 2000;1:9-18.

71. Yen PM. Physiological and molecular basis of thyroid hormone action. *Physiol Rev.* 2001;81:1097-1142.

72. Olateju TO, Vanderpump MP. Thyroid hormone resistance. *Ann Clin Biochem.* 2006;43:431-440.

73. Yen PM. Molecular basis of resistance to thyroid hormone. *Trends Endocrinol Metab.* 2003;14:327-333.

74. Weiss RE, Refetoff S. Resistance to thyroid hormone. *Rev Endocr Metab Disord.* 2000;1:97-108.

75. Sorensen HG, van der Deure WM, Hansen PS, et al. Identification and consequences of polymorphisms in the thyroid hormone receptor alpha and beta genes. *Thyroid.* 2008;18:1087-1094.

76. Tinnikov A, Nordstrom K, Thoren P, et al. Retardation of post-natal development caused by a negatively acting thyroid hormone receptor alpha1. *Embo J.* 2002;21:5079-5087.

77. Venero C, Guadano-Ferraz A, Herrero AI, et al. Anxiety, memory impairment, and locomotor dysfunction caused by a mutant thyroid hormone receptor alpha1 can be ameliorated by T3 treatment. *Genes Dev.* 2005;19:2152-2163.

78. Kaneshige M, Suzuki H, Kaneshige K, et al. A targeted dominant negative mutation of the thyroid hormone alpha 1 receptor causes increased mortality, infertility, and dwarfism in mice. *Proc Natl Acad Sci U S A.* 2002;98:15095-15100.

79. Liu YY, Schultz JJ, Brent GA. A thyroid hormone receptor alpha gene mutation (P398H) is associated with visceral adiposity and impaired catecholamine-stimulated lipolysis in mice. *J Biol Chem.* 2003;278:38913-38920.

80. Robbins J, Bartalena L. Plasma transport of thyroid hormone. In: Hennemann G, ed. *Thyroid Hormone Metabolism.* New York, NY: Marcel Dekker; 1986:3-38.

81. Hennemann G, Visser TJ. Thyroid hormone synthesis, plasma membrane transport and metabolism. In: Grossman A, ed. *Handbook of Experimental Pharmacology.* Berlin, Germany: Springer; 1997:75-117.

82. Hennemann G, Docter R. Plasma transport proteins and their role in tissue delivery of thyroid hormone. In: Greer MA, ed. *The Thyroid Gland.* New York, NY: Raven Press; 1990:221-232.

83. Mannavola D, Vannucchi G, Fugazzola L, et al. TBG deficiency: description of two novel mutations associated with complete TBG deficiency and review of the literature. *J Mol Med.* 1990;84:864-871.

84. Refetoff S. Inherited thyroxine-binding globulin abnormalities in man. *Endocr Rev.* 1989;10:275-293.

85. Mori Y, Jing P, Kayama M, et al. Gene amplification as a common cause of inherited thyroxine-binding globulin excess: analysis of one familial and two sporadic cases. *Endocr J.* 1999;46:613-619.

86. Saraiva MJ. Transthyretin mutations in hyperthyroxinemia and amyloid diseases. *Hum Mutat.* 2001;17:493-503.

87. Moses AC, Rosen HN, Moller DE, et al. A point mutation in transthyretin increases affinity for thyroxine and produces euthyroid hyperthyroxinemia. *J Clin Invest.* 2001;86:2025-2033.

88. Cameron SJ, Hagedorn JC, Sokoll LJ, Caturegli P, Ladenson PW. Dysprealbuminemic hyper-thyroxinemia in a patient with hyperthyroid graves disease. *Clin Chem.* 2001;51:1065-1069.
89. Bartalena L, Robbins J. Variations in thyroid hormone transport proteins and their clinical implications. *Thyroid.* 1992;2:237-245.
90. Hennemann G, Docter R, Krenning EP, Bos G, Otten M, Visser TJ. Raised total thyroxine and free thyroxine index but normal free thyroxine. A serum abnormality due to inherited increased affinity of iodothyronines for serum binding protein. *Lancet.* 1979;1:639-642.
91. Pannain S, Feldman M, Eiholzer U, Weiss RE, Scherberg NH, Refetoff S. Familial dysalbu-minemic hyperthyroxinemia in a Swiss family caused by a mutant albumin (R218P) shows an apparent discrepancy between serum concentration and affinity for thyroxine. *J Clin En-docrinol Metab.* 2000;85:2786-2792.
92. Hennemann G, Docter R, Friesema EC, de Jong M, Krenning EP, Visser TJ. Plasma mem-brane transport of thyroid hormones and its role in thyroid hormone metabolism and bio-availability. *Endocr Rev.* 2001;22:451-476.
93. Friesema EC, Ganguly S, Abdalla A, Manning Fox JE, Halestrap AP, Visser TJ. Identifi-cation of monocarboxylate transporter 8 as a specific thyroid hormone transporter. *J Biol Chem.* 2003;278:40128-40135.
94. Friesema EC, Grueters A, Biebermann H, et al. Association between mutations in a thyroid hormone transporter and severe X-linked psychomotor retardation. *Lancet.* 2004;364:1435-1437.
95. Dumitrescu AM, Liao XH, Best TB, Brockmann K, Refetoff S. A novel syndrome combining thyroid and neurological abnormalities is associated with mutations in a monocarboxylate transporter gene. *Am J Hum Genet.* 2004;74:168-175.
96. Dominguez-Gerpe LF-IM, Vieitez-Rodriguez O, Areal-Mendez C, Eiras-Martinez A, San-Jose E, Lado-Abeal J. Study of a possible association between serum levels of T4, T3 or TSH and the SNP S33P of the monocarboxylate transporter 8 (MCT8). *Thyroid.* 2006;16:883-884, 878.
97. van der Deure WM, Peeters RP, Visser TJ. Genetic variation in thyroid hormone transporters. *Best Pract Res Clin Endocrinol Metab.* 2007;21:339-350.
98. Lago-Leston R, Iglesias MJ, San-Jose E, et al. Prevalence and functional analysis of the S107P polymorphism (rs6647476) of the monocarboxylate transporter 8 (SLC16A2) gene in the male population of Northwest Spain (Galicia). *Clin Endocrinol.* 2009;70(4):636-643.
99. Kim DK, Kanai Y, Matsuo H, et al. The human T-type amino acid transporter-1: characteriza-tion, gene organization, and chromosomal location. *Genomics.* 2002;79:95-103.
100. Friesema EC, Jansen J, Jachtenberg JW, Visser WE, Kester MH, Visser TJ. Effective cellular uptake and efflux of thyroid hormone by human monocarboxylate transporter 10. *Mol Endo-crinol.* 2008;22:1357-1369.
101. Heuer H, Maier MK, Iden S, et al. The monocarboxylate transporter 8 linked to human psy-chomotor retardation is highly expressed in thyroid hormone sensitive neuron populations. *Endocrinology.* 2005;146(4):1701-1706.
102. Heuer H, Visser TJ. Minireview: pathophysiological importance of thyroid hormone trans-porters. *Endocrinology.* 2009;150:1078-1083.
103. Dumitrescu AM, Liao XH, Weiss RE, Millen K, Refetoff S. Tissue-specific thyroid hormone deprivation and excess in monocarboxylate transporter (mct) 8-deficient mice. *Endocrinol-ogy.* 2006;147:4036-4043.
104. Konig J, Seithel A, Gradhand U, Fromm MF. Pharmacogenomics of human OATP transport-ers. *Naunyn Schmiedebergs Arch Pharmacol.* 2006;372:432-443.
105. Kullak-Ublick GA, Ismair MG, Stieger B, et al. Organic anion-transporting polypeptide B (OATP-B) and its functional comparison with three other OATPs of human liver. *Gastroen-terology.* 2001;120:525-533.
106. Fujiwara K, Adachi H, Nishio T, et al. Identification of thyroid hormone transporters in humans: different molecules are involved in a tissue-specific manner. *Endocrinology.* 2001;142:2005-2012.

107. Abe T, Kakyo M, Tokui T, et al. Identification of a novel gene family encoding human liver-specific organic anion transporter LST-1. *J Biol Chem.* 1999;274:17159-17163.

108. Pizzagalli F, Hagenbuch B, Stieger B, Klenk U, Folkers G, Meier PJ. Identification of a novel human organic anion transporting polypeptide as a high affinity thyroxine transporter. *Mol Endocrinol.* 2002;16:2283-2296.

109. Mikkaichi T, Suzuki T, Onogawa T, et al. Isolation and characterization of a digoxin transporter and its rat homologue expressed in the kidney. *Proc Natl Acad Sci U S A.* 2004;101:3569-3574.

110. van der Deure WM, Peeters RP, Visser TJ. Molecular aspects of thyroid hormone transporters, including MCT8, MCT10 and OATPs, and the effects of genetic variation in these transporters. *J Mol Endocrinol.* 2010;44(1):1-11.

111. Abe T, Unno M, Onogawa T, et al. LST-2, a human liver-specific organic anion transporter, determines methotrexate sensitivity in gastrointestinal cancers. *Gastroenterology.* 2001;120:1689-1699.

112. van der Deure WM, Friesema EC, de Jong FJ, et al. OATP1B1: an important factor in hepatic thyroid hormone and estrogen transport and metabolism. *Endocrinology.* 2008;149(9):4695-4701.

113. Smith NF, Figg WD, Sparreboom A. Role of the liver-specific transporters OATP1B1 and OATP1B3 in governing drug elimination. *Expert Opin Drug Metab Toxicol.* 2005;1:429-445.

114. Niemi M, Backman JT, Kajosaari LI, et al. Polymorphic organic anion transporting polypeptide 1B1 is a major determinant of repaglinide pharmacokinetics. *Clin Pharmacol Ther.* 2005;77:468-478.

115. van der Deure WM, Hansen PS, Peeters RP, et al. Thyroid hormone transport and metabolism by organic anion transporter 1C1 and consequences of genetic variation. *Endocrinology.* 2008;149:5307-5314.

116. Sugiyama D, Kusuhara H, Taniguchi H, et al. Functional characterization of rat brain-specific organic anion transporter (Oatp14) at the blood-brain barrier: high affinity transporter for thyroxine. *J Biol Chem.* 2003;278:43489-43495.

117. van der Deure WM, Appelhof BC, Peeters RP, et al. Polymorphisms in the brain-specific thyroid hormone transporter OATP1C1 are associated with fatigue and depression in hypothyroid patients. *Clin Endocrinol (Oxford).* 2008;69:804-811.

118. Canani LH, Capp C, Dora JM, et al. The type 2 deiodinase A/G (Thr92Ala) polymorphism is associated with decreased enzyme velocity and increased insulin resistance in patients with type 2 diabetes mellitus. *J Clin Endocrinol Metab.* 2005;90:3472-3478.

119. Mentuccia D, Proietti-Pannunzi L, Tanner K, et al. Association between a novel variant of the human type 2 deiodinase gene Thr92Ala and insulin resistance: evidence of interaction with the Trp64Arg variant of the beta-3-adrenergic receptor. *Diabetes.* 2002;51:880-883.

120. Dayan CM, Panicker V. Novel insights into thyroid hormones from the study of common genetic variation. *Nat Rev Endocrinol.* 2009;5:211-218.

121. Bianco AC, Salvatore D, Gereben B, Berry MJ, Larsen PR. Biochemistry, cellular and molecular biology, and physiological roles of the iodothyronine selenodeiodinases. *Endocr Rev.* 2002;23:38-89.

122. Hernandez A, Martinez ME, Fiering S, Galton VA, St Germain D. Type 3 deiodinase is critical for the maturation and function of the thyroid axis. *J Clin Invest.* 2006;116:476-484.

123. Hernandez A, Fiering S, Martinez E, Galton VA, St Germain D. The gene locus encoding iodothyronine deiodinase type 3 (Dio3) is imprinted in the fetus and expresses antisense transcripts. *Endocrinology.* 2002;143:4483-4486.

124. Schneider MJ, Fiering SN, Pallud SE, Parlow AF, St Germain DL, Galton VA. Targeted disruption of the type 2 selenodeiodinase gene (DIO2) results in a phenotype of pituitary resistance to T4. *Mol Endocrinol.* 2001;15:2137-2148.

125. Berry MJ, Grieco D, Taylor BA, et al. Physiological and genetic analyses of inbred mouse strains with a type I iodothyronine 5'-deiodinase deficiency. *J Clin Invest.* 1993;92:1517-1528.

126. Dumitrescu AM, Liao XH, Abdullah MS, et al. Mutations in SECISBP2 result in abnormal thyroid hormone metabolism. *Nat Genet.* 2005;37:1247-1252.
127. Galton VA, Schneider MJ, Clark AS, St Germain DL. Life without thyroxine to 3,5,3'-triiodothyronine conversion: studies in mice devoid of the 5'-deiodinases. *Endocrinology.* 2009;150:2957-2963.
128. Peeters RP, van der Deure WM, Visser TJ. Genetic variation in thyroid hormone pathway genes; polymorphisms in the TSH receptor and the iodothyronine deiodinases. *Eur J Endocrinol.* 2006;155:655-662.
129. Panicker V, Cluett C, Shields B, et al. A common variation in deiodinase 1 gene DIO1 is associated with the relative levels of free thyroxine and triiodothyronine. *J Clin Endocrinol Metab.* 2008;93:3075-3081.
130. de Jong FJ, Peeters RP, den Heijer T, et al. The association of polymorphisms in the type 1 and 2 deiodinase genes with circulating thyroid hormone parameters and atrophy of the medial temporal lobe. *J Clin Endocrinol Metab.* 2007;92:636-640.
131. Cooper-Kazaz R, van der Deure WM, Medici M, et al. Preliminary evidence that a functional polymorphism in type 1 deiodinase is associated with enhanced potentiation of the antidepressant effect of sertraline by triiodothyronine. *J Affect Disord.* 2009;116:113-116.
132. Peeters RP, van den Beld AW, Attalki H, et al. A new polymorphism in the type II deiodinase gene is associated with circulating thyroid hormone parameters. *Am J Physiol Endocrinol Metab.* 2005;289:E75-E81.
133. Panicker V, Wilson SG, Spector TD, et al. Genetic loci linked to pituitary-thyroid axis setpoints: a genome-wide scan of a large twin cohort. *J Clin Endocrinol Metab.* 2008;93(9):3519-3523.
134. Arnaud-Lopez L, Usala G, Ceresini G, et al. Phosphodiesterase 8B gene variants are associated with serum TSH levels and thyroid function. *Am J Hum Genet.* 2008;82:1270-1280.
135. van der Deure WM, Hansen PS, Peeters RP, et al. The effect of genetic variation in the type 1 deiodinase gene on the inter-individual variation in serum thyroid hormone levels. An investigation in healthy Danish twins. *Clin Endocrinol (Oxford).* 2009;70(6):954-960.

Chapter 3
Influence of Iodine Deficiency and Excess on Thyroid Function Tests

Maria Andersson and Michael B. Zimmermann

3.1 Introduction

Iodine is an essential component of the thyroid hormones, and adequate iodine intake is necessary for normal thyroid function. The iodine intake of populations is assessed by measuring urinary iodine concentration (UIC) in a spot urine sample [1]. The recommendations for daily iodine intake and the recommended levels for optimal iodine nutrition by age and population group are shown in Table 3.1 [1, 2]. The epidemiological criteria for classifying the degree of iodine status in a population based on median or range of UIC or both UIC cutoffs are listed in Table 3.2.

The optimal range of iodine intake to prevent thyroid disease is relatively narrow [1, 3]. Both low and high iodine intakes may interfere with thyroid function. The relationship between iodine intake and thyroid function has been assessed in cross-sectional, longitudinal, and intervention studies by measuring UIC and thyroid hormones in populations with different iodine status. However, interpretation of epidemiological studies on iodine intake and thyroid function is challenging for several reasons [4, 5]. One should consider not only the present iodine intake level, but also the history of iodine intake of the population. Many studies include hospital or clinic-based cohorts rather than true population cohorts. Diseases, medications, ethnicity, and age of studied cohorts vary. Diagnostic methods also vary, and differing cutoffs for thyroid function tests have been applied. Finally, environmental factors and genes may contribute to differences in thyroid function seen between regions [5]. In the following chapter, we discuss the effect of variations in iodine status on thyroid function tests in four age/population groups: adults, pregnant women, newborns and children, considering first the cross-sectional and then the longitudinal data.

M. B. Zimmermann (✉)
Institute of Food, Nutrition and Health,
Swiss Federal Institute of Technology Zurich (ETH Zurich)
Human Nutrition Laboratory, Zurich, Switzerland
e-mail: michael.zimmermann@ilw.agrl.ethz.ch

G. A. Brent (ed.), *Thyroid Function Testing,*
DOI 10.1007/978-1-4419-1485-9_3, © Springer Science+Business Media, LLC 2010

Table 3.1 Recommended nutrient intake for iodine intake by age or population group and epidemiological criteria for assessing adequate iodine intake based on median urinary iodine concentrations (UIC) of populations [1, 2]

WHO recommendations	Iodine intake (μg/day)	UIC for adequate intake (μg/L)
Children 0–5 years	90	≥100
Children 6–12 years	120	100–199
Children ≥12 years + adults	150	100–199
Pregnancy	250	150–249
Lactation	250	≥100

Table 3.2 Epidemiological criteria for assessment of iodine nutrition in a population based on median or range of urinary iodine concentrations (UIC) or both UIC cutoffs [1, 2]

	Iodine intake	Iodine nutrition
School-aged children		
<20 μg/L	Insufficient	Severe iodine deficiency
20–49 μg/L	Insufficient	Moderate iodine deficiency
50–99 μg/L	Insufficient	Mild iodine deficiency
100–199 μg/L	Adequate	Optimum
200–299 μg/L	More than adequate	Risk of iodine-induced hyperthyroidism in susceptible groups
>300 μg/L	Excessive	Risk of adverse health consequences (iodine-induced hyperthyroidism, autoimmune thyroid disease)
Pregnant women		
<150 μg/L	Insufficient	
150–249 μg/L	Adequate	
250–499 μg/L	More than adequate	
≥500 μg/L[a]	Excessive	
Lactating women[b]		
<100 μg/L	Insufficient	
≥100 μg/L	Adequate	
Children less than 2 years of age		
<100 μg/L	Insufficient	
≥100 μg/L	Adequate	

There is no information about iodine nutrition for pregnant and lactating women in the WHO assessment table [1]

[a] The term excessive means in excess of the amount needed to prevent and control iodine deficiency

[b] In lactating women, the numbers for median UIC are lower than the iodine requirements because of the iodine excreted in breastmilk

3.2   Iodine Metabolism and Thyroid Function

Iodine deficiency remains a public-health problem in 47 countries worldwide, and approximately one-third of the global population has low iodine intake [6]. In iodine deficiency, thyroid function is maintained by increasing clearance of circulating iodine by the thyroid. Low iodine intake triggers thyroid stimulating hormone (TSH) secretion from the pituitary gland and increases the expression of the sodium/iodide symporter (NIS) to maximize the iodine uptake into the thyroid cell. The thyroid accumulates a larger percentage of ingested iodine (as iodide), reuses the iodine from the degradation of thyroid hormones more efficiently, and reduces the amount of iodine excreted in the urine [7]. In chronic iodine deficiency, the thyroid uptake of iodine from the circulation can increase from 10 to 80% [8, 9]. Under normal circumstances, plasma iodine has a half-life of ≈10 hours, but this is reduced in iodine deficiency. The body of a healthy adult contains 15–20 mg of iodine, of which 70–80% is in the thyroid [8]. In chronic iodine deficiency, the iodine content of the thyroid may fall to <20 μg. In iodine-sufficient areas, the adult thyroid traps ≈60 μg of iodine/day to balance losses and maintain thyroid hormone synthesis. The NIS transfers iodide into the thyroid at a concentration gradient 20–50 times that of plasma [10]. Iodine comprises 65% and 59% of the weights of thyroxine (T4) and triiodothyronine (T3), respectively. Turnover is relatively slow: the half-life of T4 is ≈5 days and for T3, 1.5–3 days. The released iodine enters the plasma iodine pool and can be taken up again by the thyroid or excreted by the kidney. More than 90% of ingested iodine is ultimately excreted in the urine.

3.3   Thyroid Adaptation to Iodine Deficiency

In mild iodine deficiency, the thyroid-pituitary axis is usually able to adapt to low dietary iodine supply by increasing TSH secretion from the pituitary [7] (discussed in Chap. 4). Circulating TSH concentrations may be slightly increased, usually within the normal range, while T4 and T3 concentrations typically remain within the normal range. Moderate iodine deficiency often results in a mild increase in the TSH concentration with normal T3 and T4 concentrations, a pattern consistent with subclinical hypothyroidism [11, 12]. As iodine deficiency becomes severe, TSH concentrations may rise further while T3 increases or remains unchanged and serum T4 decreases. The preferential secretion of T3 is an adaptation to low iodine supply, as the metabolic potency of T3 is much greater than that of T4, but T3 requires only 75% as much iodine for its synthesis. However, in severe iodine deficiency euthyroidism cannot be maintained despite preferential T3 secretion, as the half-life for T4 is 7 days but less than 1 day for T3 [13]. In severe iodine deficiency, serum TSH is inversely associated with total and free T4, but not with total or free T3, suggesting stronger feedback control of TSH secretion by

T4 than by T3 [12, 14–18]. In persistent severe deficiency, both serum T4 and T3 will decrease, and overt hypothyroidism develops. In myxedematous cretins, the thyroid is atrophic, TSH is dramatically elevated and T4 and T3 are low [7]. In contrast, in neurological cretins, thyroid function and goiter are similar to that found in the surrounding population.

In iodine deficiency, serum thyroglobulin (Tg) concentrations predictably increase due to hyperstimulation of the thyroid by TSH [19–25] (also discussed in Chap. 7). Serum Tg often correlates with serum TSH, but is not necessarily higher in goitrous as compared to nongoitrous subjects [18]. Elevated serum Tg concentration in iodine deficiency respond rapidly to iodine repletion [25–27]. In chronically iodine deficient populations with elevated TSH concentrations [12, 16, 28, 29], a combination of factors determines whether goiter develops. These include the duration of high TSH concentrations, the efficiency of the thyroidal response in converting T3 to T4, as well as other hormonal factors [30]. In adult populations, TSH concentrations usually do not correlate with the presence of goiter [12, 16].

Table 3.3 shows the thyroid function indicators recommended for the assessment of iodine status by age group.

Table 3.3 Thyroid function indicators recommended for the assessment of iodine status by age group

	Age group	Advantages	Disadvantages	Application
TSH (mU/L)	Newborn babies	Measures thyroid function at particularly susceptible age Minimum costs if congenital hypothyroidism screening program is already in place Heel-stick method to obtain sample, and storage on filter paper is simple	Not useful if iodine antiseptics used during delivery [70] Needs standardized sensitive assay Should be taken by heel-prick at least 48 h after birth to avoid physiological newborn surge	<3% frequency of TSH values >5 mU/L indicates iodine sufficiency in a population [72]
Serum or whole blood thyroglobulin (µg/L)	School-aged children and adults	Finger-stick approach to obtain sample, and storage on filter paper is simple International reference range available [27] Measures improvement in thyroid function within several months after iodine repletion	Expensive immunoassay Standard reference material is available, but needs validation	Reference interval in iodine sufficient children is 4–40 µg/L [27]

3.4 Epidemiology of Thyroid Function in Areas of Low Iodine Intake

3.4.1 Adults

3.4.1.1 Cross-Sectional Studies

In areas of mild and moderate iodine deficiency, the prevalence of hypothyroidism is generally low in the adult population [3, 31–34]. In mild iodine deficiency there are no, or only weak, associations between iodine status and thyroid hormone concentrations. In France, a nationally representative cross-sectional study of the adult population identified mild iodine deficiency by a median UIC of 85 µg/L in men (n = 4,860) and 82 µg/L in women (n = 7,154) [35]. TSH and free T4 concentrations were measured in men 45–60 years, women 35–44 years, and women 45–60 years without previous or present thyroid diseases [34]. The prevalence of abnormal TSH values in these three groups were TSH < 0.4 mU/L of 7.0%, 5.3%, and 4.4%; TSH 4.0–9.9 mU/L of 4.0%, 7.2%, and 11.1%; and TSH ≥ 10.0 mU/L of 0.2%, 0.4%, and 0.7%, respectively. The mean ± SD free T4 concentration was 13.8 ± 2.2 pmol/L for men and 14.0 ± 2.3 pmol/L for women. A cross-sectional study in Denmark compared serum TSH, free T4, and free T3 concentrations in adults (n = 4,649) from two regions with different iodine intake before introduction to iodine fortification: Copenhagen, an area of mild iodine deficiency with median UIC of 61 µg/L and Aalborg, an area of moderate iodine deficiency with median UIC of 45 µg/L [32]. Lower TSH levels were found in the area with moderate iodine deficiency than in the area with mild iodine deficiency [32]. This difference was explained by declining TSH with age in moderate iodine deficiency, a decline not observed in mild iodine deficiency [32]. The incidence of hypothyroidism was 40.1/100,000 per year in Copenhagen and 26.5/100,000 per year in Aalborg [3, 36]. The observed differences in the incidence of overt hypothyroidism between the two areas and the change in thyroid disease after the introduction to iodization are described in Sect. 3.5.3.

In a mild-to-moderate iodine-deficient adult population (n = 233) in New Zealand, with median 24 hour urinary iodine excretion (UIE) of 75 µg/day (median UIC 54 µg/L) significant inverse correlations were found for the relationship between UIE and Tg, but not for TSH or T4 [37]. Aghini-Lombardi et al. assessed thyroid status in a cross-sectional study of the population of Pescopagano (n = 1,411), an iodine-deficient village of Southern Italy with long standing mild-to-moderate iodine deficiency and no iodine prophylaxis [31]. The overall median UIC in all age groups combined was 55 µg/L and the goiter prevalence in the adult population >15 years (n = 992) was 58.8%. Thyroid functional autonomy, defined by normal serum concentrations of free T4 and free T3 and subnormal serum TSH concentrations (<0.4 mU/L), was found in 6.4% of adults. Subclinical hypothyroidism, defined as elevated serum TSH (>3.7 mU/L) and normal serum levels of free T4 and free T3, was found in 3.8%. There was no difference between females (4.4%) and males (3.1%).

In contrast, severe iodine deficiency strongly influences thyroid function in adults. A study of adults ($n = 502$) in seven villages in Senegal, an area with severe iodine deficiency and high goiter prevalence (62%), showed clear alterations in thyroid function [38]. The median UIC was 10 µg/L and the mean ± SD free T4 of 11.9 ± 3.5 pmol/L and elevated free T3 to free T4 ratios [38]. In chronic severe iodine deficiency, elevated serum TSH levels have been repeatedly but not systematically reported in adults [12, 24, 39, 40]. In adults ($n = 488$) in an area of endemic goiter (goiter prevalence 80.1%) in Tuscany, Italy, Tg concentrations were increased but did not correlate with TSH [24].

3.4.1.2   Longitudinal Studies

Andersen et al. evaluated 24 hour UIE and thyroid hormone concentrations monthly for 1 year in a longitudinal study of 16 healthy adult men [41]. Negative correlation between UIE and serum TSH was found in subjects with an annual average daily UIE below 50 µg/day (moderately iodine deficient) but no correlation or a positive correlation was found between UIE and TSH in subjects with UIE above 50 µg/day (mildly iodine deficient). Subjects with moderate iodine deficiency showed significantly lower T4 and T3 concentrations compared to subjects with mild iodine deficiency. The results suggest altered thyroid function in adult men at UIE of 50 µg/day [41].

3.4.1.3   Summary

Although serum TSH, Tg, and free T3 may be slightly increased and free T4 slightly decreased in iodine deficiency, values in adult populations often remain within the normal range, and overlap with iodine-sufficient populations [8]. New and narrower reference intervals for TSH and free T4 may assist in detecting mild-to-moderate degrees of iodine deficiency [42]. However, with the exception of severe iodine deficiency, significant correlation between individual UIC and thyroid hormone concentrations is rarely found in adults.

3.4.2   Pregnancy

3.4.2.1   Cross-Sectional Studies

Iodine requirements are increased during pregnancy (Table 3.1) because of an increase in maternal T4 production, transfer of T4 and iodine to the fetus, and possibly also to compensate for an increase in maternal renal iodine clearance [43–47] (discussed in depth in Chap. 11). Population-based studies have shown that women with an iodine intake <100 μg/day before pregnancy may become hypothyroxinemic during pregnancy [48–51]. In South Wales in the United Kingdom, iodine intake was measured in a subgroup ($n = 626$) of pregnant women in weeks 11–15, participating in an ongoing study on thyroid function during early gestation. Their iodine intake was low: 60% of the pregnant women had UIC <150 μg/L [52]. However, no significant difference in the concentration of either TSH or free T4 was found between five subgroups of women classified according to their UIC [52]. In Switzerland, in a representative national sample of pregnant women ($n = 365$) in the third trimester who were borderline iodine deficient (median UIC 139 μg/L), 16% had a total T4 <100 nmol/L, and 6% had a TSH >4.0 mU/L. In Danish pregnant women not taking iodine supplements, the median UIC was only 33 μg/g creatinine [50] and TSH and Tg concentrations were increased in late pregnancy [53]. Moderate iodine deficiency with mean UIC of 69 ± 4 μg/L in the first trimester and alterations in thyroid function have been reported in pregnant women in southwestern France [48].

3.4.2.2 Longitudinal Studies

Controlled trials of iodine supplementation in mildly iodine-deficient-pregnant women suggest beneficial effects on maternal serum Tg, but no effects on maternal total or free T4 and T3 [54]. In Europe, six randomized controlled trials of iodine supplementation in pregnancy, involving 450 women with mild-to-moderate iodine deficiency, have been published. [53, 55–59]. Supplementation significantly increased maternal UIC in all studies. Iodine doses varied between 50 and 230 μg/day, and the data indicate no clear dose–response relationship for UIC, TSH, Tg, thyroid hormones, or thyroid volume. In three of the five trials that measured maternal thyroid volume, supplementation was associated with significantly reduced maternal thyroid size, and the data also suggest an increase in newborn thyroid volume and Tg can be prevented or minimized by supplementation. The data are equivocal for an effect on maternal TSH; values are generally lower (within the normal reference range) with iodine supplementation. In these mild-to-moderately iodine-deficient pregnant women, supplementation had no effect on maternal and newborn total or free T4 and T3 concentrations.

However, in regions with severe iodine deficiency and endemic goiter, randomized controlled trials of iodine supplements given to iodine-deficient mothers before pregnancy or during early pregnancy have shown improved motor and cognitive performance of their offspring, suggesting improved thyroid function [60–62]. However, thyroid hormone concentrations were not measured in these studies. In a recent Italian study, thyroid function was measured in 100 pregnant women from a mildly iodine-deficient area: 62 women who had regularly used iodized salt for at least 2 years prior to becoming pregnant and 38 who commenced iodized salt consumption when becoming pregnant [63]. The prevalence of maternal thyroid failure during pregnancy was 6.4% and 36.8%, respectively [63].

3.4.2.3 Summary

Iodine deficiency during pregnancy may be associated with elevated TSH and Tg concentrations and reduced maternal T4 levels [64, 65]. However, Laurberg et al. suggest cautious interpretation of a low free T4 concentration in late pregnancy and its ascription to low iodine intake [66]. Nonetheless, abnormalities in thyroid function in pregnant women with mild iodine deficiency can be apparent before changes in thyroid function are detected in the general population of the same area [44, 48].

3.4.3 Newborns

3.4.3.1 Cross-Sectional Studies

Neonatal Serum TSH

Neonates have lower thyroid iodine stores and higher iodine turnover compared to adults [67] (also discussed in Chap. 9). At low maternal iodine intake, Tg concentrations rise and TSH stimulation increases to maintain high iodine turnover [68, 69]. Thus, in iodine deficient infants, serum TSH concentrations increase for the first few weeks of life. This condition is termed transient newborn hyperthyrotropinemia, and newborn TSH obtained in whole blood collected 3–4 days after birth is a sensitive indicator of iodine status in the newborn period [70–73]. The World Health Organization (WHO) recommends measurement of the prevalence of neonates with elevated TSH levels as a sensitive indicator of the severity of iodine deficiency in a given population [1]. Typically, a few drops of whole blood are collected on filter paper from the cord or by heel prick. Newborn TSH screening is not specific enough to use as an individual test to diagnose iodine deficiency, but can provide an estimate of overall population iodine status. Alterations in neonatal thyroid function with high serum TSH and low T4 have been reported in areas where thyroid function in adults or school-age children was normal [74].

Elevated newborn serum TSH levels (>5 mU/L) have been observed in several areas of mild iodine deficiency as well as in areas of presumed iodine-sufficiency [75]. Mild iodine deficiency has been identified in two cross-sectional studies of pregnant women and newborns in Australia [76, 77]. In Sydney, the prevalence of elevated newborn TSH values ranged from 5.4 to 8.1% and the median UIC in mothers was 109 µg/L [76]. In the Central Coast area of New South Wales, median UIC in 815 third trimester pregnant women was 85 µg/L and 2.2% of 824 newborns had whole-blood TSH values >5 mU/L [77]. Mothers with a UIC <50 µg/L were 2.6 times (RR = 2.65; 95% CI 1.49–4.73; $p < 0.01$) more likely to have a child with elevated TSH level. In Estonia, where median UIC in school children was 65 µg/L [78] neonatal TSH screening of 20,021 newborns revealed a prevalence of elevated TSH of 17.7% [79].

Neonatal Cord-Blood TSH

Normal physiologic concentrations of TSH in cord blood collected at birth during the physiologic newborn surge in TSH secretion are typically higher than those for heel-prick blood, as heel pricks are often done a few days after birth, when the surge of TSH has subsided. Thus, if a TSH cutoff value >5 mU/L for heel-prick blood is applied for cord blood [1], an elevated value is less likely to reflect iodine deficiency in the mother or in the neonate [66]. For this reason, transiently elevated TSH in cord blood is much less specific than heel-stick samples taken 3–4 days after birth for assessing iodine status in populations [80].

Elevated TSH levels (>5 mU/L) are common in cord blood in areas of mild, moderate, and severe iodine deficiency. In Hong Kong, an area with mild iodine deficiency, infants with iodine-deficient mothers had higher cord-blood TSH than iodine-sufficient mothers [81]. In Burdwan district of West Bengal, a hospital-based cross-sectional study of 267 third trimester pregnant mothers with median UIC of 144 µg/L reported elevated cord-blood TSH levels in 2.9% of the neonates [82]. Cross-sectional studies in regions of Bangladesh and Guatemala found elevated cord-blood TSH concentrations in two areas of moderate maternal iodine deficiency [83]. In Bangladesh, the maternal median UIC was 96 µg/L and the proportion of cord bloods with elevated TSH levels was 84%. In Guatemala, the maternal median UIC was 120 µg/L and the proportion of cord bloods with elevated TSH levels was 58%.

In populations with severe iodine deficiency, high prevalences of elevated newborn TSH levels are commonly reported. A cross-sectional, hospital-based study measured neonatal cord-blood TSH at birth in eight urban populations of Malaysia, Philippines, Pakistan, and Kyrgyzstan between 1992 and 1994 [70]. UIC obtained from the mothers of the infants tested or from school children at the time of cord-blood sampling showed severe iodine deficiency with median UIC <50 µg/L in all sites. The prevalence of elevated TSH values ranged between 32 and 80% in the eight cities. In an area of severe iodine deficiency in the Democratic Republic of Congo [84–86], thyroid failure in neonates was reported due to a combination of iodine deficiency and thiocyanate overload with elevated cord-serum TSH >100 mU/L and cord-serum T4 <40 nmol/L.

Because of the newborn TSH surge, cord-blood TSH and Tg concentrations in newborns are often higher than in maternal blood [87–89]. In two randomized prospective iodine intervention studies of pregnant women with mild-to-moderate iodine deficiency, iodine supplementation decreased serum TSH concentration in women in late pregnancy, but iodine had no significant effect on the concentration of TSH in cord blood [53, 56]. In an observational study of women living in an area with mild-to-moderate iodine deficiency, mothers supplemented with iodine had a lower serum TSH concentration than nonsupplemented, control mothers [90]. However, the mothers taking iodine supplements had higher TSH concentration in cord-blood serum compared to the controls [90]. Neonates with higher serum TSH concentration did not have lower cord-serum free T4 concentration [90].

3.4.3.2   Longitudinal Studies

Studies performed in iodine-sufficient populations suggest the cutoff for defining iodine deficiency in a population is a prevalence of >3% of newborn TSH values above 5 mU/L [1, 72, 75]. In Switzerland, a prospective population-based, national study evaluated UIC in pregnant women and the frequency of elevated TSH concentrations in the newborn screening program 5 years after increase in salt iodine concentration [72]. Before the salt iodine increase, the median UIC among pregnant women was 138 µg/L ($n = 511$), suggesting mild iodine deficiency and the prevalence of newborn TSH concentrations >5 mU/L was 2.9%. Five years later, after the increase in salt iodine concentration, median UIC in pregnancy had increased significantly to 249 µg/L, indicating sufficiency, and the prevalence of elevated newborn TSH decreased to 1.7%.

3.4.3.3   Summary

Thyroid function in neonates is highly vulnerable to low iodine intake and even mild iodine deficiency can increase newborn TSH and Tg concentrations. An increasing frequency of term newborn TSH concentrations >5 mU/L taken 3–4 days after birth is correlated with the severity of iodine deficiency in a population [91].

3.4.4   Children

3.4.4.1   Cross-Sectional Studies

Children may be more vulnerable to fluctuations in iodine intake due to lower thyroid stores of iodine and higher iodine turnover than adults [7]. However, in areas of iodine deficiency and endemic goiter, children often have TSH, T3, and T4 concentrations within the normal range. In such areas, the Tg concentration is typically elevated [92–96], and the prevalence of elevated Tg increases with the degree of deficiency [25, 95]. Measurement of Tg in children is thus a sensitive indicator of iodine status and improving thyroid function after iodine repletion. A standardized dried blood spot Tg assay has been developed [26, 27] and is recommended for assessing and monitoring iodine nutrition in the field [1]. An international reference range for dried blood spot Tg has been established in iodine-sufficient 5–14-year-old children that can be used for monitoring iodine nutrition [27].

   In a cross-sectional study in mildly iodine-deficient, school-age children 6–16 years old ($n = 1221$) with a median UIC of 90 µg/L in Jean province, Spain, the prevalence of serum TSH concentrations >5 mU/L and Tg >10 µg/L was 1.2% and 36.7%, respectively [97]. The UIC correlated with TSH ($r = 0.13$; $p < 0.0003$) in both boys and girls and with Tg ($r = 0.13$; $p < 0.01$) in the boys, but not with free T3 or free T4 concentrations. In Sardinia, Italy, no alterations in thyroid hormone concentrations were found in school-age children in an urban area with borderline iodine sufficiency (mean UIC of 105 μg/L) and a goiter prevalence of 12%, nor in provinces with moderate iodine deficiency (mean UIC <60 μg/L) and goiter prevalence up to 61% [98].

Studies in children with moderate-to-severe iodine deficiency and endemic goiter in Algeria, Albania, India, Indonesia, Morocco, and South Africa have reported normal TSH, T3, and T4 concentrations but elevated Tg concentrations in both children and adolescents [92–95, 99]. In contrast, several studies comparing children with or without goiter indicate altered thyroid function in goitrous children. A case-control study of children (mean age 8.6 years) with and without goiter and low iodine intake in the Gulbahar area in Afghanistan showed a significant association between goiter and TSH concentration [100]. Amongst the children with goiter ($n = 101$), 35% had abnormal TSH levels (>2.6 mU/L) as compared with 14% of children without goiter ($n = 110$) (OR = 3.10; 95% CI 1.6–6.1; $p < 0.001$). In a study of 8–15-year-old children with goiter and a median UIC of 84 μg/L in Northwestern Greece ($n = 97$), 11% of the children showed signs of subclinical hypothyroidism [101]. In areas of severe iodine deficiency, such as in Sudan and Northern Zaire, a combination of iodine deficiency and thiocyanate overload has been associated with decreased serum T4 concentrations and elevated TSH concentrations in children [102, 103].

3.4.4.2 Longitudinal Studies

Randomized controlled iodine-intervention studies show improved thyroid function after iodine repletion in moderate-to-severe iodine-deficient children, but not in mildly iodine deficient children [95, 104]. In South Africa, mildly iodine-deficient children 5–14 years old with a median UIC of 70–78 μg/L and normal total T4 concentration received 191 mg iodine as oral iodized oil or placebo [95, 96]. After 6 months, median UIC increased to 149 μg/L ($p < 0.001$) in the treated group, without significant change in the mean total T4 concentration. In Albania, 310 moderately iodine-deficient children 10–12 years old with median UIC of 42–44 μg/L received 400 mg of iodine as oral iodized oil [95, 104]. Although mean total T4 was within the normal range, nearly one third of the children had low levels of total T4 because of chronic iodine deficiency at baseline. Treatment with iodine significantly improved both iodine status ($p < 0.001$) and thyroid status ($p < 0.01$). The median UIC increased to 172 μg/L at 6 months, mean total T4 concentration increased ≈40%, and the prevalence of hypothyroxinemia was reduced to <1%. In Iran, 198 school children 8–14 years old with a mean UIC of 11.4 ± 19.8 μg/g creatinine were treated with 480 mg iodine as iodized oil [105]. Iodine treatment significantly improved mean UIC, T4, and TSH concentrations and reduced mean serum Tg concentration at 2 and 3 years after injection ($p < 0.001$).

In Morocco, 159 severely iodine-deficient children 6–16 years old with median UIC of 14–18 μg/L were enrolled to receive iodized salt [26, 106]. Before iodization, median UIC was 18 μg/L, median serum was TSH 0.8 mU/L, mean total T4 was 82.4 ± 17.4 nmol/L, and median Tg was 24.2 µg/L with 88% of children having an elevated Tg. Mean total T4 concentration was in the low-normal range, and 21% of children were hypothyroxinemic at baseline. One year after the introduction of iodized salt, median UIC had normalized to 181 µg/L, median serum TSH and mean total T4 improved to 0.6 mU/L and 92.3 ± 12.6 nmol/L, Tg normalized to 4.5 µg/L and prevalence of elevated Tg decreased to 12%. Because of practical and financial constraints, including a lack of infrastructure and electricity at the production site, salt iodization abruptly ceased. The children were followed for another 14 months, and concentrations of urinary iodine, TSH, total T4, and Tg were measured. Fourteen months after the discontinuation of salt iodization, median UIC had fallen to the preiodization concentration 20 µg/L, median serum TSH, mean total T4 and median Tg were sharply higher than before the introduction of iodized salt ($p < 0.001$) with concentrations of 1.9 mU/L, 85.4 ± 19.0 nmol/L, and 49.1 µg/L, respectively. The prevalence of elevated Tg was 89%, similar to that before the intervention [106].

In northern Benin, 198 children, 6–12 years old with severe iodine deficiency (median UIC of 20 µg/L and goiter prevalence between 20–60%) were supplemented with iodized oil and iodized salt. Initial mean serum concentrations of TSH and free T4 were within the normal range, whereas serum Tg concentrations were elevated. After 10 months, all indicators significantly improved and the serum concentrations of TSH decreased in 33%, free T4 increased in 18%, and Tg decreased in 56% of the cases [25].

3.4.4.3 Summary

Mild-to-moderate iodine deficiency does commonly not have a large effect on thyroid hormone concentrations in children; TSH, T3, and T4 concentrations often remain within the normal range. In contrast, Tg concentrations rise in iodine-deficient children and population-based monitoring in children has been simplified by the recent development of a standardized dried blood spot Tg assay. The impact of severe iodine deficiency on thyroid hormone concentrations in children may be age dependent [7, 107–110].

3.5 Introducing/Increasing Iodine Intakes and/or Iodine Excess: Effects on Thyroid Function in Populations

Over two-thirds of the 5 billion people living in countries affected by iodine deficiency now have access to iodized salt [1, 111]. Iodine excess is occurring more frequently, particularly when salt iodine levels are too high or are poorly monitored [111]. For example, in Brazil, Armenia, and Uganda, median UIC is >300 µg/L, while in Chile it is >500 µg/L [6]. High dietary iodine can also rarely come from natural sources, such as seaweed in coastal Japan [112, 113], iodine-rich drinking

Table 3.4 Tolerable upper intake level for iodine (μg/day)

Age group	European Commission/Scientific Committee on Food [120]	US Institute of Medicine [121]
1–3 years	200	200
4–6 years	250	300
7–10 years	300	300
11–14 years	450	300
15–17 years	500	900
Adult	600	1100
Pregnant women	600	1100

water in China [114, 115], and iodine-rich meat and milk in Iceland from fish products used for animal feed [116]. The median UIC in primary-school-age children in the United States is 229 μg/L [117], as a result of iodine-containing agents used in dairying and food preparation [118, 119], together with iodine from fortified salt.

European [120] and US [121] expert committees have recommended tolerable upper intake levels for iodine (Table 3.4), but caution that individuals with chronic iodine deficiency may respond adversely to intakes lower than these. In monitoring populations consuming iodized salt, the World Health Organization/International Council for Control of Iodine Deficiency Disorders (WHO/ICCIDD) recommendations [1] for the median UIC that indicates more-than-adequate and excess iodine intake are shown in Table 3.2.

In areas of iodine sufficiency, most healthy adults are remarkably tolerant to iodine intakes up to 1 mg/day, as the thyroid is able to adjust to a wide range of intakes to regulate the synthesis and release of thyroid hormones [122]. Large amounts of iodine given for days to months in small groups of healthy subjects have shown few adverse effects [123].

However, doses of iodine in the microgram range may cause hyper- or hypothyroidism in those with past or present thyroid abnormalities. This occurs because, in a damaged thyroid gland, the normal down-regulation of iodine transport into the gland may not occur. Thus, even in so-called iodine-sufficient populations, because many individuals will have past or present thyroid disorders, it is to be expected that changes in population iodine intake will be an important determinant of the pattern of thyroid diseases. This has been demonstrated in epidemiological studies that have studied the relationship between iodine intake and the incidence and prevalence of thyroid diseases, as discussed below.

3.5.1 Cross-Sectional Studies: The Epidemiology of Thyroid Function in Areas of Low and High Iodine Intakes

Danish investigators compared the incidence and prevalence of hyperthyroidism and hypothyroidism in Jutland, Denmark, an area with low iodine intake (approximately

40–70 µg/day) and Iceland, an area of high iodine intake (approximately 400–450 µg/day, based on urinary iodine excretion around 300 µg/24 hours in young subjects) [4]. It was assumed these levels of iodine intake were present for the lifetime of the inhabitants. The two areas have similar genetic backgrounds, economic development, and healthcare systems, and the same thyroid assays were used. There was a distinctly different pattern of thyroid dysfunction in the two areas: compared to Iceland, there was a higher prevalence of hyperthyroidism but a lower prevalence of hypothyroidism in Jutland. The lifetime risk for developing hyperthyroidism was 2.3 times higher in Jutland than in Iceland. Multinodular toxic goiter was the most common cause of hyperthyroidism in Jutland, but relatively rare in Iceland. In contrast, nearly all cases of hyperthyroidism in Iceland were Graves' disease in young and middle-aged subjects [4].

Other populations with long-standing mild-to-moderate iodine deficiency demonstrate a similar pattern of a high prevalence of thyroid hyperfunction with low serum TSH and a low prevalence of thyroid hypofunction with elevated serum TSH [31, 124–127]. Moreover, studies [128–133] have demonstrated a similar pattern of more cases of hyperthyroidism in mild iodine deficiency and more cases of thyroid hypofunction with high iodine intake. The increase in frequency of thyroid multinodularity with advancing age in mildly iodine-deficient areas is associated with a decrease in serum TSH in females [32, 134]. In contrast, there is a mild increase in serum TSH in older females in the United Kingdom [135] and Sweden [136] with higher iodine intakes. These data argue that the high rates of hyperthyroidism in populations with mild iodine deficiency are due to multifocal autonomous function of a nodular thyroid. Thus, like diffuse goiter, thyroid hyperfunction should be included in the spectrum disorders associated with mild-to-moderate iodine deficiency disorders.

Two mechanisms may be responsible for the increase in hypothyroidism in a population where the iodine intake is chronically high. One mechanism is the inhibitory effect of iodine on thyroid hormone synthesis and secretion, the Wolff-Chaikoff effect. This autoregulatory process is thought to protect against thyroid hormone hypersecretion in the face of high iodine intake. However, this autoregulation is not perfect and commonly induces some degree of thyroid hypofunction. In Japanese adults with chronic excess iodine intakes, many with overt hypothyroidism will become euthyroid if their iodine intakes are normalized [137, 138]. The other proposed mechanism is induction of thyroid hypofunction due to autoimmune thyroiditis. In animal models, increasing iodine intake is associated with a progressive increase in thyroiditis [139, 140]. After an increase in iodine intake in human populations, the histology of surgical thyroid specimens shows an increase in the prevalence of thyroiditis [141].

3.5.2 High Iodine Intake Produces Thyroid Dysfunction in Children

In children, excess dietary iodine has been associated with goiter and thyroid dysfunction. In the reports of 'endemic coast goiter' in Hokkaido, Japan [5], the traditional local diet was high in iodine-rich seaweed. UIE in children consuming the local diet was ≈23,000 μg/day. The overall prevalence of visible goiter in children was 3–9%, but in several villages ≈25% had visible goiter. Most of the goiters responded to administration of thyroid hormone and/or restriction of dietary iodine intake. TSH assays were not available, but it was suggested an increase in serum TSH was involved in generation of goiter. No cases of clinical hypo- or hyperthyroidism were reported.

Goiter in children may also be precipitated by iodine intake well below the many milligrams per day in the studies from Hokkaido. Li et al. [114] examined thyroid status in Chinese children ($n = 171$) from two villages, where the iodine concentrations in drinking water were 462 μg/L and 54 μg/L, and the mean UICs were 1,235 μg/g and 428 μg/g creatinine, respectively. Mean serum TSH (7.8 mU/L) was increased in the first village, and was high-to-normal (3.9 mU/L) in the second village. In the first village, the goiter rate was >60% and mean ± SD Tvol was 13.3 ± 2.7, compared to a goiter rate of 15–20% and a mean ± SD Tvol of 5.9 ± 1.8 in the second village. There were no signs of neurologic deficits in the children. In other reports from China, drinking water with iodine concentrations >300 μg/L resulted in UIC >900 μg/L and a goiter rate >10% [115]. These Chinese studies suggest goiter and thyroid dysfunction may occur in children at iodine intakes in the range of 400–1300 μg/day.

This contention is supported by the findings of a recent study in an international cohort of 6–12-year-old children, where chronic iodine intakes ≥500 μg/day in children were associated with an increase in thyroid size as determined by ultrasonography [142]. Although overall these findings suggest moderately high dietary intakes of iodine—in the range of 300–500 μg/day—are well-tolerated by healthy children, iodine intakes in this range are of no benefit and may have adverse effects not detected in these studies.

3.5.3   Longitudinal Studies: The Effects of Increasing Iodine Intakes in Populations on Thyroid Function

In an effort to control iodine deficiency, iodine intakes of many populations around the world have been increased. Increasing iodine intakes in iodine-deficient populations is typically accompanied by a clear rise in the incidence of hyperthyroidism; the magnitude of the increase depending on the amount of iodine administered and the severity of the preexisting iodine deficiency. Most patients who develop iodine-induced hyperthyroidism (IIH) have preexisting multinodular thyroid disease [143]. Thyrocytes in nodules often become insensitive to TSH control, and if iodine supply is suddenly increased, these autonomous nodules may overproduce thyroid hormones. Before iodine administration, although most are euthyroid, they may have radioactive iodine uptakes that are not suppressible, low serum TSH concentration values, and a serum TSH that does not respond to thyrotropin-releasing hormone [143]. Although only 3% of iodine deficient, goitrous adult Sudanese developed hyperthyroidism after receiving iodized oil, serum TSH concentrations were <0.1 mU/L in 5.9–16.7% of subjects 12 months after iodine [144]. After iodized salt was introduced to adult subjects with nodular goiter in Zaire, 7.4% developed severe thyrotoxicosis, and in many subjects the disorder persisted longer than 1 year [145, 146]. Similarly, in Zimbabwe, introduction of over-iodized salt produced a threefold increase in IIH [147]. The increase in the incidence of IIH after a properly monitored introduction of iodine is transient, because the resulting iodine sufficiency in the population reduces the future risk of developing autonomous thyroid nodules [148]. In Switzerland in 1980, when the iodine content of salt was raised from 7.5 to 15 ppm, the UIC increased from ≈80–150 µg/g creatinine. In the first 2 years after this increase, the incidence of toxic nodular goiter rose by 12%, but gradually regressed to a stable level of only 25% of the initial incidence [149].

To investigate the effects of iodine intake on thyroid disorders in China [150, 151], a 5-year, prospective community-based survey was done in three rural Chinese communities with mildly deficient, more-than-adequate (previously mild iodine deficiency corrected by iodized salt), and excessive iodine intake from environmental sources; the median UICs were 88, 214, and 634 µg/L, respectively. For the three communities, the cumulative incidence of hyperthyroidism was 1.4, 0.9, and 0.8%; of overt hypothyroidism, 0.2, 0.5, and 0.3%; of subclinical hypothyroidism, 0.2, 2.6, and 2.9%; and of autoimmune thyroiditis, 0.2, 1.0, and 1.3%, respectively. In most individuals, these latter two disorders were not sustained. Among subjects with euthyroidism and antithyroid antibodies at baseline, the 5-year incidence of elevated serum TSH levels was greater among those with more-than-adequate or excessive iodine intake than among those with mildly deficient iodine intake. In all three communities, independent of iodine intake, either positive TPOAb (OR = 4.2; 95% CI 1.7–8.8) or goiter (OR = 3.1; 95% CI 1.4–6.8) in original healthy participants was associated with the occurrence of hyperthyroidism.

Denmark has documented the pattern of thyroid disease after careful introduction of iodized salt [152, 153]. New cases of overt hypothyroidism were identified in two areas of Denmark with previous moderate and mild iodine deficiency, respectively (Aalborg, median UIC = 45 µg/L; and Copenhagen, median UIC = 61 µg/L) before and for the first 7 years after introduction of a national program of salt iodization. The overall incidence rate of hypothyroidism modestly increased during the study period: baseline, 38.3/100,000 per year; after salt iodization, 47.2/100,000 (vs. baseline, RR = 1.23; 95% CI 1.07–1.42). There was a geographic difference because hypothyroidism increased only in the area with previous moderate iodine deficiency. The increase occurred in young and middle-aged adults. Similarly, new cases of overt hyperthyroidism in these two areas of Denmark before and for the first 6 years after iodine fortification were identified. The overall incidence rate of hyperthyroidism increased (baseline, 102.8/100,000 per year; after salt iodization, 138.7/100,000 [p for trend < 0.001]). Hyperthyroidism increased in both sexes and in all age groups, but in contrast to IIH, where most cases occur in older individuals, many of the new cases were observed in young subjects—the increase was highest in adults aged 20–39 years—and were presumably of autoimmune origin. The authors suggested that further monitoring is expected to show a decrease in the number of elderly subjects suffering from nodular hyperthyroidism.

3.6 Conclusions

Concerns about potential increases in iodine-induced thyroid disease continue to delay or limit the implementation of iodine prophylaxis in iodine-deficient populations. Are these concerns justified? Looking at the benefits versus the risks of iodine prophylaxis, it is clear that severe iodine deficiency in pregnancy can cause hypothyroidism, poor pregnancy outcome, cretinism, and irreversible mental retardation. Mild-to-moderate iodine deficiency *in utero* and in childhood results in less severe learning disability, poor growth, and diffuse goiter. In adults, mild-to-moderate iodine deficiency appears to be associated with higher rates of more aggressive subtypes of thyroid cancer, and increases risk for nontoxic and toxic nodular goiter and associated hyperthyroidism.

However, increasing iodine intakes in deficient populations is not without risk. Mild iodine deficiency may be associated with a decreased risk of overt and subclinical hypothyroidism, as well as autoimmune thyroiditis. In China, chronic excess iodine intakes are associated with a small increase in subclinical hypothyroidism and autoimmune thyroiditis, but not overt hypo- or hyperthyroidism. In contrast, in Denmark, correcting mild-to-moderate deficiency modestly increased rates of hypo- and hyperthyroidism. The differing effects of varying iodine intakes in these studies may be related to differences in underlying thyroid autonomy, genetic susceptibility, or other environmental variables.

More prospective data on the epidemiology of thyroid disorders caused by changes in iodine intake in other countries would be valuable. But it appears achieving optimal iodine intakes (in the range of 150–250 µg/day) can minimize the amount of thyroid dysfunction in populations [154]. Iodine prophylaxis with periodic monitoring is an extremely cost-effective approach to help control thyroid disorders, compared to clinical diagnosis and treatment. If programs of iodine prophylaxis are carefully monitored for both iodine deficiency and excess, the relatively small risks of iodine excess are far outweighed by the substantial risks of iodine deficiency—pregnancy loss, goiter, and mental retardation, which continue to affect up to a third of the global population [8].

References

1. World Health Organization, United Nations Children's Fund, International Council for the Control of Iodine Deficiency Disorders. *Assessment of Iodine Deficiency Disorders and Monitoring Their Elimination. A Guide for Programme Managers.* 3rd ed. Geneva, Switzerland: World Health Organization; 2007.

2. WHO Secretariat on behalf of the participants to the Consultation, Andersson M, de Benoist B, Delange F, Zupan J. Prevention and control of iodine deficiency in pregnant and lactating women and in children less than 2-years-old: conclusions and recommendations of the Technical Consultation. *Public Health Nutr.* 2007;10:1606-1611.

3. Bulow PI, Knudsen N, Jorgensen T, Perrild H, Ovesen L, Laurberg P. Large differences in incidences of overt hyper- and hypothyroidism associated with a small difference in iodine intake: a prospective comparative register-based population survey. *J Clin Endocrinol Metab.* 2002;87:4462-4469.

4. Laurberg P, Bulow PI, Knudsen N, Ovesen L, Andersen S. Environmental iodine intake affects the type of nonmalignant thyroid disease. *Thyroid.* 2001;11:457-469.

5. Laurberg P. Global or Gaelic epidemic of hypothyroidism? *Lancet.* 2005;365:738-740.

6. de Benoist B, McLean E, Andersson M, Rogers L. Iodine deficiency in 2007: global progress since 2003. *Food Nutr Bull.* 2008;29:195-202.

7. Delange FD, Dunn JT. Iodine deficiency. In: Braverman LE, Utiger RD, eds. *The Thyroid: A Fundamental and Clinical Text.* 9th ed. Philadelphia, PA: Lippincott Williams & Wilkins; 2005.

8. Zimmermann MB, Jooste PL, Pandav CS. Iodine-deficiency disorders. *Lancet.* 2008;372 (9645):1251-1262.

9. Rousset BA, Dunn JT. Thyroid hormone synthesis and secretion. In: DeGroot LE, Hannemann G, eds. *The Thyroid and Its Diseases,* 2004. Internet: http://www.thyroidmanager.org/Chapter2/2-frame.htm. Accessed September 9, 2008.

10. Eskandari S, Loo DD, Dai G, Levy O, Wright EM, Carrasco N. Thyroid Na+/I- symporter. Mechanism, stoichiometry, and specificity. *J Biol Chem.* 1997;272:27230-27238.

11. Chopra IJ, Hershman JM, Hornabrook RW. Serum thyroid hormone and thyrotropin levels in subjects from endemic goiter regions of New Guinea. *J Clin Endocrinol Metab.* 1975;40:326-333.

12. Delange F, Hershman JM, Ermans AM. Relationship between the serum thyrotropin level, the prevalence of goiter and the pattern of iodine metabolism in Idjwi Island. *J Clin Endocrinol Metab.* 1971;33:261-268.

13. Vanderpas J. Nutritional epidemiology and thyroid hormone metabolism. *Annu Rev Nutr.* 2006;26:293-322.

14. Stevenson C, Silva E, Pineda G. Thyroxine (T4) and triiodothyronine (T3): effects of iodine on the serum concentrations and disposal rates in subjects from an endemic goiter area. *J Clin Endocrinol Metab.* 1974;38:390-393.

15. Chopra IJ, Sack J, Fisher DA. Circulating 3,3',5'-triiodothyronine (reverse T3) in the human newborn. *J Clin Invest.* 1975;55:1137-1141.

16. Patel YC, Pharoah PO, Hornabrook RW, Hetzel BS. Serum triiodothyronine, thyroxine and thyroid-stimulating hormone in endemic goiter: a comparison of goitrous and nongoitrous subjects in New Guinea. *J Clin Endocrinol Metab.* 1973;37:783-789.

17. Pharaoh PO, Lawton NF, Ellis SM, Williams ES, Ekins RP. The role of triiodothyronine (T3) in the maintenance of euthyroidism in endemic goitre. *Clin Endocrinol (Oxford).* 1973;2:193-199.

18. Ingenbleek Y, Luypaert B, De Nayer P. Nutritional status and endemic goitre. *Lancet.* 1980;1:388-391.

19. Spencer CA, Wang CC. Thyroglobulin measurement. Techniques, clinical benefits, and pitfalls. *Endocrinol Metab Clin North Am.* 1995;24:841-863.

20. Dunn JT, Dunn AD. Thyroglobulin: chemistry, biosynthesis and proteolysis. In: Braverman LE, Rutiger RD, eds. *Werner and Ingbar's the Thyroid: A Fundamental and Clinical Text.* 8th ed. Philadelphia, PA: Lippincott Williams & Wilkins; 2000.

21. Van Herle AJ, Hershman JM, Hornabrook RW, Chopra IJ. Serum thyroglobulin in inhabitants of an endemic goiter region of New Guinea. *J Clin Endocrinol Metab.* 1976;43:512-516.

22. Pezzino V, Vigneri R, Squatrito S, Filetti S, Camus M, Polosa P. Increased serum thyroglobulin levels in patients with nontoxic goiter. *J Clin Endocrinol Metab.* 1978;46:653-657.

23. Hershman JM, Due DT, Sharp B, et al. Endemic goiter in Vietnam. *J Clin Endocrinol Metab.* 1983;57:243-249.
24. Fenzi GF, Ceccarelli C, Macchia E, et al. Reciprocal changes of serum thyroglobulin and TSH in residents of a moderate endemic goitre area. *Clin Endocrinol (Oxford).* 1985;23:115-122.
25. van den Briel T, West CE, Hautvast JG, Vulsma T, de Vijlder JJ, Ategbo EA. Serum thyroglobulin and urinary iodine concentration are the most appropriate indicators of iodine status and thyroid function under conditions of increasing iodine supply in schoolchildren in Benin. *J Nutr.* 2001;131:2701-2706.
26. Zimmermann MB, Moretti D, Chaouki N, Torresani T. Development of a dried whole-blood spot thyroglobulin assay and its evaluation as an indicator of thyroid status in goitrous children receiving iodized salt. *Am J Clin Nutr.* 2003;77:1453-1458.
27. Zimmermann MB, de Benoist B, Corigliano S, et al. Assessment of iodine status using dried blood spot thyroglobulin: development of reference material and establishment of an international reference range in iodine-sufficient children. *J Clin Endocrinol Metab.* 2006;91:4881-4887.
28. Hennemann G, Djokomoeljanto R, Docter R, et al. The relationship between serum protein-bound iodine levels and urinary iodine excretion and serum thyrotrophin concentrations in subjects from an endemic goitre area in central Java. *Acta Endocrinol (Copenhagen).* 1978;88:474-481.
29. Dumont JE, Ermans AM, Maenhaut C, Coppee F, Stanbury JB. Large goitre as a maladaptation to iodine deficiency. *Clin Endocrinol (Oxford).* 1995;43:1-10.
30. Dumont JE, Lamy F, Roger P, Maenhaut C. Physiological and pathological regulation of thyroid cell proliferation and differentiation by thyrotropin and other factors. *Physiol Rev.* 1992;72:667-697.
31. Aghini-Lombardi F, Antonangeli L, Martino E, et al. The spectrum of thyroid disorders in an iodine-deficient community: the Pescopagano survey. *J Clin Endocrinol Metab.* 1999;84:561-566.
32. Knudsen N, Bulow I, Jorgensen T, Laurberg P, Ovesen L, Perrild H. Comparative study of thyroid function and types of thyroid dysfunction in two areas in Denmark with slightly different iodine status. *Eur J Endocrinol.* 2000;143:485-491.
33. Laurberg P, Nohr SB, Pedersen KM, et al. Thyroid disorders in mild iodine deficiency. *Thyroid.* 2000;10:951-963.
34. Valeix P, Dos Santos C, Castetbon K, Bertrais S, Cousty C, Hercberg S. Thyroid hormone levels and thyroid dysfunction of French adults participating in the SU.VI.MAX study. *Ann Endocrinol (Paris).* 2004;65:477-486.
35. Valeix P, Zarebska M, Preziosi P, Galan P, Pelletier B, Hercberg S. Iodine deficiency in France. *Lancet.* 1999;353:1766-1767.
36. Rasmussen LB, Ovesen L, Bulow I, et al. Dietary iodine intake and urinary iodine excretion in a Danish population: effect of geography, supplements and food choice. *Br J Nutr.* 2002;87:61-69.
37. Thomson CD, Woodruffe S, Colls AJ, Joseph J, Doyle TC. Urinary iodine and thyroid status of New Zealand residents. *Eur J Clin Nutr.* 2001;55:387-392.
38. Lazarus JH, Parkes AB, John R, N'Diaye M, Prysor-Jones SG. Endemic goitre in Senegal—thyroid function etiological factors and treatment with oral iodized oil. *Acta Endocrinol (Copenhagen).* 1992;126:149-154.
39. Buttfield IH, Black ML, Hoffmann MJ, et al. Studies of the control of thyroid function in endemic goiter in Eastern New Guinea. *J Clin Endocrinol Metab.* 1966;26:1201-1207.
40. Delange F. The disorders induced by iodine deficiency. *Thyroid.* 1994;4:107-128.
41. Andersen S, Pedersen KM, Pedersen IB, Laurberg P. Variations in urinary iodine excretion and thyroid function. A 1-year study in healthy men. *Eur J Endocrinol.* 2001;144:461-465.
42. Soldin OP, Tractenberg RE, Pezzullo JC. Do thyroxine and thyroid-stimulating hormone levels reflect urinary iodine concentrations? *Ther Drug Monit.* 2005;27:178-185.
43. Aboul-Khair SA, Crooks J, Turnbull AC, Hytten FE. The physiological changes in thyroid function during pregnancy. *Clin Sci.* 1964;27:195-207.

44. Glinoer D. The regulation of thyroid function in pregnancy: pathways of endocrine adaptation from physiology to pathology. *Endocr Rev.* 1997;18:404-433.
45. Liberman CS, Pino SC, Fang SL, Braverman LE, Emerson CH. Circulating iodide concentrations during and after pregnancy. *J Clin Endocrinol Metab.* 1998;83:3545-3549.
46. Lazarus JH. Epidemiology and prevention of thyroid disease in pregnancy. *Thyroid.* 2002;12:861-865.
47. Glinoer D. The importance of iodine nutrition during pregnancy. *Public Health Nutr.* 2007;10:1542-1546.
48. Caron P, Hoff M, Bazzi S, et al. Urinary iodine excretion during normal pregnancy in healthy women living in the southwest of France: correlation with maternal thyroid parameters. *Thyroid.* 1997;7:749-754.
49. Kung AW, Lao TT, Chau MT, Tam SC, Low LC. Goitrogenesis during pregnancy and neonatal hypothyroxinaemia in a borderline iodine sufficient area. *Clin Endocrinol (Oxford).* 2000;53:725-731.
50. Nohr SB, Laurberg P, Borlum KG, et al. Iodine deficiency in pregnancy in Denmark. Regional variations and frequency of individual iodine supplementation. *Acta Obstet Gynecol Scand.* 1993;72:350-353.
51. Vermiglio F, Lo Presti VP, Castagna MG, et al. Increased risk of maternal thyroid failure with pregnancy progression in an iodine deficient area with major iodine deficiency disorders. *Thyroid.* 1999;9:19-24.
52. Lazarus JH. Comments. *Public Health Nutr.* 2007;10:1553.
53. Pedersen KM, Laurberg P, Iversen E, et al. Amelioration of some pregnancy-associated variations in thyroid function by iodine supplementation. *J Clin Endocrinol Metab.* 1993;77:1078-1083.
54. Zimmermann MB. The adverse effects of mild-to-moderate iodine deficiency during pregnancy and childhood: a review. *Thyroid.* 2007;17:829-835.
55. Romano R, Jannini EA, Pepe M, et al. The effects of iodoprophylaxis on thyroid size during pregnancy. *Am J Obstet Gynecol.* 1991;164:482-485.
56. Glinoer D, De Nayer P, Delange F, et al. A randomized trial for the treatment of mild iodine deficiency during pregnancy: maternal and neonatal effects. *J Clin Endocrinol Metab.* 1995;80:258-269.
57. Liesenkotter KP, Gopel W, Bogner U, Stach B, Gruters A. Earliest prevention of endemic goiter by iodine supplementation during pregnancy. *Eur J Endocrinol.* 1996;134:443-448.
58. Nohr SB, Jorgensen A, Pedersen KM, Laurberg P. Postpartum thyroid dysfunction in pregnant thyroid peroxidase antibody-positive women living in an area with mild to moderate iodine deficiency: is iodine supplementation safe? *J Clin Endocrinol Metab.* 2000;85:3191-3198.
59. Antonangeli L, Maccherini D, Cavaliere R, et al. Comparison of two different doses of iodide in the prevention of gestational goiter in marginal iodine deficiency: a longitudinal study. *Eur J Endocrinol.* 2002;147:29-34.
60. Pharoah PO, Connolly KJ. A controlled trial of iodinated oil for the prevention of endemic cretinism: a long-term follow-up. *Int J Epidemiol.* 1987;16:68-73.
61. Cao XY, Jiang XM, Dou ZH, et al. Timing of vulnerability of the brain to iodine deficiency in endemic cretinism. *N Engl J Med.* 1994;331:1739-1744.
62. Connolly KJ, Pharoah PO, Hetzel BS. Fetal iodine deficiency and motor performance during childhood. *Lancet.* 1979;2:1149-1151.
63. Moleti M, Lo Presti VP, Campolo MC, et al. Iodine prophylaxis using iodized salt and risk of maternal thyroid failure in conditions of mild iodine deficiency. *J Clin Endocrinol Metab.* 2008;93:2616-2621.
64. Weeke J, Dybkjaer L, Granlie K, et al. A longitudinal study of serum TSH, and total and free iodothyronines during normal pregnancy. *Acta Endocrinol (Copenhagen).* 1982;101:531-537.
65. Glinoer D. Maternal and fetal impact of chronic iodine deficiency. *Clin Obstet Gynecol.* 1997;40:102-116.

66. Laurberg P, Andersen S, Bjarnadottir RI, et al. Evaluating iodine deficiency in pregnant women and young infants-complex physiology with a risk of misinterpretation. *Public Health Nutr.* 2007;10:1547-1552.

67. Delange F. Screening for congenital hypothyroidism used as an indicator of the degree of iodine deficiency and of its control. *Thyroid.* 1998;8:1185-1192.

68. Glinoer D, Delange F, Laboureur I, et al. Maternal and neonatal thyroid function at birth in an area of marginally low iodine intake. *J Clin Endocrinol Metab.* 1992;75:800-805.

69. Delange F. Iodine requirements during pregnancy, lactation and the neonatal period and indicators of optimal iodine nutrition. *Public Health Nutr.* 2007;10:1571-1580.

70. Sullivan KM, May W, Nordenberg D, Houston R, Maberly GF. Use of thyroid stimulating hormone testing in newborns to identify iodine deficiency. *J Nutr.* 1997;127:55-58.

71. Delange F. Neonatal screening for congenital hypothyroidism: results and perspectives. *Horm Res.* 1997;48:51-61.

72. Zimmermann MB, Aeberli I, Torresani T, Burgi H. Increasing the iodine concentration in the Swiss iodized salt program markedly improved iodine status in pregnant women and children: a 5-y prospective national study. *Am J Clin Nutr.* 2005;82:388-392.

73. Zimmermann MB. Methods to assess iron and iodine status. *Br J Nutr.* 2008;99(suppl 3):S2-S9.

74. Sava L, Delange F, Belfiore A, Purrello F, Vigneri R. Transient impairment of thyroid function in newborn from an area of endemic goiter. *J Clin Endocrinol Metab.* 1984;59:90-95.

75. Nordenberg D, Sullivan K, Maberly G, et al. Congenital hypothyroid screening programs and the sensitive thyrotropin assay: strategies for the surveillance of iodine deficiency disorders. In: Delange F, Dunn J, Glinoer D, eds. *Iodine Deficiency in Europe: A Continuing Concern.* New York, NY: Plenum Publishing; 1993:211-217.

76. McElduff A, McElduff P, Gunton JE, Hams G, Wiley V, Wilcken BM. Neonatal thyroid-stimulating hormone concentrations in northern Sydney: further indications of mild iodine deficiency? *Med J Aust.* 2002;176:317-320.

77. Travers CA, Guttikonda K, Norton CA, et al. Iodine status in pregnant women and their newborns: are our babies at risk of iodine deficiency? *Med J Aust.* 2006;184:617-620.

78. Veinpalu M, Ambos A, Velbri S, Vaher Y, Podar T. Urinary iodine excretion in Estonian children. *Eur J Endocrinol.* 1996;135:248.

79. Mikelsaar RV, Viikmaa M. Neonatal thyroid-stimulating hormone screening as an indirect method for the assessment of iodine deficiency in Estonia. *Horm Res.* 1999;52:284-286.

80. Guibourdenche J, Noel M, Chevenne D, et al. Biochemical investigation of foetal and neonatal thyroid function using the ACS-180SE analyser: clinical application. *Ann Clin Biochem.* 2001;38:520-526.

81. Kung AW, Lao TT, Low LC, Pang RW, Robinson JD. Iodine insufficiency and neonatal hyperthyrotropinaemia in Hong Kong. *Clin Endocrinol (Oxford).* 1997;46:315-319.

82. Chakraborty I, Chatterjee S, Bhadra D, Mukhopadhyaya BB, Dasgupta A, Purkait B. Iodine deficiency disorders among the pregnant women in a rural hospital of West Bengal. *Indian J Med Res.* 2006;123:825-829.

83. Copeland DL, Sullivan KM, Houston R, et al. Comparison of neonatal thyroid-stimulating hormone levels and indicators of iodine deficiency in school children. *Public Health Nutr.* 2002;5:81-87.

84. Delange F, Thilly C, Camus M, et al. Evidence for fetal hhypothyroidism and maternal thyroid status in severe endemic goiter. In: Robbins J, Braverman LE, eds. *Thyroid Research.* Amsterdam, The Netherlands: Excerpta Medica; 1976:493-496.

85. Thilly CH, Delange F, Lagasse R, et al. Fetal hypothyroidism and maternal thyroid status in severe endemic goiter. *J Clin Endocrinol Metab.* 1978;47:354-360.

86. Delange F, Thilly C, Bourdoux P, et al. Influence of dietary goitroogens during pregnancy in humans on thyroid function of newborn. In: Delange F, Iteke FB, Ermans AM, eds. *Nutritional Factors Involved in the Goitrogenic Action of Cassava.* Ottawa, Canada: International Development Research Centre; 1982:40-50.

87. Burrow GN, Fisher DA, Larsen PR. Maternal and fetal thyroid function. *N Engl J Med.* 1994;331:1072-1078.
88. Eltom A, Eltom M, Idris M, Gebre-Medhin M. Thyroid function in the newborn in relation to maternal thyroid status during labour in a mild iodine deficiency endemic area in Sudan. *Clin Endocrinol (Oxford).* 2001;55:485-490.
89. Morreale de Escobar G, Obregon MJ, Escobar del Rey F. Role of thyroid hormone during early brain development. *Eur J Endocrinol.* 2004;151(suppl 3):U25-U37.
90. Nohr SB, Laurberg P. Opposite variations in maternal and neonatal thyroid function induced by iodine supplementation during pregnancy. *J Clin Endocrinol Metab.* 2000;85:623-627.
91. Gruneiro-Papendieck L, Chiesa A, Mendez V, Bengolea S, Prieto L. Neonatal TSH levels as an index of iodine sufficiency: differences related to time of screening sampling and methodology. *Horm Res.* 2004;62:272-276.
92. Benmiloud M, Chaouki ML, Gutekunst R, Teichert HM, Wood WG, Dunn JT. Oral iodized oil for correcting iodine deficiency: optimal dosing and outcome indicator selection. *J Clin Endocrinol Metab.* 1994;79:20-24.
93. Pardede LV, Hardjowasito W, Gross R, et al. Urinary iodine excretion is the most appropriate outcome indicator for iodine deficiency at field conditions at district level. *J Nutr.* 1998;128:1122-1126.
94. Zimmermann M, Adou P, Torresani T, Zeder C, Hurrell R. Persistence of goiter despite oral iodine supplementation in goitrous children with iron deficiency anemia in Cote d'Ivoire. *Am J Clin Nutr.* 2000;71:88-93.
95. Zimmermann MB, Jooste PL, Mabapa NS, et al. Treatment of iodine deficiency in school-age children increases insulin-like growth factor (IGF)-I and IGF binding protein-3 concentrations and improves somatic growth. *J Clin Endocrinol Metab.* 2007;92:437-442.
96. Zimmermann MB, Jooste PL, Mabapa NS, et al. Vitamin A supplementation in iodine-deficient African children decreases thyrotropin stimulation of the thyroid and reduces the goiter rate. *Am J Clin Nutr.* 2007;86:1040-1044.
97. Santiago-Fernandez P, Torres-Barahona R, Muela-Martinez JA, et al. Intelligence quotient and iodine intake: a cross-sectional study in children. *J Clin Endocrinol Metab.* 2004;89:3851-3857.
98. Martino E, Loviselli A, Velluzzi F, et al. Endemic goiter and thyroid function in central-southern Sardinia. Report on an extensive epidemiological survey. *J Endocrinol Invest.* 1994;17:653-657.
99. Dodd NS, Samuel AM. Iodine deficiency in adolescents from Bombay slums. *Natl Med J India.* 1993;6:110-113.
100. Oberlin O, Plantin-Carrenard E, Rigal O, Wilkinson C. Goitre and iodine deficiency in Afghanistan: a case-control study. *Br J Nutr.* 2006;95:196-203.
101. Tsatsoulis A, Johnson EO, Andricula M, et al. Thyroid autoimmunity is associated with higher urinary iodine concentrations in an iodine-deficient area of Northwestern Greece. *Thyroid.* 1999;9:279-283.
102. Vanderpas J, Bourdoux P, Lagasse R, et al. Endemic infantile hypothyroidism in a severe endemic goitre area of central Africa. *Clin Endocrinol (Oxford).* 1984;20:327-340.
103. Moreno-Reyes R, Boelaert M, el Badawi S, Eltom M, Vanderpas JB. Endemic juvenile hypothyroidism in a severe endemic goitre area of Sudan. *Clin Endocrinol (Oxford).* 1993;38:19-24.
104. Zimmermann MB, Connolly K, Bozo M, Bridson J, Rohner F, Grimci L. Iodine supplementation improves cognition in iodine-deficient schoolchildren in Albania: a randomized, controlled, double-blind study. *Am J Clin Nutr.* 2006;83:108-114.
105. Mirmiran P, Kimiagar M, Azizi F. Three-year survey of effects of iodized oil injection in schoolchildren with iodine deficiency disorders. *Exp Clin Endocrinol Diabetes.* 2002;110:393-397.
106. Zimmermann MB, Wegmuller R, Zeder C, Torresani T, Chaouki N. Rapid relapse of thyroid dysfunction and goiter in school-age children after discontinuation of salt iodization. *Am J Clin Nutr.* 2004;79:642-645.

107. Bourdoux P, Ermans AM. Factors influencing the levels of circulating T4, T3 and TSH in human beings submitted to severe iodine deficiency. *Ann Endocrinol (Paris).* 1981;42:40A.
108. Bachtarzi H, Benmiloud M. TSH-regulation and goitrogenesis in severe iodine deficiency. *Acta Endocrinol (Copenhagen).* 1983;103:21-27.
109. Malvaux P. Thyroid function during the neonatal period, infancy and childhood. In: Delange F, Fisher DA, Malvaux P, eds. *Pediatric Thyroidology.* Basel, Switzerland: S. Karger AG; 1985:33-43.
110. Delange F. Adaptation to iodine deficiency during growth: etiopathogenesis of endemic goiter abd cretinism. In: Delange F, Fisher AG, Glinoer D, eds. *Pediatric Thyrology.* Basel, Switzerland: S. Karger AG; 1985:295-326.
111. Delange F, de Benoist B, Pretell E, Dunn JT. Iodine deficiency in the world: where do we stand at the turn of the century? *Thyroid.* 2001;11:437-447.
112. Suzuki H, Higuchi T, Sawa K, Ohtaki S, Horiuchi Y. "Endemic coast goitre" in Hokkaido, Japan. *Acta Endocrinol (Copenhagen).* 1965;50:161-176.
113. Nagataki S. The average of dietary iodine intake due to the ingestion of seaweeds is 1.2 mg/day in Japan. *Thyroid.* 2008;18:667-668.
114. Li M, Liu DR, Qu CY, et al. Endemic goitre in central China caused by excessive iodine intake. *Lancet.* 1987;2:257-259.
115. Zhao J, Chen Z, Maberly G. Iodine-rich drinking water of natural origin in China. *Lancet.* 1998;352:2024.
116. Sigurdsson G, Franzson L. Urine excretion of iodine in an Icelandic population. *Icelandic Med J.* 1988;74:179-181.
117. Caldwell KL, Miller GA, Wang RY, Jain RB, Jones RL. Iodine status of the U.S. population, National Health and Nutrition Examination Survey 2003–2004. *Thyroid.* 2008;18:1207-1214.
118. London WT, Vought RL, Brown FA. Bread—dietary source of large quantities of iodine. *N Engl J Med.* 1965;273:381.
119. Pearce EN, Pino S, He X, Bazrafshan HR, Lee SL, Braverman LE. Sources of dietary iodine: bread, cows' milk, and infant formula in the Boston area. *J Clin Endocrinol Metab.* 2004;89:3421-3424.
120. Scientific Committee on Food, Health and Consumer Protection Directorate-General. *Opinion of the Scientific Committee on Food on the Tolerable Upper Intake Level of Iodine.* Brussels, Belgium: European Commission; 2002.
121. Institute of Medicine, Academy of Sciences, USA. *Dietary Reference Intakes for Vitamin A, Vitamin K, Arsenic, Boron, Chromium, Copper, Iodine, Iron, Manganese, Molybdenum, Nickel, Silicon, Vanadium and Zinc.* Washington, DC: National Academy Press; 2001.
122. Chow CC, Phillips DI, Lazarus JH, Parkes AB. Effect of low dose iodide supplementation on thyroid function in potentially susceptible subjects: are dietary iodide levels in Britain acceptable? *Clin Endocrinol (Oxford).* 1991;34:413-416.
123. Gardner DF, Centor RM, Utiger RD. Effects of low dose oral iodide supplementation on thyroid function in normal men. *Clin Endocrinol (Oxford).* 1988;28:283-288.
124. Laurberg P, Pedersen KM, Hreidarsson A, Sigfusson N, Iversen E, Knudsen PR. Iodine intake and the pattern of thyroid disorders: a comparative epidemiological study of thyroid abnormalities in the elderly in Iceland and in Jutland, Denmark. *J Clin Endocrinol Metab.* 1998;83:765-769.
125. Seck T, Scheidt-Nave C, Ziegler R, Pfeilschifter J. Prevalence of thyroid gland dysfunctions in 50- to 80-year-old patients. An epidemiologic cross-sectional study in a southwestern community. *Med Klin (Munich).* 1997;92:642-646.
126. Hintze G, Burghardt U, Baumert J, Windeler J, Kobberling J. Prevalence of thyroid dysfunction in elderly subjects from the general population in an iodine deficiency area. *Aging (Milano).* 1991;3:325-331.
127. Hintze G, Windeler J, Baumert J, Stein H, Kobberling J. Thyroid volume and goitre prevalence in the elderly as determined by ultrasound and their relationships to laboratory indices. *Acta Endocrinol (Copenhagen).* 1991;124:12-18.

128. Szabolcs I, Podoba J, Feldkamp J, et al. Comparative screening for thyroid disorders in old age in areas of iodine deficiency, long-term iodine prophylaxis and abundant iodine intake. *Clin Endocrinol (Oxford)*. 1997;47:87-92.

129. Konno N, Makita H, Yuri K, Iizuka N, Kawasaki K. Association between dietary iodine intake and prevalence of subclinical hypothyroidism in the coastal regions of Japan. *J Clin Endocrinol Metab*. 1994;78:393-397.

130. Roti E, Gardini E, Minelli R, Bianconi L, Braverman LE. Prevalence of anti-thyroid peroxidase antibodies in serum in the elderly: comparison with other tests for anti-thyroid antibodies. *Clin Chem*. 1992;38:88-92.

131. Ozbakir O, Dogukan A, Kelestimur F. The prevalence of thyroid dysfunction among elderly subjects in an endemic goiter area of Central Anatolia. *Endocr J*. 1995;42:713-716.

132. Nygaard B, Gideon P, Dige-Petersen H, Jespersen N, Solling K, Veje A. Thyroid volume and morphology and urinary iodine excretion in a Danish municipality. *Acta Endocrinol (Copenhagen)*. 1993;129:505-510.

133. Knudsen N, Jorgensen T, Rasmussen S, Christiansen E, Perrild H. The prevalence of thyroid dysfunction in a population with borderline iodine deficiency. *Clin Endocrinol (Oxford)*. 1999;51:361-367.

134. Knudsen N, Bulow I, Jorgensen T, Laurberg P, Ovesen L, Perrild H. Goitre prevalence and thyroid abnormalities at ultrasonography: a comparative epidemiological study in two regions with slightly different iodine status. *Clin Endocrinol (Oxford)*. 2000;53:479-485.

135. Tunbridge WM, Evered DC, Hall R, et al. The spectrum of thyroid disease in a community: the Whickham survey. *Clin Endocrinol (Oxford)*. 1977;7:481-493.

136. Petersen K, Lindstedt G, Lundberg PA, Bengtsson C, Lapidus L, Nystrom E. Thyroid disease in middle-aged and elderly Swedish women: thyroid-related hormones, thyroid dysfunction and goitre in relation to age and smoking. *J Intern Med*. 1991;229:407-413.

137. Tajiri J, Higashi K, Morita M, Umeda T, Sato T. Studies of hypothyroidism in patients with high iodine intake. *J Clin Endocrinol Metab*. 1986;63:412-417.

138. Sato K, Okamura K, Hirata T, et al. Immunological and chemical types of reversible hypothyroidism; clinical characteristics and long-term prognosis. *Clin Endocrinol (Oxford)*. 1996;45:519-528.

139. Sundick RS, Bagchi N, Brown TR. The role of iodine in thyroid autoimmunity: from chickens to humans: a review. *Autoimmunity*. 1992;13:61-68.

140. Safran M, Paul TL, Roti E, Braverman LE. Environmental factors affecting autoimmune thyroid disease. *Endocrinol Metab Clin North Am*. 1987;16:327-342.

141. Harach HR, Escalante DA, Onativia A, Lederer Outes J, Saravia Day E, Williams ED. Thyroid carcinoma and thyroiditis in an endemic goiter region before and after iodine prophylaxis. *Acta Endocrinol (Copenhagen)*. 1985;108:55-60.

142. Zimmermann MB, Ito Y, Hess SY, Fujieda K, Molinari L. High thyroid volume in children with excess dietary iodine intakes. *Am J Clin Nutr*. 2005;81:840-844.

143. Roti E, Uberti ED. Iodine excess and hyperthyroidism. *Thyroid*. 2001;11:493-500.

144. Elnagar B, Eltom M, Karlsson FA, Ermans AM, Gebre-Medhin M, Bourdoux PP. The effects of different doses of oral iodized oil on goiter size, urinary iodine, and thyroid-related hormones. *J Clin Endocrinol Metab*. 1995;80:891-897.

145. Ermans AM, Gullo D, Mugisho SG, et al. Iodine supplementation must be monitored at the population level in iodine deficient areas [abstract]. *Thyroid*. 1995;5(suppl 1):S137.

146. Bourdoux PP, Ermans AM, Mukalay wa Mukalay A, Filetti S, Vigneri R. Iodine-induced thyrotoxicosis in Kivu, Zaire. *Lancet*. 1996;347:552-553.

147. Todd CH, Allain T, Gomo ZA, Hasler JA, Ndiweni M, Oken E. Increase in thyrotoxicosis associated with iodine supplements in Zimbabwe. *Lancet*. 1995;346:1563-1564.

148. Delange F, de Benoist B, Alnwick D. Risks of iodine-induced hyperthyroidism after correction of iodine deficiency by iodized salt. *Thyroid*. 1999;9:545-556.

149. Burgi H, Kohler M, Morselli B. Thyrotoxicosis incidence in Switzerland and benefit of improved iodine supply. *Lancet*. 1998;352:1034.

150. Yang F, Shan Z, Teng X, et al. Chronic iodine excess does not increase the incidence of hyperthyroidism: a prospective community-based epidemiological survey in China. *Eur J Endocrinol.* 2007;156:403-408.
151. Teng W, Shan Z, Teng X, et al. Effect of iodine intake on thyroid diseases in China. *N Engl J Med.* 2006;354:2783-2793.
152. Pedersen IB, Laurberg P, Knudsen N, et al. An increased incidence of overt hypothyroidism after iodine fortification of salt in Denmark: a prospective population study. *J Clin Endocrinol Metab.* 2007;92:3122-3127.
153. Bulow PI, Laurberg P, Knudsen N, et al. Increase in incidence of hyperthyroidism predominantly occurs in young people after iodine fortification of salt in Denmark. *J Clin Endocrinol Metab.* 2006;91:3830-3834.
154. Zimmermann MB. Iodine requirements and the risks and benefits of correcting iodine deficiency in populations. *J Trace Elem Med Biol.* 2008;22:81-92.

Chapter 4
Regulation of Thyroid Hormone Production and Measurement of Thyrotropin

Jerome M. Hershman

4.1 Introduction

The hypothalamic-pituitary axis regulates the production of thyroid hormones so that the serum concentrations of thyroxine (T4) and triiodothyronine (T3) remain in a narrow range in the euthyroid state. These hormones have essential roles in growth; development; metabolism of carbohydrate, fat, and proteins; and adaptation to the environment. This chapter will focus on the production of thyroid hormones, hypothalamic-pituitary control of the thyroid, and the use of serum thyrotropin (thyroid stimulating hormone, TSH) measurements for evaluation of thyroid function.

4.2 Production of Thyroid Hormone

4.2.1 Sodium/Iodide Symporter

Iodide is an essential substrate for the production of thyroid hormone. The source of iodide (iodine) is dietary. Since iodine is a scarce nutrient, the thyroid gland has a transport protein that concentrates iodide from the serum. This protein, located on the basolateral membrane of the thyroid follicular cell, actively transports iodide against a concentration gradient, resulting in a cell to plasma ratio of 30–40:1 (Fig. 4.1). Because sodium is cotransported with iodide, the transport protein is called the sodium/iodide symporter (NIS) [1]. The sodium/potassium ATPase, another membrane protein, provides the energy for this process. The human NIS gene has 13 exons and is located on chromosome 19. Human NIS contains 643 amino acids and has 13 transmembrane domains. The amino terminus of the molecule is in the extracellular compartment and the C-terminal end is intracellular.

J. M. Hershman (✉)
Division of Endocrinology and Diabetes, David Geffen School of Medicine at UCLA,
University of California, Los Angeles, CA 90095, USA
e-mail: jhershmn@ucla.edu

G. A. Brent (ed.), *Thyroid Function Testing*,
DOI 10.1007/978-1-4419-1485-9_4, © Springer Science+Business Media, LLC 2010

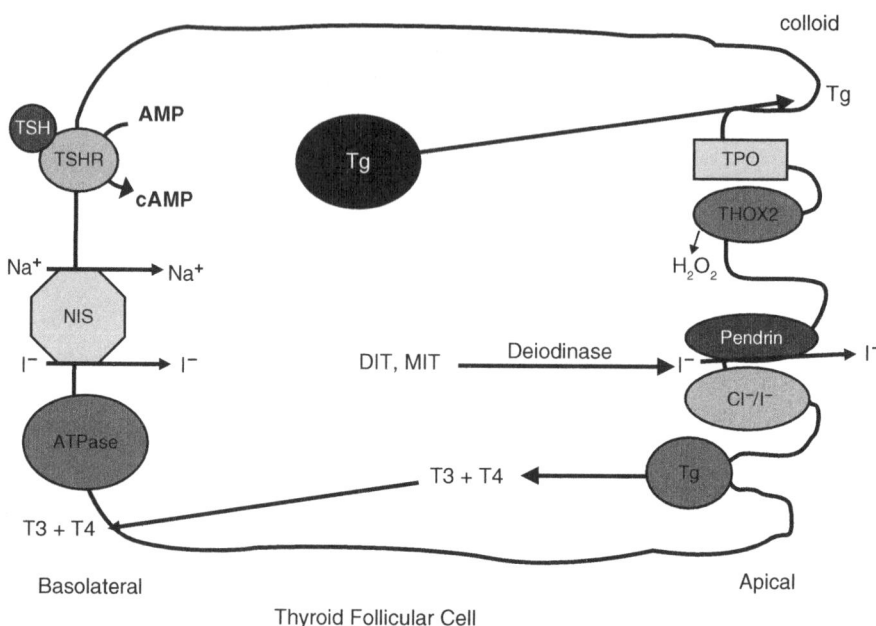

Fig. 4.1 Diagram of a thyroid cell and the biosynthetic steps in the formation and secretion of thyroid hormones

Human NIS is a glycoprotein of 108 kDa; its carbohydrate is not essential for its function.

TSH increases the gene expression of NIS by stimulating the cyclic AMP pathway. The regulation occurs through the induction of several transcription factors that bind to a far upstream enhancer in the NIS gene [2]. PAX-8 binds to its response element in the enhancer, and CREB, CREM, and ATF1 bind to a CRE-like sequence of the enhancer. The induction of NIS by TSH is a rapid process; NIS is a stable protein lasting for several days after synthesis. For NIS to function, it must translocate to the membrane.

4.2.2 Dietary Iodine Requirements

The dietary iodine requirement for adequate synthesis of thyroid hormone is at least 100 μg/day (discussed in depth in Chap. 3). This is reflected in a urine iodine of about 150 μg/g creatinine. A recent survey of urinary iodine in the United States shows mean urinary iodine was 168 μg/L, unchanged from the previous decade, and that only 11% had urinary iodine less than 50 μg/L [3]. It is estimated that worldwide one billion people live in regions with iodine deficiency. Pregnancy increases iodine requirement to 250 μg/day because of an increased renal loss in the face of a need to synthesize more thyroid hormone during pregnancy [4]. A survey of 100 pregnant women in Boston showed that 49% had suboptimal iodine intake and that

9% had iodine deficiency, which could impair thyroid hormone synthesis in the pregnant woman and fetus, possibly resulting in congenital hypothyroidism [5].

Excess iodine intake, resulting in high intrathyroidal iodide, may cause a transient blockade of the synthesis of thyroid hormone (Wolf–Chaikoff effect). Normal subjects escape from this blockade by down-regulation of iodide transport, probably by inhibition of gene expression of NIS (escape from the Wolff–Chaikoff effect), an autoregulatory process.

4.2.3   Thyroid Peroxidase

Thyroid peroxidase (TPO) is a glycoprotein located on the apical membrane of the thyroid follicular cell (Fig. 4.1) [6]. Its function is to oxidize iodide to a higher valence state for incorporation into tyrosine (organification) to produce monoiodotyrosine and diiodotyrosine within the thyroglobulin molecule. It is also responsible for the coupling of iodotyrosines to form T4 and T3. The human TPO gene is located on chromosome 2 and has 17 exons separated by 16 introns. The TPO protein contains 933 amino acids and about 10% carbohydrate. TPO contains a prosthetic heme group that is essential for its function. TSH stimulates the activity of TPO, probably through regulation of gene expression involving the transcription factors PAX-8 and TTF-1. Mutations in the TPO gene result in defective iodine oxidation and organification and cause goitrous congenital hypothyroidism [7].

4.2.4   Hydrogen Peroxide Generation

Hydrogen peroxide is essential for oxidation of iodide, organification of iodine, and coupling of iodotyrosines. The H_2O_2 generating system is located on the apical membrane where TPO also resides. The system involves oxidation of NADPH by an NADPH oxidase. There are two thyroidal NADPH oxidases, THOX1 (DUOX1) and THOX2 (DUOX2). The genes for both of the oxidases are on chromosome 15 and each consists of 33 exons. Each of them contain about 1,550 amino acids with seven transmembrane domains. The THOX proteins are glycosylated and have a molecular weight of about 189 kDa. The precise biochemical mechanism resulting in generation of H_2O_2 remains controversial. TSH stimulates the process and high concentrations of iodide inhibit it. Patients with mutations in THOX2 have congenital hypothyroidism, indicating that THOX1 cannot compensate for this deficiency [8].

4.2.5   Apical Iodide Transport

Pendrin is a protein located on the apical membrane that transports iodide from the cytoplasm to the apical lumen where it participates in iodination of thyroglobulin

(Fig. 4.1). Pendrin is also present in the endolymphatic system of the inner ear. Deficiencies in pendrin result in deafness and mild hypothyroidism called Pendred's syndrome [9]. There is a second apical iodide transporter. The relative contributions of these apical transporters to thyroid hormone synthesis is unclear.

4.2.6 Thyroglobulin

Thyroglobulin is a very large protein that serves as the matrix for synthesis of thyroid hormone [10]. Thyroglobulin resides within the follicle at the apical portion of the thyroid cell and makes up the colloid in the follicular lumen. It serves as the storage protein for thyroid hormone. The thyroglobulin gene is located on chromosome 8 and contains 48 introns. Gene expression of thyroglobulin is regulated by the transcription factors PAX-8, TTF-1, and TTF-2. The mature protein is a dimer, consisting of two 330 kDa monomers. The thyroglobulin molecule contains 132 tyrosyl residues, but only a few are used for synthesis of T4 and T3. Defects in thyroglobulin synthesis cause congenital hypothyroidism.

When there is a need for thyroid hormone, thyroglobulin is processed by reentry from the colloid into the thyroid cell by pinocytosis forming vesicles. Fusion of these vesicles with lysosomes results in proteolyic breakdown of the thyroglobulin and release of T4 and T3 as well as iodothyronines. The majority of the iodotyrosines are deiodinated by intrathyroidal dehalogenase, and the iodide is recycled so that it is available for thyroid hormone synthesis. This is an important mechanism for conservation of iodide. Patients with molecular defects in the dehalogenase have congenital hypothyroidism and goiter that can be overcome by increasing iodide intake [11].

The normal human thyroid contains a 2-month supply of thyroid hormone in thyroglobulin. Approximately 85 μg of T4 and 7 μg of T3 are secreted daily by the thyroid. However, the daily production of T3 is approximately 33 μg. Eighty percent of the daily T3 production arises from extrathyroid sources by a deiodinase system that is described in Chap. 2.

4.3 TSH Biochemistry and Physiology

Thyrotropin is produced by specialized pituitary cells called thyrotrophs. Thyrotropin is a glycoprotein composed of two subunits that are not covalently bound. The alpha subunit of TSH contains 92 amino acids and is common to three other glycoprotein hormones: follicle-stimulating hormone (FSH), luteinizing hormone (LH), and human chorionic gonadotropin (HCG). The beta subunit is unique to TSH and contains 112 amino acids. The intact molecule of human thyrotropin has a molecular weight of 28–30 kDa and contains about 15% by weight of covalently bound oligosaccharide side chains. Both subunits are synthesized and secreted in specialized pituitary cells called thyrotrophs. The human thyrotropin beta-subunit gene contains three exons and two introns, and the alpha-subunit gene contains four exons and three introns.

The secreted thyrotropin molecule has a plasma half-time of disappearance of about 30 minutes and a metabolic clearance rate of 25 ml/min/m². The secretion rate is approximately 40–150 mU/day in humans.

Thyrotropin binds to a receptor on the surface of the thyroid follicular cell. The TSH receptor (TSH-R) is a G protein-coupled receptor with seven transmembrane spanning regions and a 400 amino acid N-terminal extracellular domain that selectively binds TSH with high affinity [12]. It activates adenylyl cyclase which increases protein kinase A, resulting in an increase of cyclic adenosine monophosphate (cAMP). This in turn stimulates the synthesis and release of T4 and T3, as well as many metabolic processes, and growth of the thyroid cells. In addition, TSH may promote thyroid cell growth by activation of phopholipases, resulting in generation of inositol phosphates and diacylglycerol, in turn activating Ca^{++}/phospholipid-independent kinases, PKC. Rarely, hypothyroidism is caused by an inactivating mutation in the TSH-R, also termed TSH resistance. There may be mutations of the TSH-R, especially in hyperfunctioning adenomas, that cause constitutive activation, resulting in hyperthyroidism with suppression of serum TSH [12].

Several pituitary transcription factors influence the development of the thyrotrophs and TSH gene expression. Thyrotroph embryonic factor regulates expression of the beta-subunit gene. Pit-1 is required for the survival of the thyrotroph and for expression of the TSH beta-subunit gene. Prophet of Pit-1 (PROP-1) is required for development of cell lines that are dependent on Pit-1.

4.3.1   T3 Negative Regulation of TSH

Thyroid hormone exerts an inhibitory effect on TSH release and synthesis. T3 exerts this effect through binding to the $\beta2$ thyroid hormone receptor in the thyrotrophs, a nuclear binding receptor that transduces the action of thyroid hormone by its regulation of transcription. This negative regulation affects transcriptional control of both subunits of thyrotropin. The promoter region of the beta subunit has a negative T3 response element in its promoter region. The thyrotrophs are exquisitely sensitive to the circulating levels of thyroid hormone, both T4 and T3. Within the thyrotroph, the type 2 thyroxine deiodinase converts T4 to T3 (see Chap. 1), thereby providing the main source of T3 for the negative feedback regulation. Although there are many other factors that regulate TSH release, the dominant factor is the negative feedback modulation by thyroid hormone, as diagrammed in Fig. 4.2.

4.4   Thyrotropin-Releasing Hormone

The hypothalamus produces thyrotropin-releasing hormone (TRH) in specific nuclei in the median eminence and paraventricular regions [13]. TRH is secreted into the portal venous blood flowing directly to the pituitary (Fig. 4.2). TRH binds

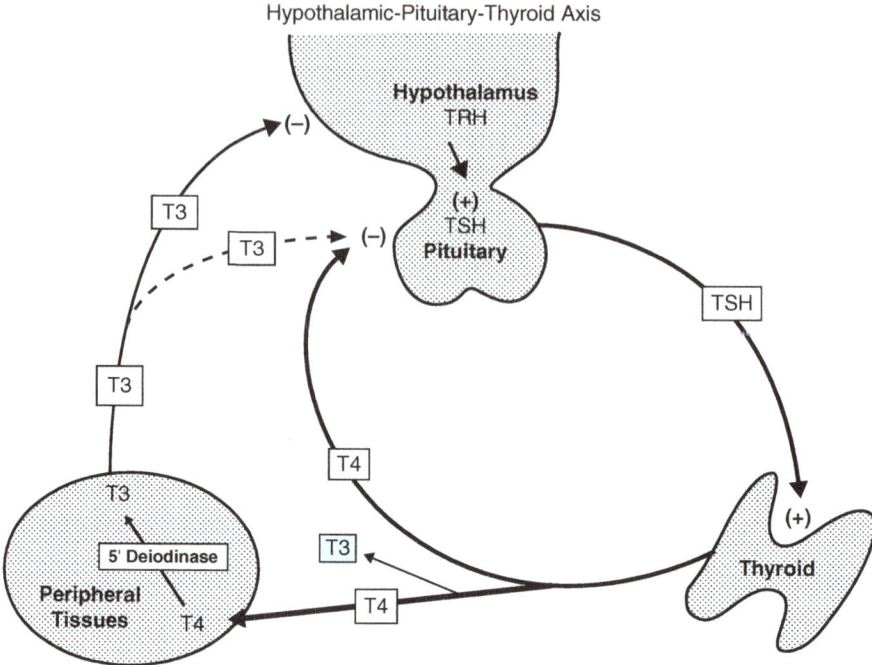

Fig. 4.2 Diagram of the hypothalamic-pituitary-thyroid axis and the negative feedback regulation by thyroid hormones

to its G protein-coupled receptor on the thyrotrophs and stimulates phospholipase C, resulting in activation of PKC as noted above. The second messenger is intracellular Ca^{++}, which causes release of TSH that is stored in granules, synthesis of more TSH, and glycosylation of TSH that is essential for its full biologic activity. TRH is a tripeptide with the structure pyroglutamyl-histidyl proline-amide. It is formed in small amounts in many parts of the central nervous system, the pancreatic islets, and other organs. It is a ubiquitous neuropeptide with many other functions.

Thyroid hormone also exerts a negative feedback effect on synthesis and probably secretion of TRH. The positive effect of TRH on release of TSH is believed to exert fine control on TSH secretion. However, knockout of TRH in mice does not cause profound hypothyroidism in contrast with the severe hypothyroidism resulting from hypophysectomy in experimental animals.

4.5   Diurnal Rhythmicity of TSH

Serum TSH levels show a diurnal rhythm with the onset of peak levels starting in the night hours shortly before the onset of sleep at about 2200 hours to midnight [14]. The peak levels occur 2–4 hours later, and there is a gradual reduction till 8 a.m., with even lower levels in the afternoon. Sleep deprivation enhances the nocturnal TSH peak, suggesting that sleep attenuates the peak. The peak is at most twofold greater than the mean based on 15 minutes sampling throughout the day. The basis for the rhythm has not been established. Recent work shows that the TSH rhythm is parallel to that of leptin. Since leptin increases TRH synthesis, the data suggest that leptin may be the basis for the TSH circadian rhythm [15]. In addition, TSH is secreted in a pulsatile manner with a periodicity of 2–3 hours, but the amplitude of the peaks is rather small. The diurnal rhythym tends to be attenuated with advanced age and is absent in most patients with primary hypothyroidism. Alcohol ingestion also attenuates the nocturnal TSH peak. From a practical point of view, the diurnal rhythm does not affect serum TSH levels when obtained during the usual hours for clinical sampling.

Studies to show whether the nocturnal peak of serum TSH causes an increase in thyroid hormone levels have generally been negative. However, a recent study showed that the level of free T3, but not free T4, increased about 0.5–2.5 hours after the nocturnal TSH peak [16]. This is most likely due to serum T3 arising from the thyroid, even though the thyroid's direct contribution to circulating T3 is believed to account for only 20% of the total in humans.

4.6   Other Factors that Regulate TSH Secretion

In addition to the negative feedback effect of thyroid hormone and the positive stimulatory effect of TRH, there are a number of other factors that affect TSH secretion. Table 4.1 summarizes these factors.

In rodents acutely exposed to the cold, serum TSH and thyroid hormone levels increase. The mechanism involves the sympathetic nervous system. Adrenergic activation increases TSH release in the rat, but it is difficult to show any modulation of TSH by cold exposure [17], adrenergic activation or inhibition in humans. However, methamphetamine usage may increase TRH, resulting in elevation of

Table 4.1 Factors that influence TSH secretion

Increase TSH	Decrease TSH
TRH	T4, T3
Leptin	Somatostatin
Cold exposure?	Dopamine
Arginine vasopressin	Cortisol
Glucagon-like peptide-1	Fasting
Galanin	Retinoid X agonists
	Pro-inflammatory cytokines
	Cholecystokinin
	Gastrin-releasing peptide
	Neuropeptide Y
	Surgical stress

serum TSH that increases thyroid hormone secretion, thereby resulting in feedback inhibition of TSH secretion [18].

The neuropeptides arginine vasopressin, glucagon-like peptide-1, galanin, and leptin stimulate TSH secretion in humans.

Dopamine, acting through the D2 receptor, inhibits TSH secretion. Somatostatin acutely inhibits TSH secretion, but chronic usage does not cause hypothyroidism in euthyroid patients. However, long-acting analogs of somatostatin are useful for reducing serum TSH levels in patients with pituitary tumors that secrete TSH and cause hyperthyroidism. Other neuropeptides that inhibit TSH secretion include cholecystokinin, gastrin-releasing peptide, and neuropeptide Y. The clinical relevance of these factors is unclear.

Retinoids impair TSH secretion through the retinoid X receptor (RXR). Targretin, a selective RXR ligand used for the treatment of cutaneous T-cell lymphoma, caused profound central hypothyroidism [19].

Proinflammatory cytokines inhibit TSH secretion. These include tumor necrosis factor-α, interleukin-1β and interleukin-6 [20]. These factors may be responsible for reducing serum TSH levels in severe nonthyroid illness, resulting in reduced serum T4 levels. In addition, these cytokines block peripheral deiodinase activity, causing low T3 levels.

4.7   Clinical Effects of TRH

Administration of TRH intravenously causes a rapid increase of serum TSH reaching a peak at 20–30 minutes (Fig. 4.3) [21]. This was used as a clinical test in a variety of settings. In general, the peak serum TSH response to TRH was proportional to the baseline serum TSH level. The principal side effects include a queasy feeling, urinary urgency, and transient hypertension. Currently TRH is not available for administration to humans in the United States.

The rapid rise of TSH was used to differentiate pituitary TSH deficiency from a hypothalmic lesion causing presumed deficiency of TRH (Fig. 4.3). When pituitary function was seriously compromised, there was no increment of TSH from a low basal level. When there was a lesion in the hypothalamus causing central hypothyroidism, there was a response of serum TSH to TRH with a peak that was normal in increment above baseline but delayed to 45–60 minutes. Unfortunately, these responses were often not so clear.

In patients with hyperthyroidism, serum TSH was suppressed by the negative feedback and there was no increment after TRH adminstration [21]. Before the current sensitive TSH assays, this failure of response was used for diagnosis of mild hyperthyroidism.

In patients with primary hypothyroidism, the TSH response to TRH was exaggerated in magnitude. A peak above approximately 30 mU/L was considered an indication of mild hypothyroidism by some experts, but this conclusion was debated by

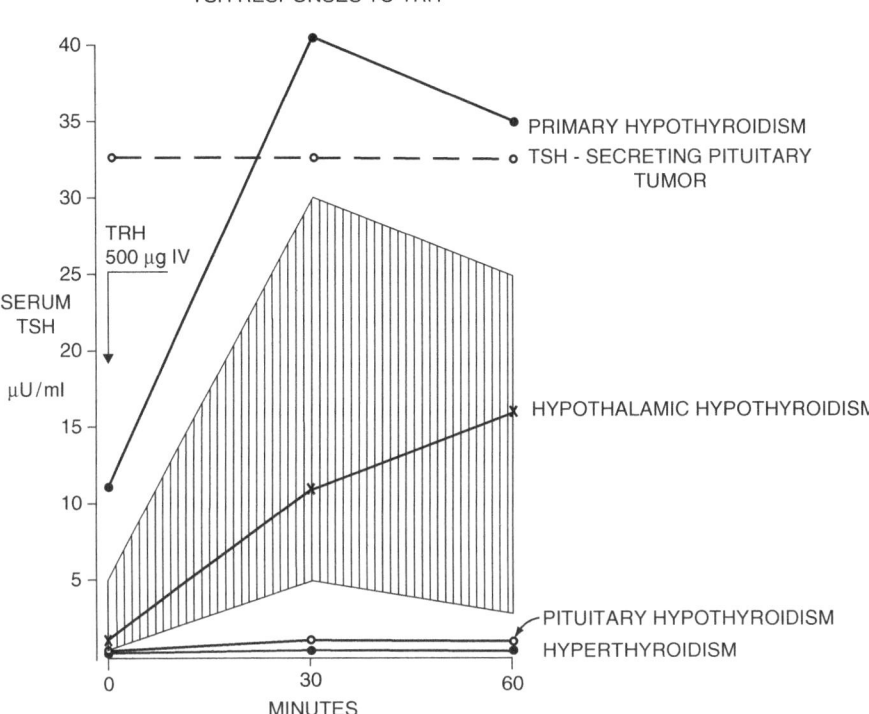

Fig. 4.3 Serum TSH response to intravenous administration of TRH in various clinical situations

others. The current precise and sensitive serum TSH assays have made this debate superfluous.

Administration of TRH intravenously also caused a rapid increment in serum prolactin, indicating that the lactotrophs had receptors for TRH. This was also used as a test of pituitary function. In addition, some patients with acromegaly had an increment in serum growth hormone after TRH.

4.8 Measurement of TSH

Sixty years ago a sensitive bioassay for TSH was developed by McKenzie [22]. This assay performed in mice could measure the very high TSH levels of primary hypothyroidism and the elevated TSH of Graves' disease, subsequently shown to be due to thyroid-stimulating immunoglobulin. The variability of these bioassays was approximately ±25%. After the development of the concept of radioimmunoassay by Yalow and Berson in 1960 [23], several investigators developed such assays for serum TSH. The initial assays were not sufficiently sensitive for precise measurement of normal

Fig. 4.4 Scheme for TSH
immunometric assay.
MAb monoclonal antibody

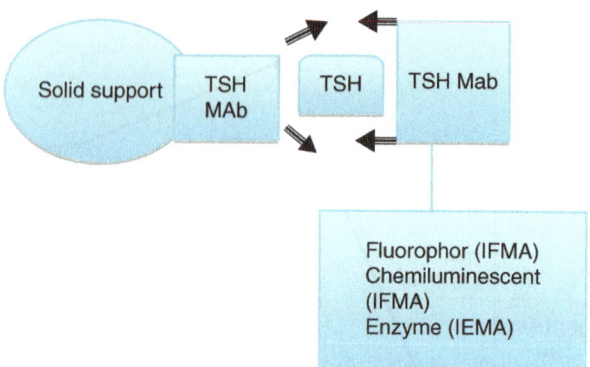

serum TSH levels [21], but subsequent improvements of the technique led to sensitive radioimmunoassays that could measure the normal serum TSH levels [24]. The assays were labor intensive and took several days for completion. In the next decade, industrial companies became involved and developed assays with enzymatic labels to avoid the difficulty of labeling TSH with radioiodine, and there was some improvement in sensitivity. However, the advent of monoclonal antibodies led to the current very sensitive immunoassays using two antibodies of TSH—the so-called sandwich assay; one antibody is directed at the alpha subunit, the other is directed at the beta subunit [25]. One antibody, immobilized to a solid support and in large amounts, binds all of the TSH. The other reporter antibody, in high concentration in solution and directed at a different epitope, has a label that is either chemiluminescent or fluorescent (Fig. 4.4). The resulting sandwich removes all of the TSH from the serum. The TSH concentration is proportional to the label in the sandwich. With these assays, the subnormal levels of TSH, down to as low as 0.01 mU/L, can be measured with good precision in 1 hour with automated analyzers. The variability of current assays is less than 5%. The true assay sensitivity is defined as the minimum concentration that can be detected in multiple assays with a coefficient of variation <20%.

Some patients have antibodies to mouse gamma globulin. These heterophilic antibodies may affect the assay results because current assays use mouse monoclonal antibodies. The heterophilic antibody may lead to either a high or low value, depending on the assay method. In one report, a mouse IgG sandwiched between the immobilized and labeled monoclonal antibodies of the TSH assay led to a raised level and an inappropriate diagnosis of hypothyroidism [26]. The paucity of new reports of this phenomenon suggests that this problem has been solved.

4.9   Normal Serum TSH Levels

The range of serum TSH in normal subjects has been defined in several studies. The largest cross-sectional study of a normal population, the NHANES 3 study, defined the 95% confidence limits as 0.45–4.1 mU/L in those with no evidence

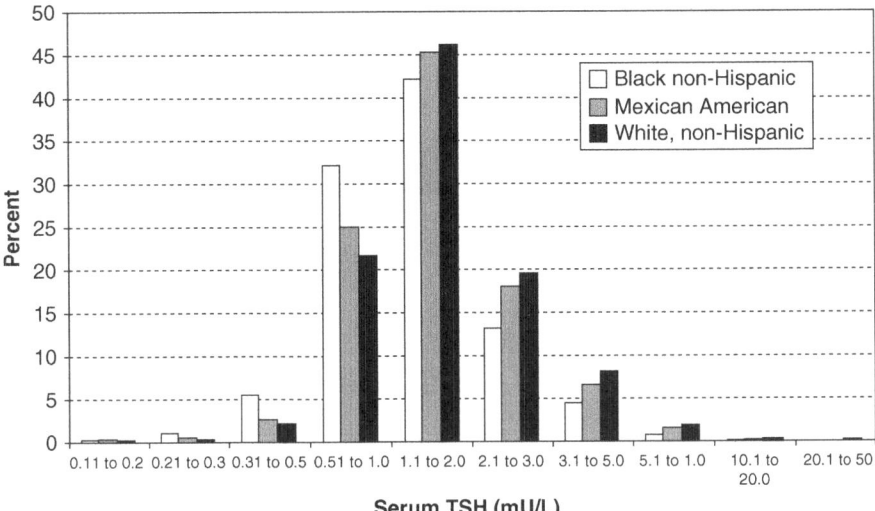

Fig. 4.5 Distribution of serum TSH levels in 13,365 euthyroid subjects in the NHANES 3 survey (reference group) [26]

of thyroid disease and also not under the influence of drugs that might influence thyroid function (Fig. 4.5) [27]. A recent study of a smaller normal population concluded that the normal range was 0.53–3.4 mU/L, but suggested an upper normal limit of 4.0 mU/L [28]. Reevaluation of the NHANES 3 data showed that the upper limit was shifted to 3.6 mU/L in those aged 20–29, 4.0 mU/L in those aged 50–59, 6.0 mU/L in those aged 70–79, and 7.5 mU/L in those over age 80 [29]. This contrasts with an earlier study of the Framingham population showing that serum TSH was not affected by age in euthyroid subjects when subjects aged 40–60 years old were compared with those over age 70 [30].

Not surprisingly, the variability of serum TSH in individual normal subjects is much less than that of the population. Monthly samples obtained over 12 months in similar circumstances showed that typical variability was approximately ±0.5 mU/L for an individual [31].

4.10   Factors Affecting TSH Clinically

Serum TSH levels are inversely proportional to the free T4 concentration. The log [TSH] level is inversely proportional to free T4. Therefore, small changes in free T4 are reflected in large changes in serum TSH, as noted in Fig. 4.6.

Serum TSH is elevated in primary hypothyroidism. In patients with severe hypothyroidism, especially children or young individuals, hyperplasia of the thyrotrophs causes pituitary enlargement. Intravenous administration of a large dose of

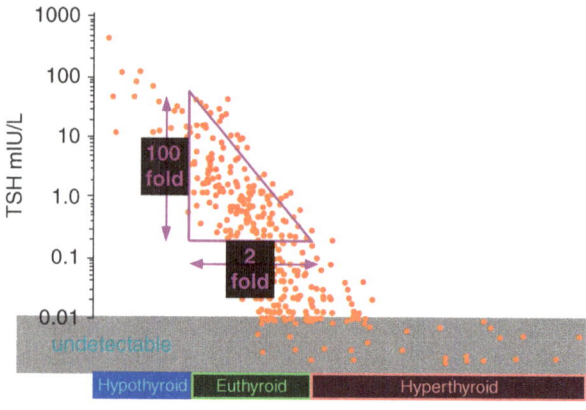

Fig. 4.6 Log–linear relationship of free T4 and TSH

T3 results in a rapid suppression of serum TSH. However, when small doses of T4 are given to patients with myxedema, there is a transient rise in serum TSH levels after a few weeks, possibly attributable to "myxedema" of the pituitary that impairs the negative feedback [32]. As the dose of T4 is increased, the serum TSH levels fall, usually reaching a stable level on a given dose of T4 after 3–6 weeks. Withdrawal of T4 therapy in both euthyroid and hypothyroid patients causes a gradual rise of serum TSH. In 3–5 weeks, the serum TSH level reflects the underlying thyroid function [33]. In contrast, patients with significant clinical hyperthyroidism will have profound suppression of serum TSH, so that TSH levels remain suppressed for many weeks after treatment of the condition, even when the treatment results in hypothyroidism. In this situation, serum TSH is not a reliable indicator of thyroid function.

Starvation and severe nonthyroid illness may result in suppression of serum TSH levels, most likely due to proinflammatory cytokines that can down-regulate TRH and TSH synthesis and release, as well as affecting the thyroid directly and peripheral thyroid hormone metabolism. This entity is discussed fully in Chap. 10. Surgical stress, probably through multiple mechanisms, reduces serum TSH [34].

References

1. Dohan O, De la Vieja A, Paroder V, et al. The sodium/iodide Symporter (NIS): characterization, regulation, and medical significance. *Endocr Rev.* 2003;24:48-77.
2. Fenton MS, Marion KM, Hershman JM. Identification of cyclic adenosine 3′,5′-monophosphate response element modulator as an activator of the human sodium/iodide symporter upstream enhancer. *Endocrinology.* 2008;149:2592-2606.
3. Caldwell KL, Jones R, Hollowell JG. Urinary iodine concentration: United States National Health and Nutrition Examination Survey 2001-2002. *Thyroid.* 2005;15:692-699.
4. Glinoer D. The importance of iodine nutrition during pregnancy. *Public Health Nutr.* 2007;10:1542-1546.

5. Pearce EN, Bazrafshan HR, He X, Pino S, Braverman LE. Dietary iodine in pregnant women from the Boston, Massachusetts area. *Thyroid.* 2004;14:327-328.
6. McLachlan SM, Rapoport B. The molecular biology of thyroid peroxidase: cloning, expression and role as autoantigen in autoimmune thyroid disease. *Endocr Rev.* 1992;13:192-206.
7. Bikker H, Baas F, De Vijlder JJ. Molecular analysis of mutated thyroid peroxidase detected in patients with total iodide organification defects. *J Clin Endocrinol Metab.* 1997;82: 649-653.
8. Ohye H, Fukata S, Hishinuma A, et al. A novel homozygous missense mutation of the dual oxidase 2 (DUOX2) gene in an adult patient with large goiter. *Thyroid.* 2008;18:561-566.
9. Kopp P. Pendred's syndrome: identification of the genetic defect a century after its recognition. *Thyroid.* 1999;9:65-69.
10. Dunn JT, Dunn AD. Update on intrathyroidal iodine metabolism. *Thyroid.* 2001;11: 407-414.
11. Stanbury JB, Kassenaar AA, Meijer JW, Terpstra J. The occurrence of mono- and di-iodotyrosine in the blood of a patient with congenital goiter. *J Clin Endocrinol Metab.* 1955;15: 1216-1227.
12. Duprez L, Parma J, Van Sande J, et al. TSH receptor mutations and thyroid disease. *Trends Endocrinol Metab.* 1998;9:133-140.
13. Hershman JM, Pittman JA Jr. Control of thyrotropin secretion in man. *N Engl J Med.* 1971;285:997-1006.
14. Parker DC, Pekary AE, Hershman JM. Effect of normal and reversed sleep-wake cycles upon nyctohemeral rhythmicity of plasma thyrotropin: evidence suggestive of an inhibitory influence in sleep. *J Clin Endocrinol Metab.* 1976;43:318-329.
15. Spiegel K, Leproult R, L'Hermite-Baleriaux M, Copinschi G, Penev PD, Van Cauter E. Leptin levels are dependent on sleep duration: relationships with sympathovagal balance, carbohydrate regulation, cortisol, and thyrotropin. *J Clin Endocrinol Metab.* 2004;89: 5762-5771.
16. Russell W, Harrison RF, Smith N, et al. Free triiodothyronine has a distinct circadian rhythm that is delayed but parallels thyrotropin levels. *J Clin Endocrinol Metab.* 2008;93: 2300-2306.
17. Hershman JM, Read DG, Bailey AL, Norman VD, Gibson TB. Effect of cold exposure on serum thyrotropin. *J Clin Endocrinol Metab.* 1970;30:430-434.
18. Morley JE, Shafer RB, Elson MK, et al. Amphetamine-induced hyperthyroxinemia. *Ann Intern Med.* 1980;93:707-709.
19. Sherman SI, Gopal J, Haugen BR, et al. Central hypothyroidism associated with retinoid X receptor-selective ligands. *N Engl J Med.* 1999;340:1075-1079.
20. Pang XP, Hershman JM, Mirell CJ, Pekary AE. Impairment of hypothalamic-pituitary-thyroid function in rats treated with human recombinant tumor necrosis factor-alpha (cachectin). *Endocrinology.* 1989;125:76-84.
21. Hershman JM, Pittman JA Jr. Utility of the radioimmunoassay of serum thyrotrophin in man. *Ann Intern Med.* 1971;74:481-490.
22. McKenzie JM. The bioassay of thyrotropin in serum. *Endocrinlogy.* 1958;63:377-382.
23. Yalow RS, Berson SA. Immunoassay of endogenous plasma insulin in man. *J Clin Invest.* 1960;39:1157-1175.
24. Pekary AE, Hershman JM, Parlow AF. A sensitive and precise radioimmunoassay for human thyroid-stimulating hormone. *J Clin Endocrinol Metab.* 1975;41:676-684.
25. Pekary AE, Hershman JM. A new monoclonal-antibody two-site solid-phase immunoradiometric assay for human thyrotropin evaluated. *Clin Chem.* 1984;30:1213-1215.
26. Kahn BB, Weintraub BD, Csako G, Zweig MH. Factitious elevation of thyrotropin in a new ultrasensitive assay: implications for the use of monoclonal antibodies in "sandwich" immunoassay. *J Clin Endocrinol Metab.* 1988;66:526-533.
27. Hollowell JG, Staehling NW, Flanders WD, et al. Serum TSH, T(4), and thyroid antibodies in the United States population (1988 to 1994): National Health and Nutrition Examination Survey (NHANES III). *J Clin Endocrinol Metab.* 2002;87:489-499.

28. Hamilton TE, Davis S, Onstad L, Kopecky KJ. Thyrotropin levels in a population with no clinical, autoantibody, or ultrasonographic evidence of thyroid disease: implications for the diagnosis of subclinical hypothyroidism. *J Clin Endocrinol Metab.* 2008;93:1224-1230.

29. Surks MI, Hollowell JG. Age-specific distribution of serum TSH and antithyroid antibodies in the United States population; implications for the prevalence of subclinical hypothyroidism. *J Clin Endocrinol Metab.* 2007;92:4575-4582.

30. Hershman JM, Pekary AE, Berg L, Solomon DH, Sawin CT. Serum thyrotropin and thyroid hormone levels in elderly and middle-aged euthyroid persons. *J Am Geriatr Soc.* 1993;41:823-828.

31. Andersen S, Pedersen KM, Bruun NH, Laurberg P. Narrow individual variations in serum T(4) and T(3) in normal subjects: a clue to the understanding of subclinical thyroid disease. *J Clin Endocrinol Metab.* 2002;87:1068-1072.

32. Pekary AE, Hershman JM, Sawin CT. Linear modulation of serum thyrotrophin by thyroid hormone treatment in hypothyroidism. *Acta Endocrinol (Copenhagen).* 1980;95:472-478.

33. Krugman LG, Hershman JM, Chopra IJ, et al. Patterns of recovery of the hypothalamic-pituitary-thyroid axis in patients taken of chronic thyroid therapy. *J Clin Endocrinol Metab.* 1975;41:70-80.

34. Sowers JR, Raj RP, Hershman JM, Carlson HE, McCallum RW. The effect of stressful diagnostic studies and surgery on anterior pituitary hormone release in man. *Acta Endocrinol (Copenhagen).* 1977;86:25-32.

Chapter 5
Measurements of Thyroxine and Triiodothyronine

Jim R. Stockigt

5.1 Introduction

The serum concentrations of thyroxine (T4) and triiodothyronine (T3) are key parameters in the assessment of thyroid function. As a thyroid disorder progresses from normality to overt dysfunction, the concentration of thyroid stimulating hormone (TSH) generally falls outside the population "normal" range before the concentration of either T4 or T3 becomes diagnostic, but a twofold change in serum T4 generally correlates better with clinical features than a twofold change in TSH. When thyroid dysfunction is corrected, the return of TSH to normal may lag some months behind the clinical response. Thus, the severity of the disorder and the initial response to treatment are often best monitored by measurement of the end-organ products, T4 and T3. Further, the diagnosis of secondary, or central hypothyroidism is likely to be missed unless end-organ function is assessed by measurement of T4. The limitations of basing initial testing for thyroid dysfunction on TSH alone have been discussed elsewhere [1, 2].

5.2 The Trophic–Target Gland Relationship

If feedback is intact, twofold changes in the concentration of T4 are generally associated with at least tenfold changes in serum TSH. Thus, logarithmic values for serum TSH can be conveniently correlated with untransformed results for serum T4. If the cause of dysfunction is central, at the pituitary or hypothalamus, deviations in TSH and T4 are generally concordant; where the abnormality is primarily in the thyroid, the changes are inverse. The general assumptions and limiting conditions that underpin the diagnostic relationship between TSH and T4 have been considered in detail elsewhere [3, 4] as summarized in Table 5.1.

J. R. Stockigt (✉)
Monash University, Melbourne, Victoria 3800, Australia
e-mail: jrs@netspace.net.au

G. A. Brent (ed.), *Thyroid Function Testing,*
DOI 10.1007/978-1-4419-1485-9_5, © Springer Science+Business Media, LLC 2010

Table 5.1 Assessment of thyroid status from the T4–TSH relationship: assumptions and limiting conditions

Assumption	Limiting conditions
1. Steady-state conditions	Difference in half-lives of TSH and T4
	Acute effects of medications
	Early response to therapy
2. Normal trophic–target hormone relationship	Alternative thyroid stimulators: immunoglobulins, chorionic gonadotrophin
	Medications: glucocorticoids, dopamine, amiodarone
	Recent thyrotoxicosis or longstanding hypothyroidism
3. Tissue response reflects hormone concentrations	Hormone resistance syndromes
4. Measurement of active hormone concentration	Alternative agonist in excess
	T3, triiodothyroacetic acid
	TSH of altered biologic activity
	Spurious assay results
	TSH assay: heterophilic antibodies
	Free T4 estimation (see text)
5. Appropriate reference ranges	Age, medications, associated illness, malnutrition
6. Adequate assay sensitivity	TSH imprecision at the limit of detection

Abnormal results that do not conform to typical disease-specific diagonal changes in the TSH–T4 relationship should be interpreted cautiously in relation to the limiting conditions given in the table. The assumption of steady-state sampling becomes insecure whenever associated illness or medications perturb the pituitary-thyroid axis (discussed in Chaps. 10 and 13); the difference in the half-lives of TSH (1 hour) and T4 (1 week) accounts for many transient anomalies in the T4–TSH relationship.

5.3 The Basis of Total and Free Thyroid Hormone Methodology

In the past two decades there has been an increasing trend for estimates of free T4 and T3 to supplant total hormone measurements. The current preference for free hormone methods is based on the fact that binding protein variations can markedly alter the total hormone concentration independent of thyroid status and that the free or unbound equilibrium concentration of the thyroid hormones reflects their biological activity, as proposed by the free hormone hypothesis [5]. The free hormone approach is clearly an advance in correcting for well-documented changes in the dominant circulating thyroid hormone binding protein, thyroxine binding globulin (TBG). However, widespread reliance on free T4 and T3 estimates has introduced a level of complexity where assessment of thyroid status is most difficult, particularly in association with critical illness or multiple medications, in late pregnancy, and with some non-TBG hereditary abnormalities of serum binding proteins [6].

While measurements of total circulating T4 and T3 are based on secure principles of competitive binding that stretch back more than five decades, efforts to estimate their free concentrations reflect great ingenuity in attempting to isolate or sample a hormone fraction that reflects the free hormone concentration. While there is broad consensus regarding the normal *total* serum concentrations (T4: 60–160 nmol/L or 5–12 μg/dL and T3: 1.1–2.8 nmol/L or 70–210 ng/dL), quoted *free* hormone concentrations vary more widely depending on the method. Situations such as critical illness, complex drug therapy, pregnancy, or binding protein variations may show marked method-dependent discrepancies in apparent free hormone concentration, sufficient to invalidate efforts to equate results or reference intervals from one method to another, or to define general estimates of sensitivity and specificity. Where free hormone estimates give divergent results, knowledge of the total hormone concentration may identify important methodological artifacts. For that reason, it is imperative to retain validated, secure total T4 and T3 methods, no matter how strong the support for the convenience of free hormone estimation.

An altered relationship between free and total thyroid hormone concentrations may be due to (1) alterations in binding protein concentration or affinity, or (2) occupancy of circulating binding sites by other ligands that displace T4 or T3. Of the acquired alterations in the serum concentration of binding proteins, the estrogen-induced increase in TBG, due to enhanced glycosylation that retards clearance, is the most common. Medications that alter the concentration of TBG are considered in Chap. 13. Numerous hereditary changes in TBG, transthyretin (TTR, or thyroxine binding prealbumin), and albumin also influence T4 binding either due to altered protein concentration, or abnormal binding affinity [7, 8]. The structural TBG variants may have either normal or reduced affinity for T4; T3 is usually similarly affected [7, 8]. In contrast, albumin variants may show *increased* affinity for either T4 or T3 [8]. In various hereditary binding protein variants, the serum total T4 concentration can vary enormously, from 25–1,800 nmol/L (2–140 μg/dL) [8], with normal free T4 and TSH concentrations.

The albumin variant responsible for familial dysalbuminemic hyperthyroxinemia (FDH), due to an Arg-His substitution at position 218 [9], has a markedly increased affinity for T4 and numerous T4-analog tracers, resulting in spuriously high serum free T4 estimates with these tracers [10]. In FDH, serum total T4 and free T4 index values and free T4 measured by several analog tracer methods give results suggestive of thyrotoxicosis, whereas serum total T3, free T3 and TSH values are normal, as is free T4 by two-step methods or equilibrium dialysis [10].

Circulating T3 or T4-binding autoantibodies can occasionally alter the distribution of circulating T4 and T3 *in vivo* [11], but they frequently result in artifactual total and free T4 and free T3 measurements [11, 12]. Tracer T4 or T3 bound to the endogenous antibody will be falsely classified as bound in adsorption separation methods, or free in double antibody methods, leading respectively to falsely low or falsely high T4 or T3 values. Notably, analog tracers may also bind to these antibodies, leading to spuriously high serum free T4 estimates [12].

5.4 Total T4 and T3 Methods

For about 35 years, serum concentrations of T4 and T3 have been measured by radioimmunoassay and, more recently, by related nonisotopic methods. Assays of total T4 and T3 in unextracted serum include a reagent such as 8-anilinonaphthalene sulfonic acid that blocks T4 and T3 binding to serum proteins, so that total hormone becomes available for competition with the assay antibody. Assays for free T4 or T3 omit this blocking reagent and may include a step, such as dialysis or ultrafiltration or immunoextraction that isolates a free hormone moiety before the assay procedure. There have been many different approaches to the estimation of serum free T4 and T3 concentrations, with detailed analysis of the theoretical basis, practical utility, and validity of these methods [5, 13].

In virtually all methods, the majority of the measured "free" hormone that is compared in the sample and standard is actually dissociated hormone derived from the *in vivo* bound moiety; provided that the assay parameter correlates closely with the free T4 concentration, the origin of the hormone that participates in the assay is only of theoretical interest. (Apart from the term "dissociation," the free T4 literature is replete with terms such as immunoextraction, sampling, sequestration, isolation, stripping or capture to describe the fact that the measured free T4 actually originates from the bound moiety). The two key questions in any method of free T4 estimation are (1) whether the dilution-dependent dissociation of bound hormone that generates "free" hormone in the assay tube occurs identically in samples and standards, and (2) whether competition for antibody binding between the assay tracer and free T4 is identical in samples and standards. If either of these conditions is breached, the assay is likely to give spurious results.

5.5 Principles of Free T4 Methods

An early example of a free hormone estimate is the time-honored free T4 index, or FT4I, computed from the serum total T4 value and the thyroid hormone-binding ratio (THBR) [14], which estimates the number of unoccupied serum protein-binding sites from the distribution of ^{125}I-T3 between a solid phase adsorbent (usually a resin) and serum-binding proteins. The THBR value, calculated as the ratio of the solid-phase radioactivity in the test serum to that of a pool of serum from normal subjects, is multiplied by the serum total T4 (or T3) concentration to yield the free T4 (or free T3) index. The THBR should be calculated as resin/serum rather than resin/total counts to improve the correction at extreme serum TBG concentrations [14]. Separate measurement of serum total T4 and binding ratio has the advantage of defining whether an abnormal free T4 estimate is due to altered total hormone concentration, anomalous protein binding, or both.

The concentration of free T4 can be estimated by two-step methods that separate a fraction of the free T4 pool from the binding proteins before the T4 assay is performed, or by one-step methods designed to give a signal that is proportional to the

Fig. 5.1 Outline of a two-step serum free T4 immunoassay. After incubation of serum or standard with the T4 antibody immobilized on solid phase, serum is removed and the antibody washed, followed by incubation with labeled T4. The higher the free hormone concentration, the lower the binding of label to the solid phase. A two-step method of this sort avoids contact of the assay tracer with serum and should be independent of differences in binding of tracer between samples and standards. (From [15] with permission)

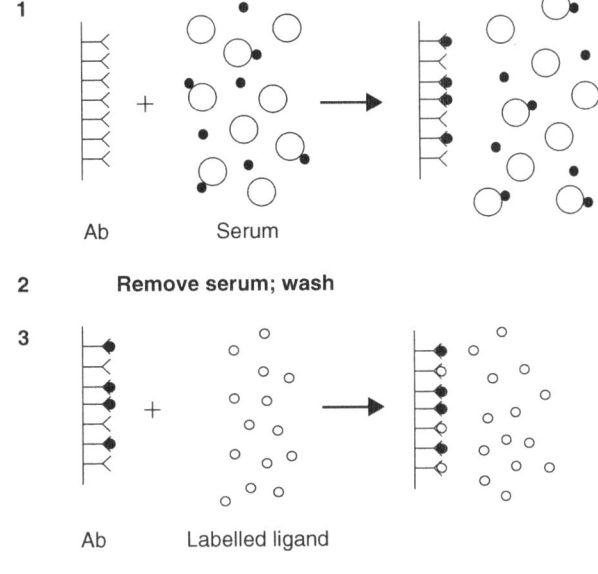

1

Ab   Serum

2   **Remove serum; wash**

3

Ab   Labelled ligand

4   **Remove labelled ligand; wash**

5   **Count Ab-bound activity**

free T4 concentration in the presence of binding proteins. (The terms "direct" and "indirect" are ambiguous, because all methods are to some degree indirect). Many of the one-step methods become invalid when the sample and standard differ in their binding of assay tracer [5, 15] but the two-step methods are less prone to artifact. A two-step free T4 method, based on back-titration of unoccupied solid-phase antibody with labeled T4, is summarized in Fig. 5.1.

It should be noted that the term T4 or T3 analog is used in two different senses. The term "analog tracer assay" is best confined to methods where a labeled, chemically modified T4 molecule and antibody are added to the serum sample; serum free T4 and the labeled analog compete for a limited number of antibody sites. (These analogs were designed to minimize their binding to serum proteins, an objective that has been achieved for TBG, but not for albumin [5, 10].) In a different sense, labeled analogs are also used to quantify unoccupied binding sites after the serum component has been removed.

The diversity and ingenuity of current methods of free thyroid hormone measurement reflects the difficulty of making a valid estimate. All methods involve comparison of samples and standards, with the assumption that differences between samples and standards are influenced solely by the analyte in question.

Some typical methods can be summarized as follows:

- In several free T4 and free T3 assay systems (Architect, Advia Centaur, Chiron ACS:180), unbound hormone present in the diluted sample binds to a limited number of antibody-coated paramagnetic particles that facilitate separation.

After washing, acridinium-labeled hormone conjugate is added; the higher the free hormone concentration, the less conjugate will be bound. Thus, chemiluminescence of the activated magnetic particles relates inversely to the free hormone concentration.

- The Amerlite MAB free T4 assay depends on the ability of serum free T4 to inhibit binding of a peroxidase-labeled anti-T4 monoclonal antibody to a T3-coated solid phase; the greater the T4 concentration, the lower the attachment of label to the solid phase.
- The Abbott AxSYM assay involves the initial binding of free T4 to anti-T4 coated microparticles immobilized on a solid phase. A T3-alkaline phosphatase conjugate then binds to the unoccupied antibody sites.
- In the Elecsys assay, free T4 in the sample binds to a ruthenium labeled anti-T4 antibody; unoccupied antibody then binds to biotinylated T4 which links to streptavidin-coated microparticles; magnetic separation of bound from free hormone is achieved in a flow chamber, followed by generation of a chemiluminescent signal that is inversely proportional to the free T4 concentration.
- In the Diagnostic Products Immulite assay, a T4 analog tracer that does not bind to TBG or TTR, competes with serum free T4 for a limited number of T4-antibody binding sites that are immobilized on a polystyrene bead. Alkaline phosphatase-labeled anti-analog then binds to the solid phase and generates a chemiluminescent signal that is inversely proportional to the sample free T4 concentration.
- In the Corning-Nichols dialysis method, undiluted serum is dialyzed against a 12-fold greater buffer volume, followed by radioimmunoassay of free T4 in the dialysate.
- A recent report [16] describes a free T4 and free T3 assay that uses on-line solid-phase extraction–liquid chromatography/tandem mass spectrometry to measure the freeT4 and T3 in protein-free dialysate after 20 hours dialysis of serum against an equal volume of buffer at pH 7.2 (effective sample dilution 1:1), using a 96 well dialysis plate. Assay standards are prepared in protein-free buffer. Detection limit, internal quality controls, assay precision and correlation with established methods appeared to be satisfactory and there appeared to be no problems with tracer impurities. Results in a wide range of thyroid disorders and assessment of potential artifacts related, for example, to heparin-induced lipolysis during sample incubation, are yet to be reported. This method has been hailed as a major step forward in the routine assessment of free thyroid hormones, subject to appropriate standardization [17]. Further assessment in selected problematic samples (see below) is awaited.

5.6   Factors that Limit the Validity of Free T4 Methods

Tracer purity is crucial whenever a labeled compound is added to serum as a marker for the natural compound. For example, in equilibrium dialysis or ultrafiltration of undiluted serum, as little as 0.1% free radioiodine in the tracer can lead to a five- to tenfold overestimate of the free T4 fraction. A laborious approach that is still valid involves the isolation of intact ^{125}I-T4 from each sample dialysate by magnesium chloride precipitation in the presence of excess unlabeled T4 [18].

Dilution effects and protein dependence   Mass action dictates that dissociation of a bound ligand occurs with progressive sample dilution, so that its free concentration will not decrease significantly with dilution until the reservoir of bound ligand becomes significantly depleted [5, 15]. In theory, the free concentration of a highly-bound ligand such as T4 should be well maintained until serum dilution is greater than 1:100. However, many commercial assays yield much lower than the predicted free T4 concentration with progressive dilution. Such protein dependence of free hormone estimates [19] reflects the extent to which the reservoir of bound T4 (or T3) is "sampled" or depleted with dilution, associated with sequestration or "stripping" of bound T4 to the assay antibody. The phenomenon of "protein dependence" of free T4 estimates will vary between samples with diverse reservoirs of TBG-bound T4, i.e., a set of serum standards may not allow valid comparison with all samples.

There has been ambiguity about the definition of dilution factor in equilibrium dialysis assays. If undiluted serum is dialysed against a volume of buffer, that volume should be included in defining the dilution factor. As emphasized by Ekins [15], the position of the dialysis membrane within a constant total volume is irrelevant in determining either the final free-ligand concentration or the effects of dialysable competitors.

Anomalous protein binding of tracer   Numerous labeled analogs of T4 that have been used as tracers in some free T4 assays interact with serum proteins, particularly albumin [10, 15]. If the labeled analog is protein-bound to a greater extent in the unknown than in the standard serum, less tracer is available to compete for the assay antibody, giving a falsely high free T4 estimate, as in FDH [10] and with iodothyronine-binding immunoglobulins [12]. Conversely, if serum albumin is subnormal, or its binding sites are occupied by other ligands, free T4 estimates by analog tracer methods tend to be low [20] because *more* tracer is available in the sample than in the standard. The early analog free T4 methods were so highly albumin-dependent that the estimated free T4 was virtually zero in euthyroid subjects with hereditary analbuminemia [10]. In renal failure, analog assays can also give low serum free T4 values by up to 40% in predialysis samples [21] (see below).

Temperature dependence   When assays are incubated at room temperature rather than at 37°C, the results in serum samples with abnormal TBG concentrations may show bias due to differences in T4 dissociation between samples and standards [22]. Incubation at 37°C accentuates the possibility of a spurious increase in free T4 due to generation of non-esterified fatty acids (NEFA) in samples from heparin-treated patients (see below). The need to standardize estimates of free T4 in terms of temperature, pH, and sample dilution has recently been emphasized [17].

Assay sensitivity   can be the limiting factor in immunoassays of the low free T4 concentration that is present in the buffer compartment after dialysis or ultrafiltration. Such assays require an antibody of high affinity to achieve acceptable precision [23].

Table 5.2 Principal medications that displace T4 from TBG binding in normal human serum

Medication	Mean percent increase in free T4 fraction*
Salicylates	
• Acetyl salicylic acid (aspirin)	62
• Salicyl salicylic acid (salsalate)	>100
Furosemide[#]	5–30
Fenclofenac	90
Mefenamic acid	31
Flufenamic acid	10
Diclofenac	7
Diflunisal	37
Phenytoin	45
Carbamazepine	30

*Determination of T4 displacement by equilibrium dialysis or ultrafiltration of undiluted or minimally-diluted serum at 37°C *in vitro*, at appropriate therapeutic concentrations of each drug
[#]Furosemide has a wide therapeutic range; effect at high doses
Data from [24, 25, 28, 74]

Effect of competitors on T4/T3 binding Compared with the binding proteins that carry steroid hormones, which show little interaction with other ligands, circulating thyroid hormone-binding sites show broad interaction with NEFA and numerous commonly-used medications that can displace T4 and T3 from TBG [8] (Table 5.2). Thyroid hormones may be displaced by these competitors *in vivo*, but it is technically very difficult to get an accurate reflection of these effects with current free T4 methods. The affinities of the important drug competitors for TBG range from three orders of magnitude less (furosemide) to almost seven orders of magnitude less than T4 itself in the case of aspirin [24, 25]. However, this parameter does not reflect *in vivo* competition, because the free serum concentration of competitors is determined by their binding to sites other than TBG, particularly albumin. The relative inhibitory potencies shown in Table 5.2 are influenced by the therapeutic concentration of each drug and its free fraction, as well as its affinity for T4-binding proteins. Thus, the hierarchy of competition at relevant therapeutic concentrations differs markedly from the affinity for TBG in isolation [24].

Free T4 assays that involve significant sample dilution generally fail to reflect the effect of binding competitors, which are usually less protein-bound than T4 itself. With progressive dilution, the free concentration of the important drug competitor declines markedly before the free T4 concentration alters [15, 26] (Fig. 5.2). If a hormone such as T4, with a free fraction of about 1:4000, is compared with a drug that has a free fraction in serum of 1:50, progressive dissociation will sustain the free T4 concentration at 1:100 dilution, while the free drug concentration will decrease markedly after only 1:10 dilution. Thus, the effect of a competitor to increase free T4 will be underestimated, the error being greatest in assays with the highest sample dilution. Ultrafiltration of undiluted serum minimizes this artifact [27, 28].

The importance of a dilution artifact was demonstrated by comparing the ability of three commercial free T4 assays to detect the T4-displacing effect of furosemide; the effect was most obvious in the method with least sample dilution [29] (Fig. 5.3).

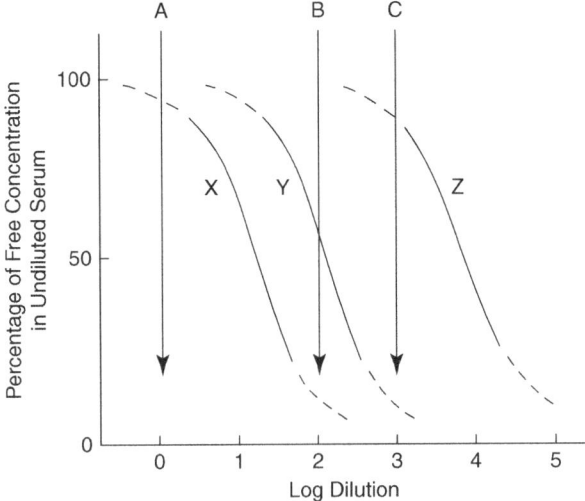

Fig. 5.2 Effect of serial dilution of serum on the relative free concentrations of three ligands that compete for the same binding site, but differ markedly in their binding in undiluted serum. A highly bound ligand (*Z*), such as T4 with free fraction about 1:4000 in undiluted serum, will maintain its free concentration at dilutions >1:100 (*C*). By contrast, a ligand (*X*) with a free fraction of 5% in undiluted serum, will show a marked decrease in its free concentration at 1:10 dilution (*B*). Ligand *Y* is intermediate. The effects of *X* and *Y* to displace *Z* will be progressively lost with increasing dilution. The effect of *X* to displace *Z* will be undetectable at dilution 1:10 or greater

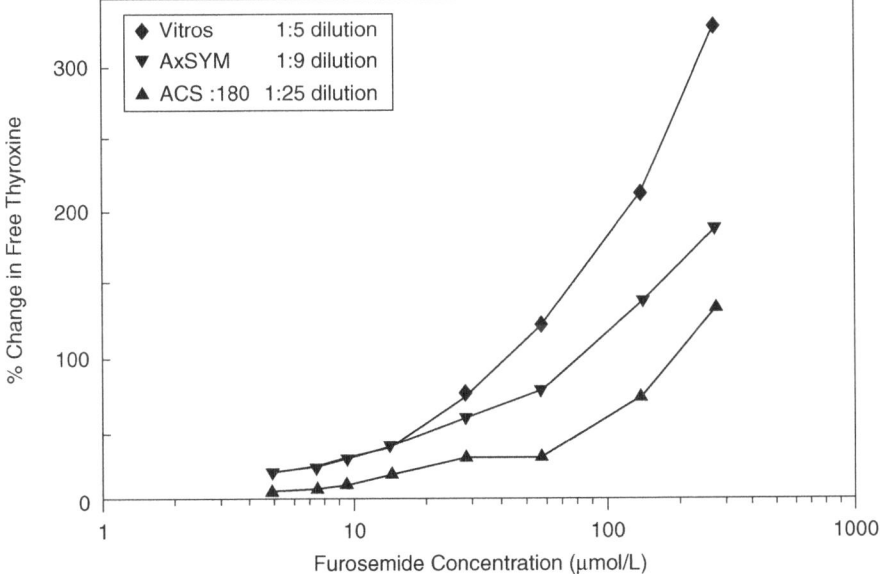

Fig. 5.3 Effect of addition of furosemide to serum on estimates of free T4 using three commercial free T4 methods that vary in sample dilution. The effect of the competitor to increase free T4 is progressively obscured with increasing sample dilution. (Redrawn from [29] with permission)

Similarly, therapeutic concentrations of phenytoin and carbamazepine increased the free concentration of T4 by 40–50% using ultrafiltration of serum that had not been diluted, but the free hormone estimate was spuriously low using a commercial single-step free T4 assay after 1:5 serum dilution [28]. During continuing drug therapy, total T4 was lowered by 25–50%; measured free T4 concentrations were normal in the ultrafiltration assay and spuriously low in the assay that used diluted serum [28].

The kinetics of the competitor itself will determine how it influences hormone binding *in vivo*. A competitor of short half-life, such as furosemide [30, 31] or salsalate [32], will show fluctuating effects on hormone binding so that free hormone estimates will vary depending on the time between dosage and sampling. In contrast, a competitor of long half-life will result in a new steady state with a normal free hormone concentration, an increased free fraction, and a lowered total hormone concentration [33].

The heparin artifact The effect of heparin is an important *in vitro* phenomenon that can lead to spuriously high estimates of circulating free T4 [34]. In the presence of a normal serum albumin concentration, NEFA concentrations >3 mmol/L will increase free T4 by displacement from TBG [24, 34], but these concentrations are uncommon *in vivo*. However, in heparin-treated patients, serum NEFA may increase

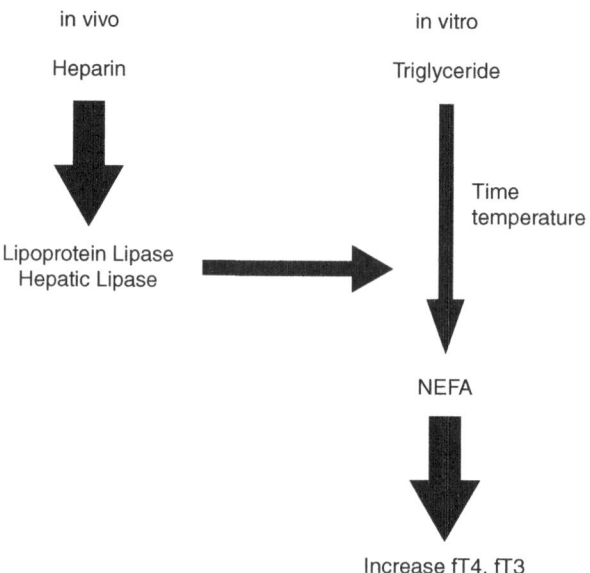

Fig. 5.4 Heparin-induced lipolysis during sample incubation can markedly increase the apparent concentration of serum free T4. Heparin acts *in vivo* (*left*) to liberate lipoprotein lipase from vascular endothelium. Lipase acts *in vitro* (*right*) to increase the concentration of non-esterified fatty acids (*NEFA*). In normal serum, NEFA concentrations >3 mmol/L, will displace T4 and T3 from TBG and thus increase apparent free T4. *In vitro* generation of NEFA is increased by incubation at 37°C and with high serum concentrations of triglyceride. The T4-displacing effect of NEFA is accentuated at low albumin concentrations

to these levels as a result of heparin-induced lipase activity during *in vitro* sample storage or incubation [34] (Fig. 5.4). This effect is accentuated if serum triglyceride concentrations are increased, serum albumin concentration is low, or incubation at 37°C is prolonged; under these conditions doses of heparin as low as 10 units may produce *in vitro* increases in serum free T4 [35]. Low molecular weight heparin preparations appear to have a similar effect [36].

5.7 Evaluation of Serum Free T4 Methods

In the past, some free T4 methods were marketed before they were rigorously assessed. There is no consensus as to how these methods should be evaluated prior to clinical use and no agreement on criteria that need to be satisfied before a free T4 method can be accepted as authentic. It is generally unsatisfactory to test a new method merely by demonstrating separation between hypothyroid, normal, and thyrotoxic values, and by showing close correlation with existing methods—any useful estimate of thyroid function will satisfy these criteria.

Methods can be tested with clinical samples, with attention to those that may challenge validity, or by manipulating a normal serum sample to examine particular theoretical issues. The latter approach includes examination of the quantitative recovery of added T4 [37], or the effect of serum dilution [38]. Criteria that assess "protein dependence" of a free hormone estimate, i.e., the degree to which free T4 is dependent on dissociation of bound hormone, give a favourable view of methods that minimize sample dilution, with adverse assessment of techniques that involve higher dilutions. Fritz et al. [39] presented further such evaluation of a commercial analog tracer free T4 method, under experimental conditions in which the free T4, total T4, and binding protein content of a normal human serum pool were independently varied by dilution, T4 loading, and addition of hormone-free serum. They concluded that the test assay reflected total rather than free T4 concentration under their experimental conditions. Midgley [40] has criticized this evaluation on the basis that a variable and unacceptably large fraction of total T4 may be sequestered or abstracted by the antibody—an effect that is progressively accentuated with dilution. Theoretical considerations aside, assessment of assays using normal serum under artificial conditions cannot test assay validity over the wide range of samples that will be encountered clinically.

The preferred alternative is to pay particular attention to samples that are likely to cause nonspecific discrepancies in assay signal as, for example, in the study reported by Docter et al. [41]. This approach requires clinical input in selecting samples that will probe a potential methodological flaw due, for example, to a binding variant, competitor, or artifact that influences the assay signal independent of thyroid status. A flaw may be due to factors such as nonspecific binding or sequestration of tracer by a variant protein, or different susceptibility to dilution in the sample and standard, or heparin-induced generation of a competitor during sample incubation (see above). The apparent free T4 concentration in unusual samples may be surprising as, for example, in hereditary analbuminemia where failure to find any detectable free T4 indicated that some analog tracer methods measured albumin-bound rather than free T4 [10].

Ultimately, as with any diagnostic method [42], the specificity of a free T4 technique will become clear only after the full diversity of the nondiseased population has been studied. An unexpected interference may only be noted after methods have been in use for some time, as in the effect of rheumatoid factor to produce spuriously high serum free T4 estimates [43].

5.8   Free T4 in Special Situations

5.8.1   *Pregnancy*

The demonstration that maternal hypothyroxinemia in the first trimester may have an adverse effect on later psychomotor development [44, 45] has focussed attention on optimal assessment of thyroid function in pregnancy (see Chap. 11). Several physiological and methodological details need to be considered to optimise interpretation of thyroid function during pregnancy. Estrogen excess progressively increases the mean serum concentration of TBG by about 60–80% up to the 20th week of pregnancy [46]: a change that tends to decrease the free concentration of T4, with an expected increase in TSH secretion, followed by an increase in total T4 so as to restore the serum free T4 concentration towards normal. Paradoxically, the increases in serum TBG and total T4 in the first trimester coincide with subnormal levels of serum TSH—a phenomenon attributable to the thyroid stimulating activity of human chorionic gonadotrophin (hCG) which has structural homology to TSH. The peak of hCG and the nadir of serum TSH occur together at 10–12 weeks gestation [46].

Interpretation of serum free T4 values during late pregnancy is complicated by inconsistencies between various assays [46, 47]. There is now consensus that serum free T4 and free T3 decrease in the third trimester, with mean levels reduced about 20–40% below the normal mean [46], although subnormal levels are uncommon. However, when Roti et al. [47] compared free T4 by seven different commercial methods in 23 euthyroid women at term, they found wide method-dependent variations (Fig. 5.5). Albumin-dependent methods gave up to 50% of subnormal values towards term [47], suggesting that such methods are unsuitable for use during pregnancy because of marked negative bias. Conversely, because of an increase in the pool of protein-bound T4 during pregnancy, methods that involve a high degree of sample dilution could be expected to show positive bias in relation to standards that contain a normal concentration of TBG. Methods that are based on dialysis of tracer to determine free fraction tend to overestimate free T4 in the presence of TBG excess; thus obscuring the normal decline in free T4 as pregnancy progresses [48]. Thus, thyroid function during pregnancy should be assessed using free T4 reference values that are both trimester-specific and method-specific.

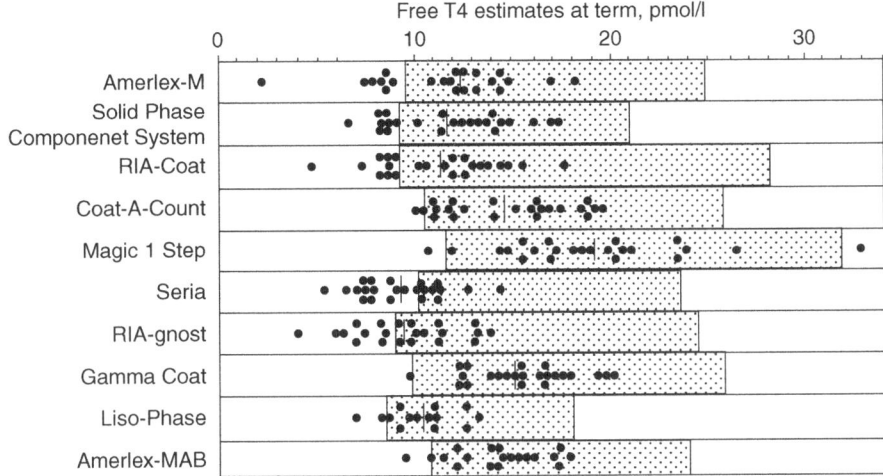

Fig. 5.5 Free T4 by ten commercial methods in normal pregnancy at term, showing marked method-dependent variation. Values are low in methods where serum albumin concentration influences the free T4 estimate. (Redrawn from [47] with permission)

A recent study has confirmed marked assay bias in free T4 estimates during pregnancy. Compared with two standard-kit free T4 methods, total serum T4 and free T4 index gave a more reliable evaluation of thyroid status in pregnancy [49]. Using trimester-specific reference values, total T4 was consistent between methods and showed the anticipated inverse relationship with serum TSH. Thus, total T4 measurement appears to be superior to free T4 estimation as a guide to therapy during pregnancy.

Method-specific free T4 intervals also need to be established for assisted reproduction procedures. One study of the effect of ovarian hyperstimulation [50] suggested that a tenfold increase in serum estradiol was associated with a mean decrease of serum free T4 of about 10%, with a 30% increase in serum TSH associated with 16% and 33% increases in total T4 and TBG respectively. This observation is supported by the finding that women on thyroxine replacement require increased thyroxine dosage during superovulation for in vitro fertilization, even in the absence of an ongoing pregnancy [51].

5.8.2 Thyrotoxicosis and Hypothyroidism

The free concentrations of T4 and T3 do not maintain a linear relationship with the total hormone levels in thyrotoxicosis or hypothyroidism. In severe thyrotoxicosis, the total concentration of T4 can be two- to threefold elevated, thus approaching or exceeding the capacity of TBG, which tends to decrease in severe thyrotoxicosis. Thus, there is a disproportionate increase in free T4 as total T4 increases [52].

Similar amplification in free T3 with increasing T4 occupancy of TBG has been reported in thyrotoxicosis [53].

The reverse phenomenon occurs in severe hypothyroidism where the occupancy of all three binding proteins will be minimal [52]. The excess of unoccupied binding sites will tend to limit the free hormone response that is achieved *in vivo* when treatment is initiated. (Thus, contrary to standard practise, it may be appropriate to use loading doses of T4 in the initial management of severe hypothyroidism to achieve low–normal circulating free T4 levels, followed by reversion to a more conservative regimen.)

5.8.3   Thyroxine Replacement

Numerous studies show that patients taking exogenous T4 show higher levels of serum total and free T4 for equivalent levels of serum TSH and T3 when compared with untreated euthyroid control subjects [54, 55]. Lack of direct secretion of T3 from the thyroid may account for this difference. The interval between tablet ingestion and blood sampling does influence measured levels of free and total T4. In athyreotic subjects who took 0.15–0.2 mg T4 orally, the serum free and total T4 concentrations were increased by about 20% 1–4 hours later, with return to baseline about 9 hours after T4 ingestion; serum TSH and T3 levels showed no time-dependent variation after ingestion of T4 [56].

5.8.4   Critical Illness

Together with the complex neuroendocrine events that accompany critical illness, assessment of thyroid function is influenced by multiple medications such as dopaminergics, furosemide, and glucocorticoids (see Chap. 13). Further, some free T4 methods are particularly vulnerable to the effects of NEFA, which may increase *in vitro* in heparin-treated patients (see above). Hence, assays that are reasonably specific in ambulatory populations diminish in value. It should be noted that no study of free T4 in critical illness can be meaningful unless free T4 methodology is specified.

Marked method-dependent differences in apparent free T4 have been demonstrated with associated illness [57–59]. Sapin et al. [57] used six commercial free T4 kits to study 20 previously euthyroid subjects on the seventh day after bone marrow transplantation, during multiple drug therapy, including heparin and glucocorticoids (Fig. 5.6). Free T4 methods that involved sample incubation at 37°C gave high free T4 values in 20–40% of their study subjects, while analog tracer methods that are influenced by tracer binding to albumin gave subnormal estimates of free T4 in 20–30%. By contrast, total T4 was normal in 19 of these 20 subjects, while serum TSH was <0.1 mU/L in half the subjects, independent of method—a change attributable to glucocorticoid treatment [58]. These free T4 methods showed an

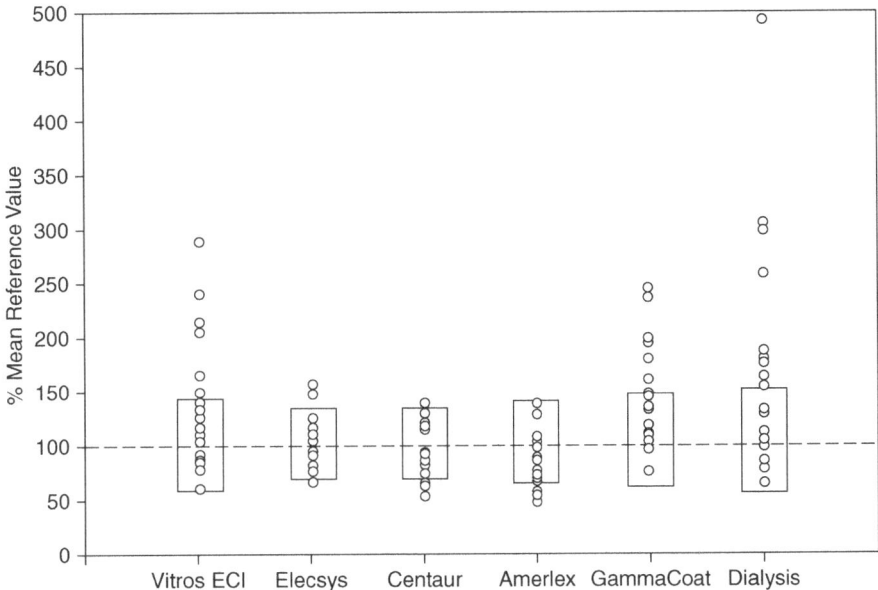

Fig. 5.6 Free T4 estimated by six different methods in 20 previously euthyroid bone marrow recipients on the seventh day after transplantation. There is a high proportion of abnormal free T4 values, either increased or decreased, depending on the type of assay. Therapy included heparin and glucocorticoids at the time of sampling. Mid-reference ranges for each method have been normalized to 100%, with the limits of the range shown by the *box*. Serum total T4 remained normal in 19 of the 20 subjects, while serum TSH was subnormal in 11, independent of the method used. (Re-drawn from [57] with permission)

unacceptable rate of false positive results in this situation; on the basis of artifacts in free T4 methodology in the face of subnormal serum TSH, findings could be falsely interpreted to indicate either thyrotoxicosis or secondary hypothyroidism.

The frequency of thyroid dysfunction is increased in renal failure [59], but assay artifacts can compromise laboratory assessment. Iitaka et al. [21] have shown marked method-dependent discrepancies in apparent free T4 concentrations in patients with renal failure (Fig. 5.7). Retained organic acids and NEFA can each displace tracer from albumin; in analog tracer methods that are albumin-dependent, more tracer is available in the sample than in the standards, leading to *lower* apparent serum free T4 values, especially if serum albumin is low. These effects were reproduced by addition to normal serum of organic acids that are retained in renal failure [21]. By contrast, dialysis methods for free T4 tend to show the opposite effect, i.e., a rise in apparent T4 as a result of NEFA generated during sample incubation, especially after heparin treatment [15, 60]. Heparinization during hemodialysis may promote NEFA-induced increases in apparent free T4 concentration during sample incubation. Concurrent medications such as furosemide or aspirin, important binding competitors [24], or dopaminergics that suppress TSH secretion may further complicate the assessment (see Chaps. 10 and 13).

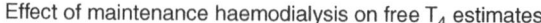

Effect of maintenance haemodialysis on free T$_4$ estimates

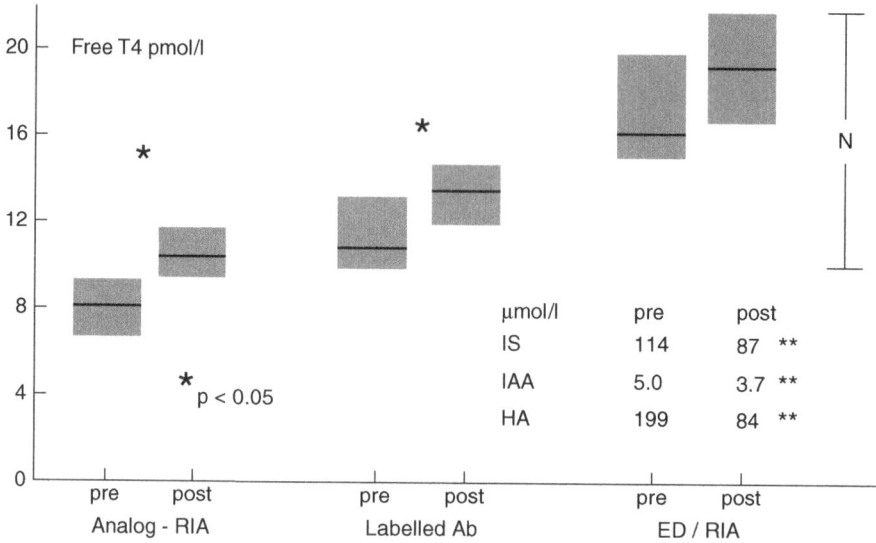

Fig. 5.7 Comparison of three methods of serum free T4 estimation, pre- and post-maintenance hemodialysis in 11 uremic subjects. The *horizontal bars* indicate the median, the *boxes* the range of values from 25–75%. Estimates of free T4 by an analog tracer method were lower than by equilibrium dialysis. With the analog tracer method, the estimate of free T4 increased after hemodialysis. Concentrations of all three organic acids, indoxyl sulphate (*IS*), indole acetic acid (*IAA*), and hippuric acid (*HA*) were lower after hemodialysis (**$p < 0.005$), but remained more than tenfold elevated above normal. NEFA increased after heparinization for hemodialysis. The effects on the free hormone estimates were reproduced by addition of organic acids to normal serum, which diminished the apparent free T4 concentration by a labeled analog method, increased the free T4 value by equilibrium dialysis, but did not alter the result by the labeled antibody method. Effects on estimation of free T3 were more marked than those on free T4. (Re-drawn from [21] with permission)

5.8.5 Premature Infants

Some premature infants at less than 28 weeks gestation have been reported to show hypothyroxinemia without the expected TSH response [61]; there is some evidence that T4 treatment may improve neurological outcome [61] (discussed in Chap. 9). By analogy with the study of Sapin et al. [57], differences in free T4 methodology may be crucial in defining this group (Fig. 5.6). Notably, Deming et al. [62] reported wide method-dependent variation in free T4 estimates in 97 infants less than 33 weeks gestational age. Although a full range of normative values was not available at this gestational age, subnormal free T4 estimates were less common with a dialysis-free T4 method than with an analog-free T4 immunoassay and with the free T4 index. Methods that are protein-dependent would tend to give low free T4 estimates [62], whereas equilibrium dialysis and related methods may be vulnerable to the heparin–NEFA effect, with a trend towards higher values. It remains uncertain whether the high free T4 values reported in some severely ill premature infants [63] are attributable to the heparin artifact.

5.9 Total T4 Measurement

Because of the preanalytical and analytical artifacts that compromise the diagnostic accuracy of free T4 estimates in critically ill patients [21, 57], especially those receiving multiple medications, there is a definite case for preferring measurement of total T4 in this group, because this parameter is generally free of assay artifact. Notably, two important studies of thyroid hormone changes during prolonged critical illness [64, 65] report total rather than free T4 and T3. Regarding the difficulties with free T4 measurement in pregnancy, it might have been wiser to retain secure measurements of total T4 as the yardstick, using modified reference intervals to accommodate the well-documented increase in TBG [49]. With the wisdom of hindsight, the methodological tangle that is a feature of free T4 estimation in the third trimester of pregnancy [47, 49] might have been avoided.

5.10 Indications for Measurement of Serum T3

While first-line assessment of thyroid status depends on assessment of the T4–TSH relationship, serum T3 is sometimes necessary to define a clinical situation (discussed in Chap. 8). Changes in serum T3 and T4 are generally concordant; the relationships between abnormal serum concentrations of T3 and T4 are summarized in Table 5.3. The reference interval for serum T3 is higher in children [66]. Serum T3 is generally a sensitive index of hyperthyroidism, although some patients may be hyperthyroid without T3 excess, especially with another severe illness [67]. Measurement of T3 is insensitive in identifying hypothyroidism because normal values may persist until the disorder is far advanced. Low values are common during febrile illness or caloric deprivation, or after surgery, without indicating any persistent thyroid abnormality (see Chap. 10). Measurement of serum T3 together with serum T4, is indicated in the following situations:

- In suspected hyperthyroidism when serum T4 is normal and serum TSH is low or undetectable, to identify "T3-toxicosis" [68] and distinguish it from the less severe entity of subclinical hyperthyroidism.
- During antithyroid drug therapy to identify patients who have persistent T3 excess, despite normal or low serum T4 values [69]. Where T4 and T3 are divergent, dose adjustment should then be based on serum T3 rather than T4.
- To detect early recurrence of hyperthyroidism after cessation of antithyroid therapy, or to detect progression from subclinical hyperthyroidism to "T3-toxicosis."

Table 5.3 Relationships between abnormal serum T3 and T4 concentrations

Serum T3 concentration	Serum T4 concentration		
	Low	Normal	High
High	Iodine deficiency T3 treatment Antithyroid drug therapy [68]	T3-thyrotoxicosis T3-binding autoantibodies	Typical thyrotoxicosis T4 overdose (T3 excess late) Thyroid hormone resistance TBG* excess
Normal	Iodine deficiency T3 treatment Hypothyroidism		T4 treatment or ingestion Euthyroid hyperthyroxinemia [3] Thyrotoxicosis with associated illness T4-binding autoantibodies
Low	Severe hypothyroidism TBG*deficiency Medications (see Chap. 13) Severe nonthyroidal illness	Many nonthyroidal illnesses Medications Fetus Restricted nutrition	Thyrotoxicosis with severe associated illness

The tabulation excludes short-term changes after commencement or cessation of antithyroid drug therapy or thyroid hormone replacement

*TBG thyroxine binding globulin; affects total T4, but free T4 estimates generally normal

- For diagnosis of amiodarone-induced hyperthyroidism which should not be based on T4 excess alone because of the frequent occurrence of euthyroid hyperthyroxinemia during amiodarone treatment [70].
- To establish the extent of hormone excess during high-dose replacement or TSH-suppressive therapy with T4, or after an intentional T4 overdose.
- For estimation of the serum T4 to T3 ratio. A high ratio (>0.024 on a molar basis or >20 ng/µg) that persists during antithyroid drug treatment may indicate that patients with hyperthyroid Graves' disease are unlikely to achieve remission [71]. Those with predominant T3 excess may be resistant to antithyroid drug and radio-iodine, so that surgery may be preferred as definitive treatment. The T4 to T3 ratio is usually lower in patients with iodide-induced hyperthyroidism [72] or thyroid hormone excess caused by thyroiditis [73], than in those with Graves' disease.

Because of its short plasma half-life, the concentration of T3 is not useful in assessing the effectiveness of replacement with oral T3; with current oral T3 preparations, serum concentration varies markedly with the interval between dosage and sampling [74].

5.11 Approach to Anomalous Results

Laboratory results may be concordant or discordant with clinical findings. With discordant results, a distinction needs to be made between an unsuspected diagnosis, subclinical disease, and anomalous assay results.

The following steps may be helpful in evaluating anomalous results:

1. Correlation with serum TSH by a method sensitive enough to identify the degree of TSH suppression, with review of the assumptions that underpin the diagnostic use of the free T4–TSH relationship (Table 5.1).
2. Reevaluation of the clinical context, with particular attention to medications.
3. Demonstration that the anomalous result persists and is not simply due to sampling under non-steady-state conditions.
4. Measurement of serum T3 with appropriate binding correction.
5. Estimation of serum free T4 by a two-step or dialysis method that is unlikely to give spuriously low results during critical illness.
6. Measurement of serum total T4 to establish whether the free T4 estimate is disproportionately high or low, possibly due to a method-dependent artifact.
7. Evaluation of the propositus and family members for an unusual binding abnormality, or hormone resistance.

5.12 Conclusion

The main purpose of free T4 and free T3 assays is to distinguish hyper- and hypothyroidism from the euthyroid state, an objective that cannot be attained with total hormone assays because of hereditary and acquired variations in the concentrations of binding proteins. Effective correction for changes in the serum concentration of TBG can be achieved with numerous types of free hormone estimates, but other changes in binding are not well accommodated. Despite remarkable analytical ingenuity, no current method reflects the free T4 concentration in undiluted serum under *in vivo* conditions. Equilibrium dialysis, widely considered the reference method for free T4 measurement, is nevertheless subject to error, either preanalytical due to generation of NEFA in the sample leading to an overestimate of free T4, or analytical, with dilution-dependent underestimation of the effect of competitors.

Current approaches to free T4 measurement are vulnerable to method-dependent artifacts: (1) when albumin binding of T4 or of the assay tracer is abnormal, (2) in the presence of medications that inhibit T4 binding to TBG, (3) during critical illness, especially in heparin-treated patients, (4) in pregnancy, and (5) in sick premature infants. Because of systematic variation between methods (i.e. whether a technique is albumin-dependent, or prone to incubation or dilution artifacts), it is essential to review methodological details whenever estimates of free T4 are clinically discordant. False positive abnormalities are more frequent than false negative results. When free T4 results are correlated with the serum TSH concentration with attention to the assumptions that define this relationship, the majority of false positive results can be readily identified. If a persistent free T4 anomaly remains unexplained, it is appropriate to use an alternative free T4 method that depends on a different assay principle and to correlate the result with an authentic *total* T4 measurement.

References

1. Beckett GJ, Toft AD. First-line thyroid function tests—TSH alone is not enough. *Clin Endocrinol.* 2003;58(1):20-21.
2. Wardle CA, Fraser WD, Squire CR. Pitfalls in the use of thyrotropin concentration as the first-line thyroid function test. *Lancet.* 2001;357(9261):1013-1014.
3. Stockigt JR. Serum thyrotropin and thyroid hormone measurements and assessment of thyroid hormone transport. In: Braverman LE, Utiger RD, eds. *The Thyroid.* 8th ed. Philadelphia, PA: Lippincott Williams & Wilkins; 2000:376-392.
4. Stockigt JR. Thyroid function tests and the effect of drugs. In: Wass WAH, Shalet SM, eds. *Oxford Textbook of Endocrinology.* New York, NY: Oxford University Press; 2002: 306-316.
5. Ekins R. The free hormone hypothesis and measurement of free hormones. *Clin Chem.* 1992;38(7):1289-1293.
6. Stockigt JR. Free thyroid hormone measurement—a critical appraisal. Endocrinology and metabolism. *Clin North Am.* 2001;30(2):265-289.
7. Bartalena L. Recent achievements in studies on thyroid hormone-binding proteins. *Endocr Rev.* 1990;11(1):47-64.
8. Stockigt JR. Thyroid hormone binding and variants of transport proteins. In: DeGroot LJ, Jameson L, eds. *Endocrinology.* 5th ed. Philadelphia, PA: WB Saunders; 2006:2215-2226.
9. Petersen CE, Scottolini AG, Cody LR, et al. A point mutation in the human serum albumin gene results in familial dysalbuminaemic hyperthyroxinaemia. *J Med Genet.* 1994;31(5): 355-359.
10. Stockigt JR, Stevens V, White EL, Barlow JW. "Unbound analog" radioimmunoassays for free thyroxin measure the albumin-bound hormone fraction. *Clin Chem.* 1983;29(7): 1408-1410.
11. Sakata S, Nakamura S, Miura K. Autoantibodies against thyroid hormones or iodothyronine. *Ann Intern Med.* 1985;103(4):579-589.
12. Beck-Peccoz P, Romelli PB, Cattaneo MG, et al. Evaluation of free T4 methods in the presence of iodothyronine autoantibodies. *J Clin Endocrinol Metab.* 1984;58(4):736-739.
13. Midgley JFM. Direct and indirect free thyroxine assay methods: theory and practice. *Clin Chem.* 2001;47(8):1353-1363.
14. Larsen PR, Alexander NM, Chopra IJ, et al. Revised nomenclature for tests of thyroid hormones and thyroid-related proteins in serum. *J Clin Endocrinol Metab.* 1987;64(5): 1089-1094.
15. Ekins R. Measurement of free hormones in blood. *Endocr Rev.* 1990;11(1):5-46.
16. Yue B, Rockwood AL, Sandrock T, et al. Free thyroid hormones in serum by direct equilibrium dialysis and on-line solid-phase extraction-liquid chromatography/tandem mass spectrometry. *Clin Chem.* 2008;54(4):642-651.
17. Thienpont LM. A major step forward in the routine measurement of serum free thyroid hormones. *Clin Chem.* 2008;54(4):625-626.
18. Sterling K, Brenner MA. Free thyroxine in human serum: simplified measurement with aid of magnesium precipitation. *J Clin Invest.* 1966;45(1):153-163.
19. Nelson JC, Weiss RM, Wilcox RB. Underestimates of serum free thyroxine (T4) concentrations by free T4 immunoassays. *J Clin Endocrinol Metab.* 1994;79(1):76-79.
20. Bayer M. Free thyroxine results are affected by albumin concentration and nonthyroidal illness. *Clin Chim Acta.* 1983;130(3):391-396.
21. Iitaka M, Kawasaki S, Sakurai S, et al. Serum substances that interfere with thyroid hormone assays in patients with chronic renal failure. *Clin Endocrinol.* 1998;48(6):739-746.
22. van der Sluis Veer, Vermes I, Bonte HE, et al. Temperature effects on free thyroxine measurements: analytical and clinical consequences. *Clin Chem.* 1992;38(7):1327-1331.
23. Nelson JC, Tomei RT. Direct determination of free thyroxine in undiluted serum by equilibrium dialysis/radioimmunoassay. *Clin Chem.* 1988;34(9):1737-1744.

24. Lim C-F, Bai Y, Topliss DJ, et al. Drug and fatty acid effects on serum thyroid hormone binding. *J Clin Endocrinol Metab.* 1988;67(4):682-688.
25. Munro SL, Lim C-F, Hall JG, et al. Drug competition for thyroxine binding to transthyretin (prealbumin): comparison with effects on thyroxine-binding globulin. *J Clin Endocrinol Metab.* 1989;68(6):1141-1147.
26. Stockigt JR, Lim C-F, Barlow JW, Topliss DJ. Thyroid hormone transport. In: Weetman AP, Grossman A, eds. *Pharmacotherapeutics of the Thyroid Gland.* Heidelberg: Springer Verlag; 1997:119-150.
27. Surks MI, Hupart KH, Chao P, Shapiro LE. Normal free thyroxine in critical nonthyroidal illnesses measured by ultrafiltration of undiluted serum and equilibrium dialysis. *J Clin Endocrinol Metab.* 1988;67(5):1031-1039.
28. Surks MI, Defesi CR. Normal free thyroxine concentrations in patients treated with phenytoin or carbamazepine: a paradox resolved. *JAMA.* 1996;275(19):1495-1498.
29. Hawkins RC. Furosemide interference in newer free thyroxine assays. *Clin Chem.* 1998;44(12):2550-2551.
30. Stockigt JR, Lim C-F, Barlow JW, et al. High concentrations of furosemide inhibit plasma binding of thyroxine. *J Clin Endocrinol Metab.* 1984;59(1):62-66.
31. Newnham HH, Hamblin PS, Long F, et al. Effect of oral frusemide on diagnostic indices of thyroid function. *Clin Endocrinol.* 1987;26(4):423-431.
32. Wang R, Nelson JC, Wilcox RB. Salsalate administration—a potential pharmacological model of the sick euthyroid syndrome. *J Clin Endocrinol Metab.* 1998;83(9):3095-3099.
33. Kurtz AB, Capper SJ, Clifford J, Humphrey MJ, Lukinac L. The effect of fenclofenac on thyroid function. *Clin Endocrinol.* 1981;15(2):117-124.
34. Mendel CM, Frost PH, Kunitake ST, Cavalieri RR. Mechanism of the heparin-induced increase in the concentration of free thyroxine in plasma. *J Clin Endocrinol Metab.* 1987;65(6): 1259-1264.
35. Jaume JC, Mendel CM, Frost PH, et al. Extremely low doses of heparin release lipase activity into the plasma and can thereby cause artifactual elevations in the serum free thyroxine concentrations as measured by equilibrium dialysis. *Thyroid.* 1996;6(2):79-83.
36. Stevenson HP, Archbold GPR, Johnston P, et al. Misleading serum free thyroxine results during low molecular weight heparin treatment. *Clin Chem.* 1998;44(5):1002-1007.
37. Wang R, Nelson JC, Weiss RM, et al. Accuracy of free thyroxine measurements across natural ranges of thyroxine binding to serum proteins. *Thyroid.* 2000;10(1):31-39.
38. Christofides ND, Wilkinson E, Stoddart M, et al. Assessment of serum thyroxine binding capacity-dependent biases in free thyroxine assays. *Clin Chem.* 1999;45(4):520-525.
39. Fritz KS, Wilcox RB, Nelson JC. A direct free thyroxine (T4) immunoassay with the characteristics of a total T4 immunoassay. *Clin Chem.* 2007;53(5):911-915.
40. Midgley JFM. Spurious conclusions on analog free thyroxine assay performance. *Clin Chem.* 2007;53(9):1714.
41. Docter R, Van Toor H, Krenning EP, et al. Free thyroxine assessed with three assays in sera of patients with nonthyroidal illness and of subjects with abnormal concentrations of thyroxine binding proteins. *Clin Chem.* 1993;39(8):1668-1674.
42. Ransohoff DF, Feinstein AR. Problems of spectrum and bias in evaluating the efficacy of diagnostic tests. *N Engl J Med.* 1978;299(17):926-930.
43. Norden AGW, Jackson RA, Norden LE, et al. Misleading results from immunoassays of serum free thyroxine in the presence of rheumatoid factor. *Clin Chem.* 1997;43(6 Pt 1):957-962.
44. Pop VJ, Kuipens JL, van Baer AL, et al. Low maternal fT4 concentrations during early pregnancy are associated with impaired psychomotor development in infancy. *Clin Endocrinol.* 1999;50(2):149-155.
45. Haddow JE, Palomaki GE, Allan WC, et al. Maternal thyroid deficiency during pregnancy and subsequent and subsequent neuropsychological development of the child. *N Engl J Med.* 1999;341(8):549-555.
46. Glinoer D. The regulation of thyroid function in pregnancy: pathways of endocrine adaptation from physiology to pathology. *Endocr Rev.* 1997;18(3):404-433.

47. Roti E, Gardini E, Minelli R, et al. Thyroid function evaluation by different commercially available free thyroid hormone measurement kits in term pregnant women and their newborns. *J Endocrinol Invest.* 1991;14(1):1-9.
48. Osathanondh R, Tulshinsky D, Chopra IJ. Total and free thyroxine and triiodothyronine in normal and complicated pregnancy. *J Clin Endocrinol Metab.* 1976;42(1):98-104.
49. Lee RH, Spencer CA, Mestman JH, et al. Free T4 assays are flawed during pregnancy. *Am J Obstet Gynecol.* 2009;260:e1-e6.
50. Muller AF, Verhoeff A, Mantel MJ, et al. Decrease of free thyroxine levels after controlled ovarian hyperstimulation. *J Clin Endocrinol Metab.* 2000;85(2):545-548.
51. Stuckey BGA. Thyroxine replacement during super-ovulation for in vitro fertilization; a potential gap in management? Fertility and Sterility 2010 in press.
52. Inada M, Sterling K. Thyroxine transport in thyrotoxicosis and hypothyroidism. *J Clin Invest.* 1967;46(9):1442-1450.
53. Nauman JA, Nauman A, Werner SC. Total and free triiodothyronine in human serum. *J Clin Invest.* 1967;46(8):1346-1355.
54. Fish LH, Schwarz HL, Cavanaugh MD, et al. Replacement dose, metabolism and bioavailability of levothyroxine in the treatment of hypothyroidism. *N Engl J Med.* 1987;316(13): 764-770.
55. Pearce CJ, Himsworth RL. Total and free thyroid hormone concentrations in patients receiving maintenance replacement treatment with thyroxine. *Br Med J (Clin Res Ed).* 1984;288(6418):693-695.
56. Ain KB, Pucino F, Shiver TM, et al. Thyroid hormone levels affected by time of blood sampling in thyroxine-treated patients. *Thyroid.* 1993;3(2):81-85.
57. Sapin R, Schlienger J-L, Gasser F, et al. Intermethod discordant free thyroxine measurements in bone marrow-transplanted patients. *Clin Chem.* 2000;46(3):418-422.
58. Surks MI, Sievert R. Drugs and thyroid function. *N Engl J Med.* 1995;333:1688-1694.
59. Kaptein EM. Thyroid hormone metabolism and thyroid diseases in chronic renal failure. *Endocr Rev.* 1996;17(1):45-63.
60. Mendel CM, Frost PH, Cavalieri RR. Effect of free fatty acids on the concentration of free thyroxine in human serum: the role of albumin. *J Clin Endocrinol Metab.* 1986;63(6): 1394-1399.
61. Fisher DA. The hypothyroxinemia of prematurity. *J Clin Endocrinol Metab.* 1997;82(6): 1701-1703.
62. Deming DD, Rabin CW, Hopper AO, et al. Direct equilibrium dialysis compared with two non-dialysis free T4 methods in premature infants. *J Pediatr.* 2007;151(4):404-408.
63. Klein RZ, Carlton EL, Faix JD. Thyroid function in very low birth weight infants. *Clin Endocrinol.* 1997;47(4):411-417.
64. Van den Berghe G, de Zegher F, Baxter RC, et al. Neuroendocrinology of prolonged critical illness: effects of exogenous thyrotropin-releasing hormone and its combination with growth hormone secretagogues. *J Clin Endocrinol Metab.* 1998;83(2):309-319.
65. Van den Berghe G, Wouters P, Weekers F, et al. Reactivation of pituitary hormone release and metabolic improvement by infusion of growth hormone releasing peptides and thyrotropin releasing hormone in patients with protracted critical illness. *J Clin Endocrinol Metab.* 1999;84(4):1311-1323.
66. Verheecke P. Free triiodothyronine concentrations in 1050 euthyroid children is inversely related to their age. *Clin Chem.* 1997;43:963-967.
67. Caplan RH, Pagliara AS, Wickus G. Thyroxine toxicosis. A common variant of hyperthyroidism. *JAMA.* 1980;244(17):1934-1938.
68. Figge J, Leinung M, Goodman AD, et al. The clinical evaluation of patients with subclinical hyperthyroidism and free triiodothyronine (T3) toxicosis. *Am J Med.* 1994;96(3):229-234.
69. Chen WW, Ladenson PW. Discordant hypothyroxinemia and hypertriiodothyroninemia in treated patients with hyperthyroid Graves' disease. *J Clin Endocrinol Metab.* 1986;63(1): 102-106.

70. Harjai KJ, Licata AA. Effects of amiodarone on thyroid function. *Ann Intern Med.* 1997;126:63-73.
71. Takamatsu J, Kuma K, Mozai T. Serum triiodothyronine to thyroxine ratio: a newly recognized predictor of the outcome of hyperthyroidism due to Graves' disease. *J Clin* Endocrinol *Metab.* 1986;62:980-983.
72. Sobrinho LG, Limbert ES, Santos MA. Thyroxine toxicosis in patients with iodine induced thyrotoxicosis. *J Clin Endocrinol Metab.* 1977;45:25-29.
73. Amino N, Yabu Y, Miki Y, et al. Serum ratio of triiodothyronine to thyroxine, and thyroxine-binding globulin and calcitonin concentrations in Graves' disease and destruction-induced thyrotoxicosis. *J Clin Endocrinol Metab.* 1981;53:113-116.
74. Surks MI, Schadlow AR, Oppenheimer JH. A new radioimmunoassay for plasma L-triiodothyronine: measurements in thyroid disease and in patients maintained on hormonal replacement. *J Clin Invest.* 1972;51:3104-3113.

Chapter 6
Thyroid Autoantibody Measurement

R. A. Ajjan and A. P. Weetman

6.1 Introduction

Thyroid dysfunction, a common condition affecting more women than men, develops in the majority secondary to a thyroid-specific autoimmune response. As with other autoimmune conditions, susceptibility to autoimmune thyroid disease (ATD) is thought to be influenced by an interaction between genetic predisposition and environmental factors, in addition to endogenous factors such as age and sex [1, 2]. Infiltration of the thyroid gland by immune cells is a characteristic finding in ATD, associated with activation of both humoral and cellular immune responses.

Autoimmune hyperthyroidism, or Graves' disease (GD), is characterized by the presence of thyroid stimulating antibodies (TSAb), which have a clear functional role; TSAb mimic the action of thyroid stimulating hormones (TSH), resulting in uncontrolled thyroid stimulation [3]. TSAb are also implicated in the extra-thyroidal manifestation of the disease, including thyroid eye disease (TED) [4], by mechanisms that remain to be fully clarified.

At the other end of the spectrum, autoimmune hypothyroidism (AH) is characterized by the presence of thyroid peroxidase (TPO) and thyroglobulin (Tg) antibodies (Ab) [5, 6]. Although the direct functional role of these antibodies is not entirely clear, they are implicated in perpetuating the intrathyroidal inflammatory reaction (see below), ultimately resulting in tissue destruction. Thyroid antibodies are also detected in postpartum thyroiditis and may be a risk factor for miscarriage in pregnant women with apparently normal thyroid function [7].

R. A. Ajjan (✉)
Division of Diabetes and Cardiovascular Research, The LIGHT Laboratories,
University of Leeds, Leeds, LS2 9JT, UK
e-mail: r.ajjan@leeds.ac.uk

G. A. Brent (ed.), *Thyroid Function Testing*,
DOI 10.1007/978-1-4419-1485-9_6, © Springer Science+Business Media, LLC 2010

6.2 Humoral Immunity in Autoimmune Thyroid Disease

As in any organ-specific autoimmune disease, an interplay between cellular and humoral immune responses is essential for the initiation and propagation of ATD. Infiltration of the thyroid gland by T cells causes tissue destruction through a direct toxic effect of these cells or indirectly through the production of various inflammatory molecules [8]. Intrathyroidal cytokine production and complement activation result in modulation of thyroid follicular cell (TFC) function and immunogenicity, in addition to perpetuation of the inflammatory reaction by recruitment of further immune cells [9]. Humoral immune responses against thyroid-specific autoantigens also contribute to the development of ATD, and this will be briefly reviewed in relation to the clinical presentation.

6.2.1 Thyroid Autoantigens

All major thyroid autoantigens are involved in thyroid hormone synthesis. The thyroid stimulating hormone receptor (TSHR), a member of the G protein-coupled receptor family, binds TSH and this causes generation of cyclic adenosine monophosphate (cAMP), stimulating both growth and function of TFC [10]. TSAb, acting on the TSHR, represent the key pathogenic mechanism in GD, whereas the contribution of TSHR blocking antibodies (TBAb) to the pathogenesis of AH is less pronounced: the epitopes for these two sets of autoantibodies with such contrasting effects are now known to largely overlap.

TPO, previously known as the microsomal antigen, is involved in iodination of tyrosine residues and their subsequent coupling to form thyroid hormones [11]. An alternatively spliced variant of TPO mRNA, termed TPO-2, has been described, which lacks enzymatic activity and is believed to have a different antibody reactivity [12]. The potential early expression of TPO-2 during the embryonic stage of thyroid development may result in immunological tolerance to this molecule but not to full length TPO, which in turn may have a role in the development of ATD in some individuals [13].

Tg serves as the storage form of thyroid hormones and is primarily secreted into the thyroid follicles, although small amounts gain access to the circulation. Several hormonogenic sites (tyrosine acceptors) are present on each subunit and seem to have a role in Tg antigenicity [14, 15]. Genetic variation in Tg has been proposed as a hypothetical mechanism for initiating thyroid autoimmunity [16].

The sodium/iodide symporter (NIS) mediates iodine uptake by the thyroid gland and studies have shown the presence of NIS antibodies in ATD but only in a minority of individuals [17], and they have no known clinical significance.

6.2.2 The Role of Thyroid Autoantibodies in Disease Pathogenesis

6.2.2.1 Graves' Disease

Production of TSAb is undoubtedly the main pathogenic mechanism in GD but a minority of these patients also have TBAb, which may be responsible for fluctuation of thyroid function in rare cases of GD, secondary to oscillating levels of TSAb and TBAb [3]. The existence of autoantibodies that increase or inhibit TFC growth (and thus causing goiter or atrophy) independently of TSHR remains debatable [18]. Around 80% of individuals with GD also exhibit antibody reactivity against TPO [19, 20], but given the number of patients who fail to mount an antibody response, the clinical diagnostic value of TPO-Ab in GD is somewhat limited.

6.2.2.2 Extrathyroidal Complications

Of the major thyroid autoantigens, TPO is effectively ruled out as a candidate by its restricted tissue distribution, but Tg, which can be detected in retrobulbar tissue from TED patients, may have a role [21]. However, the low incidence of TED in AH and the failure of Tg-immunized mice to develop TED argues against a key role for this molecule in disease pathogenesis. The close association between GD and TED is mostly likely explained by the existence of a shared thyroid and orbital autoantigen, and this makes TSHR a credible candidate. Receptor expression (both mRNA and protein) has been detected in retrobulbar-derived tissue, including fibroblasts, muscles and preadipocytes, supporting this view [22]. The increased expression of TSHR during preadipocyte maturation into adipocyte led to the hypothesis that increased adipocyte differentiation in the orbit, secondary to yet unidentified factors, may contribute to the initiation of TED [23, 24]. The importance of TSHR in TED pathogenesis is further supported by the development of orbital changes in some, but not all, animal models immunized with TSHR, although reproducing these models has been difficult [25].

A number of antibodies against eye muscle and fibroblasts have been detected in TED, including 23, 55, 64, 66, and 95 kDa antigens, as well as antibodies against collagen XIII, tubulin, and acetylcholine receptor [26–28]. These antibodies lack diagnostic sensitivity and specificity, are likely to be produced secondary to tissue damage, and probably have no role in disease initiation.

6.2.2.3 Autoimmune Hypothyroidism

AH can present clinically in a goitrous form, Hashimoto's thyroiditis, or an atrophic form without an associated goitre, termed primary myxoedema. The majority of individuals with AH have serum antibodies to Tg and TPO, and occasionally to TSHR. Low titers of Tg-Ab are commonly found in apparently normal individuals, especially in the elderly or following viral infections [29, 30]. In contrast, titers of Tg-Ab are generally high in AH, and they are mainly of the IgG class rather than IgM [5, 6]. Tg-Ab are unable to fix complement, but have the capability of mediating antibody-dependent cell-mediated cytotoxicity (ADCC) *in vitro* [31], which may have a role in tissue destruction *in vivo*. The degree of Tg iodination may influence its immunogenicity, and this may be one mechanism for increased AH in iodine-rich areas [14, 15].

TPO-Ab are present in almost all subjects with AH, but are also detected in a small percentage of clinically normal individuals. TPO-Ab may play a direct role in immunopathogenesis through ADCC (in addition to their ability to fix complement), leading to thyroid cell destruction [5, 6]. Initial work suggested a functional role for these antibodies as they may inhibit TPO activity *in vitro*, but any clinically relevant effect is doubtful [32]. Bispecific Abs interacting with both Tg and TPO have been termed TgPOAb [33]. These Abs appear to be present in sera with high Tg-Ab and TPO-Ab titers, and they are more frequently detected in patients with HT than in patients with other ATD, but recently their existence as a discrete entity has been questioned. TBAb are detected in a minority of AH sera, and these can cause hypothyroidism without long-term tissue destruction [34]. The role of thyroid autoantibodies in inducing thyroid dysfunction is summarized in Fig. 6.1.

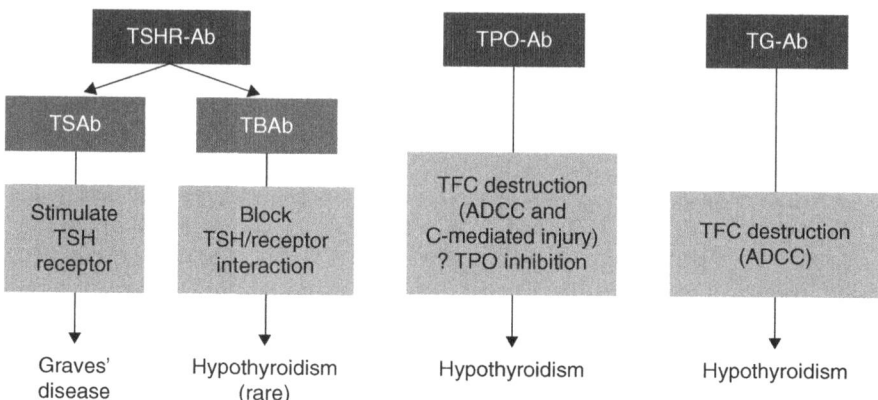

Fig. 6.1 Role of thyroid autoantibodies in gland dysfunction. *TSHR* thyroid stimulating hormone receptor, *TSAb* thyroid stimulating antibodies, *TBAb* thyroid blocking antibodies, *TPO* thyroid peroxidase, *TG* thyroglobulin, *TFC* thyroid follicular cells, *ADCC* antibody-dependent cell-mediated cytotoxicity, *C* complement

6.3 Assays for Thyroid Antibodies

6.3.1 Thyroid Stimulating Hormone Receptor

Antibodies to TSHR are detected using either a binding or a bioassay. TSH binding inhibiting immunoglobulin (TBII) assays, which measure inhibition of TSH binding to its receptor, are commercially available. TBII assays fail to determine the functionality of the antibody as they are unable to distinguish between stimulating and blocking antibodies. However, in clinical settings this is less important as clinical examination and biochemical findings allow straightforward interpretation of the functional characteristics of a positive TBII result in any individual patient.

Earlier, first generation TBII assays used porcine thyroid cell membranes and bovine labeled TSH and had a sensitivity of 50–80% [35]. Second generation TBII assays, employing recombinant human TSHR, increased sensitivity to more than 90%, without any loss in specificity [36–38]. Second generation assays are now commercially available in radiolabeled or chemiluminescence assay format and it is generally accepted that levels above 1.5 IU/L confirm the presence of TSHR-Ab, whereas values between 1 and 1.5 IU/L are classified as inconclusive. Despite some standarization, commercially available bioassays can differ in their sensitivity, which is largely dependent on the cutoff values used [39]. A third generation assay has been introduced recently based on detection of human monoclonal TSAb (instead of TSH) binding to recombinant TSHR. The sensitivity of this assay ranges between 95 and 97% with 100% specificity, compared with 89–94% sensitivity using second generation assays [40, 41].

In contrast to TBII, TSHR bioassays assess antibody functionality and rely on the detection of cAMP production in cell lines endogenously expressing or stably transfected with TSHR. The presence of TSAb leads to increased cAMP production in these cells, whereas TBAb result in inhibition of cAMP production after TSH stimulation. However, the distinction between TSAb and TBAb is not always straightforward as antibodies with TSH-blocking activity may also display stimulating activity, and some sera may have a mixture of stimulating and blocking antibodies [42]. Early bioassays used human thyrocytes or rat FRTL-5 cells [43–47], but subsequently TSHR-transfected stable cell lines have been used, which are more consistent and easier to maintain [48–51]. Bioassays have been further refined by using cell lines stably expressing both TSHR and a reporter gene luciferase, the activity of which was assessed by measuring light output from cells stimulated with patient sera [52–54], but have no present clinical application. Other techniques include the use of flow cytometry in cells expressing the holoreceptor or the extracellular domain (ECD), which are technically difficult to undertake [55, 56].

Although TSHR bioassays have expanded and improved in sensitivity and specificity over the years, the techniques involved are both demanding and expensive, making their use difficult. Furthermore, they have limited clinical value as the simpler TBII assay, in combination with the clinical picture and biochemical testing, is often enough to make an accurate diagnosis. Therefore, bioassays remain largely limited to research purposes, but there may be exceptions in rare clinical scenarios as discussed below.

6.3.2 Thyroid Peroxidase

TPO-Ab were initially assayed using crude preparations of thyroid cell membranes in agglutination or immunofluorescence tests. Czarnocka and colleagues subsequently identified TPO as the microsomal antigen [57], leading to the development of more sophisticated quantitative immunoassays. However, differences in TPO preparations may affect assay sensitivity, and the use of recombinant TPO, which is guaranteed to be free of contaminants, remains the best option to ensure consistency and reproducibility of the results. The majority of TPO-Ab assays currently report using international units and the standard preparation MRC 66/387 as a reference [58, 59]. TPO antibodies are detected in around 10% of the population without apparent thyroid disease [60], a percentage that can dramatically increase if low cutoff values are used [61]. Therefore, establishing an accurate reference range for individual laboratories, which varies according to the sensitivity and specificity of the methodology employed, is important for reliable interpretation of TPO-Ab results. TPO-Ab, detectable in almost all AH patients and around 80% of individuals with GD [62], are routinely used to help with clinical management decisions.

6.3.3 Thyroglobulin

Earlier tests to detect Tg-Ab relied on immunofluorescent techniques on thyroid tissue sections. This was followed by red cell agglutination methods and more recently by sensitive immunoassays, which are more reliable. In general, it is difficult to standardize Tg-Ab measurements due to the great variability of Tg preparations, and to address this problem a common practice is to calibrate against the primary standard MRC 65/93 [58, 59]. However, the use of this standard still does not ensure similar quantitative or qualitative results with the different methodologies. This may be an explanation for the different reporting methods used for Tg-Ab; some methods report below detection limit as a "normal" result, whereas others have a "normal range" above which the results are regarded as positive.

Up to 27% of individuals without evidence of thyroid autoimmunity have elevated levels of Tg-Ab [30], thus questioning the specificity of these antibodies and their usefulness in clinical settings. Furthermore, a significant number of patients with ATD exhibit TPO but not Tg antibody reactivity, while the reverse is unusual [63]. Therefore, Tg-Ab estimation is probably not routinely necessary for the diagnosis of ATD and the main clinical application is following treatment of individuals with differentiated thyroid cancer (DTC).

6.3.4 Sodium/Iodide Symporter

An early report using Western blotting suggested the presence of NIS antibodies in the majority of GD and a minority of AH patients [64]. More sophisticated techniques using *in vitro* translation and transcription showed that less than a quarter of patients with ATD have antibodies against the symporter [65, 66]. Bioassays have also been developed using cell lines stably transfected with NIS and these showed the presence of antibodies that can modify the function of the symporter in some ATD patients, although this concept is not shared by all [66–68].

Due to the low frequency of NIS-Ab in ATD, a commercial test has not been developed and, therefore, measurement of these antibodies remains purely of research interest.

6.4 Clinical Applications of Antibody Measurement

6.4.1 Graves' Disease

In many cases, the clinical features alone suffice to make the diagnosis of GD. However, in atypical cases, or if the physician has limited experience in thyroid disease, measuring TSHR antibodies can be of value to confirm the diagnosis. One should bear in mind, however, that the diagnostic accuracy is only important as far as it has an effect on clinical management. If a decision is taken to treat hyperthyroidism with radioactive iodine (RAI), then the underlying diagnosis is generally of academic interest.

Some argue that TSHR antibody testing can be useful in predicting relapse after a course of antithyroid drugs, and this has been an area of hot debate for the past decade [69]. In general, detection of TSHR-Ab following medical treatment of GD, particularly if levels are high, is associated with significant risk of relapse and this may be useful to plan follow-up. However, the converse is not true: a negative TSHR-Ab post treatment is still associated with a significant risk of relapse, making long-term clinical predictions uncertain.

TPO-Ab measurement in hyperthyroidism is undertaken in some centers, mainly due to ease of testing and low cost. However, around 20% of confirmed GD patients test negative for TPO-Ab, and therefore the role of these antibodies in the clinical management of hyperthyroidism is debatable [19, 20, 70]. It should also be noted that a very small minority of GD patients test negative for TBII, even using modern assays [71]; the most likely explanation is that there is purely intrathyroidal production of TSAb or that the most modern assays are still too insensitive to detect these antibodies in the circulation.

6.4.2   Graves' Ophthalmopathy

TSHR is believed to be one of the antigens involved in TED as it can be found in retrobulbar tissue, and antibody levels correlate with activity and severity of the disease [72, 73]. TSHR-Ab can be useful for the diagnosis of rare cases of euthyroid TED, as most of these patients have detectable antibodies using a sensitive second or third generation TBII assay [74]. However, a negative test does not rule out the diagnosis and orbital imaging becomes essential to confirm the condition and rule out other causes of the orbital symptoms.

Although TSHR-Ab levels correlate with disease outcome in some patients with TED, no prediction is possible in half the individuals, and therefore there is little practical role for TSHR-Ab measurement for assessing TED severity or for planning future therapy [75]. Clinical judgment in each patient with individually tailored therapy remains the best option in clinical practice.

6.4.3   Autoimmune Hypothyroidism

TPO-Ab, detected in almost all AH patients, are routinely used to confirm the autoimmune nature of hypothyroidism. Detection of these antibodies can also predict the development of AH. The Whickham survey has shown that almost 30% of individuals with positive TPO-Ab and normal thyroid function develop frank hypothyroidism in the following 20 years, whereas this percentage doubles in those who additionally have marginally raised plasma TSH [29, 76]. Therefore, in subclinical hypothyroidism, characterized by elevated TSH and normal thyroid hormones, TPO-Ab reactivity is associated with high risk of future hypothyroidism and treatment, rather than monitoring, can be advocated [77]. Furthermore, elevated TPO-Ab titers can also predict the development of amiodarone-induced hypothyroidism; therefore measurement of these antibodies is mandatory before starting amiodarone treatment [78, 79]. Similar considerations also apply in the case of treatment with alpha-interferon and lithium.

The existence of TBAb in hypothyroidism is best demonstrated by the rare development of transient neonatal hypothyroidism in babies secondary to transplacental transfer of these antibodies [34, 80]. Furthermore, a study of ten patients has shown the association of TBAb with 90% of newly diagnosed patients [81]. Tissue destruction is clearly evident in histopathology thyroid specimens from individuals with AH, and this remains the main pathogenic mechanism for thyroid failure in this condition. However, in the early stages of the disease, TBAb may play a role in inducing clinical hypothyroidism before widespread tissue destruction takes place. Also, TBAb may be the explanation for the occurrence of transient hypothyroidism before the development of autoimmune hyperthyroidism in rare clinical cases [82].

6.4.4 Pregnancy and Postpartum Thyroiditis

Hyperthyroidism, found in around 0.2% of pregnancies, is usually due to GD [83, 84] (pregnancy discussed in depth in Chap. 11). TSHR-Ab levels, which are typically higher in the earlier stages of pregnancy, are usually detected in these individuals and help to make the diagnosis. Neonatal thyrotoxicosis occurs in 1% of newborns to mothers with active GD, secondary to transplacental passage of TSAb. The fetal thyroid is unresponsive to TSAb before the 20th week of gestation and this, together with enhanced transplacental transfer of TSAb in the third trimester, explains the occurrence of fetal hyperthyroidism in the second half of pregnancy. Measurement of TSHR-Ab at 28 weeks in pregnant mothers with active GD is helpful in predicting neonatal thyrotoxicosis [85, 86]. In patients who have previously been treated with RAI or surgery, TSHR-Ab measurement is indicated in the first trimester of pregnancy and repeat testing should be performed at 28 weeks in those with positive antibodies. TSHR-Ab measurement is not required in euthyroid GD patients who have had previous treatment with antithyroid drugs.

A higher percentage of pregnant women (around 2.5%) have evidence of hypothyroidism—manifested as raised TSH levels [87]—and TPO-Ab measurement is required to establish the presence of thyroid autoimmunity. Furthermore, detection of TPO-Ab during pregnancy, with otherwise normal thyroid function, is associated with increased rate of miscarriage, intellectual dysfunction, and hearing deficit in the newborn [88–90]. The exact mechanism leading to pregnancy loss in women with elevated TPO-Ab levels remains speculative [91], but treatment with levothyroxine may have a beneficial effect, particularly in those with TSH levels above 2 mIU/L [90]. Therefore, thyroid function should be monitored carefully in pregnant women with detectable TPO-Ab, and a policy of a low threshold for levothyroxine treatment should probably be adopted in those with borderline thyroid function.

Postpartum thyroiditis (PPT) has a prevalence of 1–20% (the wide range reflecting racial differences), and results in thyroid dysfunction, which occurs during the first year after delivery [7]. Classically, PPT runs a biphasic course of a hyperthyroid phase followed by temporary or permanent hypothyroidism, although thyrotoxicosis or hypothyroidism may occur in isolation. TPO-Ab levels are positive in most women with PPT and measurement of these antibodies helps in making the diagnosis. Additionally, raised TPO-Ab levels during pregnancy predict the development of PPT in up to 50% of patients [7, 84]. TSHR-Ab measurement can be useful to differentiate PPT from GD in the postpartum period, although TSHR-Ab can be detected in a small minority of individuals during the hyperthyroid phase of PPT [92, 93]. Equally, detection of TSHR-Ab in presumed PPT may simply represent early GD, which can develop following PPT in some individuals [94, 95].

Table 6.1 Role of thyroid antibody measurement in clinical practice

Antibody measurement	Useful	Probably not useful
TSHR-Ab	Determine the etiology of hyperthyroidism in uncertain cases	Prediction of relapse following medical treatment
	Diagnosis of euthyroid TED	Prediction of TED outcome
	Prediction of neonatal thyrotoxicosis	
TPO-Ab	Hypothyroidism (particularly in subclinical disease)	Diagnosis of GD
	Diagnosis of PPT	
Tg-Ab	Following ablative therapy for DTC	Diagnosis of ATD

TSHR thyroid stimulating hormone receptor, *TPO* thyroid peroxidase, *Tg* thyroglobulin, *Ab* antibody, *GD* Graves' disease, *TED* thyroid eye disease, *ATD* autoimmune thyroid disease, *PPT* postpartum thyroiditis, *DTC* differentiated thyroid cancer

6.4.5 Differentiated Thyroid Cancer

DTC is usually treated with thyroidectomy followed by RAI ablation. Tg is a specific marker for thyroid tissue and one tool used to monitor DTC recurrence [96] (discussed in depth in Chap. 7). However, Tg-Ab can interfere with Tg estimation, and therefore levels of these antibodies should be assessed in all patients prior to undertaking Tg analysis. The persistence, or the new emergence, of Tg-Ab following ablative therapy indicates the presence of thyroid tissue and can itself be a marker of disease recurrence. It should be noted that some Tg tests differ in their susceptibility to interference from Tg-Ab, and this should be taken into account when managing patients with DTC [97].

The role of thyroid autoantibody testing in clinical practice is summarized in Table 6.1.

6.5 Recommendation for the Use of Thyroid Autoantibodies in Clinical Practice

Although TSHR-Ab are detected in the majority of individuals with GD, it is mainly useful in difficult cases where the diagnosis is uncertain. TSHR-Ab measurement is unnecessary in hyperthyroid TED but can be useful in rare cases of euthyroid ophthalmopathy. Furthermore, these antibodies should be measured in pregnant women with active GD and in those who have had definitive treatment (i.e., surgery or RAI) for the condition; high levels of TSHR-Ab in pregnant women predict the possible development of neonatal thyrotoxicosis and careful fetal monitoring becomes mandatory. TSHR-Ab can also be measured in women with postpartum hyperthyroidism to help differentiate PPT from GD, although a minority of PPT patients may display antibody positivity during the hyperthyroid phase. Detection of TSHR-Ab is relatively easy using TBII, especially with a modern assay, but a functional bioassay, which is technically more demanding, can be definitive in rare cases, such as GD in pregnancy, particularly if maternal thyroid status cannot be assessed due to previous thyroidectomy or RAI treatment. At present, TSHR-Ab measurement unfortunately has little use in planning the clinical management of GD or predicting outcome of TED.

Almost all individuals with AH have TPO-Ab, so this is a helpful tool to make the correct diagnosis and rule out other causes of hypothyroidism, such as non-autoimmune thyroiditis. Also, TPO-Ab can be used to plan clinical management; levothyroxine replacement therapy is worth considering in individuals with sub-clinical hypothyroidism who also have raised TPO-Ab levels, given the lifelong chance of these patients developing overt hypothyroidism. TPO-Ab levels should be measured in women with postpartum thyroid dysfunction and are consistent with PPT. Furthermore, detection of TPO-Ab in pregnancy is associated with higher risk of fetal loss, which may be prevented by thyroxine treatment, particularly in those with TSH > 2 mIU/L, although concrete evidence supporting such a practice is still lacking. Measurement of TPO-Ab in hyperthyroid individuals has a limited value, as only 80% of GD patients display antibody reactivity.

Tg-Ab have little role in the management of ATD due to their low sensitivity and specificity; therefore they are not routinely requested for suspected ATD. However, measurement of Tg-Ab is important in individuals who have had treatment for DTC, as these antibodies can interfere with Tg measurement—a marker of residual thyroid tissue and disease recurrence. Furthermore, the persistent elevation, or the emergence of Tg-Ab, following ablative treatment, may also be indicative of DTC relapse.

In summary, TSHR-Ab testing is advocated in unclear cases of hyperthyroidism, suspected euthyroid ophthalmopathy, and to predict neonatal thyrotoxicosis. Measurement of TPO-Ab levels is helpful to confirm the autoimmune nature of hypothyroidism (particularly subclinical disease) and the diagnosis of PPT, whereas Tg-Ab levels are used to exclude interference with Tg plasma measurements in individuals who have undergone thyroid ablative therapy for DTC.

6.6 Conclusion

Thyroid dysfunction is a common condition and is usually due to thyroid autoimmunity, where both cellular and humoral immune responses play a role in disease pathogenesis. Markers of the humoral immune response have been used to aid the clinical diagnosis and management plan of individuals with ATD. The increase in sensitivity and specificity, coupled with the relative ease of thyroid autoantibody analysis, paved the way for the routine use of antibody testing in clinical practice.

Thus far, measurement of thyroid autoantibodies has only been used for diagnostic purposes. However, further characterization of these antibodies may help to devise new treatment strategies, particularly in individuals having side effects with the medical treatment or in those with severe extrathyroidal manifestations. For example, antibodies against TSAb can be developed that neutralise the

TSHR-stimulating activity, thereby directly targeting the pathogenic mechanism of the disease. Future research in this area should be directed at fully elucidating the exact role of thyroid autoantibodies in ATD as this will help to develop novel tactics that might target the thyroid-specific humoral immune responses, potentially resulting in reversal of the disease process.

References

1. Ajjan RA, Weetman AP. Autoimmune thyroid disease and autoimmune polyglandular syndrome. In: Austin KF, Frank MM, Canton HI, Atkinson JP, Samter M, eds. *Samter's Immunological Diseases*. London, United Kingdom: Wolters Kulwar Company; 2001:605-626.
2. Weetman AP. Autoimmune thyroid disease: propagation and progression. *Eur J Endocrinol.* 2003;148:1-9.
3. Weetman AP. Graves' disease. *N Engl J Med.* 2000;343:1236-1248.
4. Khoo TK, Bahn RS. Pathogenesis of Graves' ophthalmopathy: the role of autoantibodies. *Thyroid.* 2007;17:1013-1018.
5. Weetman AP, McGregor AM. Autoimmune thyroid disease: developments in our understanding. *Endocr Rev.* 1984;5:309-355.
6. Weetman AP, McGregor AM. Autoimmune thyroid disease: further developments in our understanding. *Endocr Rev.* 1994;15:788-830.
7. Muller AF, Drexhage HA, Berghout A. Postpartum thyroiditis and autoimmune thyroiditis in women of childbearing age: recent insights and consequences for antenatal and postnatal care. *Endocr Rev.* 2001;22:605-630.
8. Weetman AP. Cellular immune responses in autoimmune thyroid disease. *Clin Endocrinol (Oxford).* 2004;61:405-413.
9. Ajjan RA, Weetman AP. Cytokines in thyroid autoimmunity. *Autoimmunity.* 2003;36: 351-359.
10. Paschke R, Van Sande J, Parma J, Vassart G. The TSH receptor and thyroid diseases. *Baillieres Clin Endocrinol Metab.* 1996;10:9-27.
11. McLachlan SM, Rapoport B. The molecular biology of thyroid peroxidase: cloning, expression and role as autoantigen in autoimmune thyroid disease. *Endocr Rev.* 1992;13:192-206.
12. Niccoli P, Fayadat L, Panneels V, Lanet J, Franc JL. Human thyroperoxidase in its alternatively spliced form (TPO2) is enzymatically inactive and exhibits changes in intracellular processing and trafficking. *J Biol Chem.* 1997;272:29487-29492.
13. Gardas A, Lewartowska A, Sutton BJ, Pasieka Z, McGregor AM, Banga JP. Human thyroid peroxidase (TPO) isoforms, TPO-1 and TPO-2: analysis of protein expression in Graves' thyroid tissue. *J Clin Endocrinol Metab.* 1997;82:3752-3757.
14. Vali M, Rose NR, Caturegli P. Thyroglobulin as autoantigen: structure-function relationships. *Rev Endocr Metab Disord.* 2000;1:69-77.
15. Gentile F, Conte M, Formisano S. Thyroglobulin as an autoantigen: what can we learn about immunopathogenicity from the correlation of antigenic properties with protein structure? *Immunology.* 2004;112:13-25.
16. McLachlan SM, Rapoport B. Why measure thyroglobulin autoantibodies rather than thyroid peroxidase autoantibodies? *Thyroid.* 2004;14:510-520.
17. Dohan O, De la Vieja A, Paroder V, et al. The sodium/iodide Symporter (NIS): characterization, regulation, and medical significance. *Endocr Rev.* 2003;24:48-77.
18. Drexhage HA. Autoimmunity and thyroid growth. Where do we stand? *Eur J Endocrinol.* 1996;135:39-45.
19. Gilmour J, Brownlee Y, Foster P, et al. The quantitative measurement of autoantibodies to thyroglobulin and thyroid peroxidase by automated microparticle based immunoassays in

Hashimoto's disease, Graves' disease and a follow-up study on postpartum thyroid disease. *Clin Lab.* 2000;46:57-61.

20. Guilhem I, Massart C, Poirier JY, Maugendre D. Differential evolution of thyroid peroxidase and thyrotropin receptor antibodies in graves' disease: thyroid peroxidase antibody activity reverts to pretreatment level after carbimazole withdrawal. *Thyroid.* 2006;16:1041-1045.
21. Marino M, Chiovato L, Lisi S, Altea MA, Marcocci C, Pinchera A. Role of thyroglobulin in the pathogenesis of Graves' ophthalmopathy: the hypothesis of Kriss revisited. *J Endocrinol Invest.* 2004;27:230-236.
22. Bahn RS. TSH receptor expression in orbital tissue and its role in the pathogenesis of Graves' ophthalmopathy. *J Endocrinol Invest.* 2004;27:216-220.
23. Valyasevi RW, Erickson DZ, Harteneck DA, et al. Differentiation of human orbital preadipocyte fibroblasts induces expression of functional thyrotropin receptor. *J Clin Endocrinol Metab.* 1999;84:2557-2562.
24. Kumar S, Coenen MJ, Scherer PE, Bahn RS. Evidence for enhanced adipogenesis in the orbits of patients with Graves' ophthalmopathy. *J Clin Endocrinol Metab.* 2004;89:930-935.
25. Many MC, Costagliola S, Detrait M, Denef F, Vassart G, Ludgate MC. Development of an animal model of autoimmune thyroid eye disease. *J Immunol.* 1999;162:4966-4974.
26. Prabhakar BS, Bahn RS, Smith TJ. Current perspective on the pathogenesis of Graves' disease and ophthalmopathy. *Endocr Rev.* 2003;24:802-835.
27. Mizokami T, Salvi M, Wall JR. Eye muscle antibodies in Graves' ophthalmopathy: pathogenic or secondary epiphenomenon? *J Endocrinol Invest.* 2004;27:221-229.
28. Bahn RS. Clinical review 157: pathophysiology of Graves' ophthalmopathy: the cycle of disease. *J Clin Endocrinol Metab.* 2003;88:1939-1946.
29. Tunbridge WM, Evered DC, Hall R, et al. The spectrum of thyroid disease in a community: the Whickham survey. *Clin Endocrinol (Oxford).* 1977;7:481-493.
30. Tomer Y. Anti-thyroglobulin autoantibodies in autoimmune thyroid diseases: cross-reactive or pathogenic? *Clin Immunol Immunopathol.* 1997;82:3-11.
31. Bogner U, Hegedus L, Hansen JM, Finke R, Schleusener H. Thyroid cytotoxic antibodies in atrophic and goitrous autoimmune thyroiditis. *Eur J Endocrinol.* 1995;132:69-74.
32. Song YH, Li Y, Maclaren NK. The nature of autoantigens targeted in autoimmune endocrine diseases. *Immunol Today.* 1996;17:232-238.
33. Ruf J, Feldt-Rasmussen U, Hegedus L, Ferrand M, Carayon P. Bispecific thyroglobulin and thyroperoxidase autoantibodies in patients with various thyroid and autoimmune diseases. *J Clin Endocrinol Metab.* 1994;79:1404-1409.
34. Wilson BE, Netzloff ML. Congenital hypothyroidism and transient thyrotropin excess: differential diagnosis of abnormal newborn thyroid screening. *Ann Clin Lab Sci.* 1982;12: 223-233.
35. Smith BR, Hall R. Thyroid-stimulating immunoglobulins in Graves' disease. *Lancet.* 1974;2:427-431.
36. Costagliola S, Morgenthaler NG, Hoermann R, et al. Second generation assay for thyrotropin receptor antibodies has superior diagnostic sensitivity for Graves' disease. *J Clin Endocrinol Metab.* 1999;84:90-97.
37. Villalta D, Orunesu E, Tozzoli R, et al. Analytical and diagnostic accuracy of "second generation" assays for thyrotrophin receptor antibodies with radioactive and chemiluminescent tracers. *J Clin Pathol.* 2004;57:378-382.
38. Paunkovic J, Paunkovic N. Does autoantibody-negative Graves' disease exist? A second evaluation of the clinical diagnosis. *Horm Metab Res.* 2006;38:53-56.
39. Preissner CM, Wolhuter PJ, Sistrunk JW, Homburger HA, Morris JC III. Comparison of thyrotropin-receptor antibodies measured by four commercially available methods with a bioassay that uses Fisher rat thyroid cells. *Clin Chem.* 2003;49:1402-1404.
40. Smith BR, Bolton J, Young S, et al. A new assay for thyrotropin receptor autoantibodies. *Thyroid.* 2004;14:830-835.
41. Kamijo K, Ishikawa K, Tanaka M. Clinical evaluation of 3rd generation assay for thyrotropin receptor antibodies: the M22-biotin-based ELISA initiated by Smith. *Endocr J.* 2005;52: 525-529.

42. Atger M, Misrahi M, Young J, et al. Autoantibodies interacting with purified native thyrotropin receptor. *Eur J Biochem.* 1999;265:1022-1031.
43. Zakarija M, McKenzie JM. Effect of thyrotropin and of LATS on mouse thyroid cyclic AMP. *Metabolism.* 1973;22:1185-1191.
44. Stockle G, Wahl R, Seif FJ. Micromethod of human thyrocyte cultures for detection of thyroid-stimulating antibodies and thyrotrophin. *Acta Endocrinol (Copenhagen).* 1981;97: 369-375.
45. Toccafondi RS, Aterini S, Medici MA, Rotella CM, Tanini A, Zonefrati R. Thyroid-stimulating antibody (TSab) detected in sera of Graves' patients using human thyroid cell cultures. *Clin Exp Immunol.* 1980;40:532-539.
46. Vitti P, Rotella CM, Valente WA, et al. Characterization of the optimal stimulatory effects of graves' monoclonal and serum immunoglobulin G on adenosine 3',5'-monophosphate production in fRTL-5 thyroid cells: a potential clinical assay. *J Clin Endocrinol Metab.* 1983;57:782-791.
47. Kasagi K, Konishi J, Iida Y, et al. A new in vitro assay for human thyroid stimulator using cultured thyroid cells: effect of sodium chloride on adenosine 3',5'-monophosphate increase. *J Clin Endocrinol Metab.* 1982;54:108-114.
48. Vitti P, Elisei R, Tonacchera M, et al. Detection of thyroid-stimulating antibody using Chinese hamster ovary cells transfected with cloned human thyrotropin receptor. *J Clin Endocrinol Metab.* 1993;76:499-503.
49. Chiovato L, Vitti P, Bendinelli G, et al. Detection of antibodies blocking thyrotropin effect using Chinese hamster ovary cells transfected with the cloned human TSH receptor. *J Endocrinol Invest.* 1994;17:809-816.
50. Murakami M, Miyashita K, Kakizaki S, et al. Clinical usefulness of thyroid-stimulating antibody measurement using Chinese hamster ovary cells expressing human thyrotropin receptors. *Eur J Endocrinol.* 1995;133:80-86.
51. Takano T, Sumizaki H, Amino N. Detection of thyroid-stimulating antibody using frozen stocks of Chinese hamster ovary cells transfected with cloned human thyrotropin receptor. *Endocr J.* 1997;44:431-435.
52. Watson PF, Ajjan RA, Phipps J, Metcalfe R, Weetman AP. A new chemiluminescent assay for the rapid detection of thyroid stimulating antibodies in Graves' disease. *Clin Endocrinol (Oxford)* 1998;49:577-581.
53. Hovens GC, Buiting AM, Karperien M, et al. A bioluminescence assay for thyrotropin receptor antibodies predicts serum thyroid hormone levels in patients with de novo Graves' disease. *Clin Endocrinol (Oxford).* 2006;64:429-435.
54. Evans C, Morgenthaler NG, Lee S, et al. Development of a luminescent bioassay for thyroid stimulating antibodies. *J Clin Endocrinol Metab.* 1999;84:374-377.
55. Costagliola S, Khoo D, Vassart G. Production of bioactive amino-terminal domain of the thyrotropin receptor via insertion in the plasma membrane by a glycosylphosphatidylinositol anchor. *FEBS Lett.* 1998;436:427-433.
56. Chazenbalk GD, Latrofa F, McLachlan SM, Rapoport B. Thyroid stimulation does not require antibodies with identical epitopes but does involve recognition of a critical conformation at the N terminus of the thyrotropin receptor A-subunit. *J Clin Endocrinol Metab.* 2004;89: 1788-1793.
57. Czarnocka B, Ruf J, Ferrand M, Carayon P, Lissitzky S. Purification of the human thyroid peroxidase and its identification as the microsomal antigen involved in autoimmune thyroid diseases. *FEBS Lett.* 1985;190:147-152.
58. Sinclair D. Clinical and laboratory aspects of thyroid autoantibodies. *Ann Clin Biochem.* 2006;43:173-183.
59. Sinclair D. Analytical aspects of thyroid antibodies estimation. *Autoimmunity.* 2008;41: 46-54.
60. Hollowell JG, Staehling NW, Flanders WD, et al. Serum TSH, T(4), and thyroid antibodies in the United States population (1988 to 1994): National Health and Nutrition Examination Survey (NHANES III). *J Clin Endocrinol Metab.* 2002;87:489-499.

61. Zophel K, Saller B, Wunderlich G, et al. Autoantibodies to thyroperoxidase (TPOAb) in a large population of euthyroid subjects: implications for the definition of TPOAb reference intervals. *Clin Lab.* 2003;49:591-600.
62. Feldt-Rasmussen U, Hoier-Madsen M, Bech K, et al. Anti-thyroid peroxidase antibodies in thyroid disorders and non-thyroid autoimmune diseases. *Autoimmunity.* 1991;9:245-254.
63. Nordyke RA, Gilbert FI Jr, Miyamoto LA, Fleury KA. The superiority of antimicrosomal over antithyroglobulin antibodies for detecting Hashimoto's thyroiditis. *Arch Intern Med.* 1993;153:862-865.
64. Endo T, Kogai T, Nakazato M, Saito T, Kaneshige M, Onaya T. Autoantibody against Na+/I− symporter in the sera of patients with autoimmune thyroid disease. *Biochem Biophys Res Commun.* 1996;224:92-95.
65. Seissler J, Wagner S, Schott M, et al. Low frequency of autoantibodies to the human Na(+)/I(−) symporter in patients with autoimmune thyroid disease. *J Clin Endocrinol Metab.* 2000;85:4630-4634.
66. Ajjan RA, Kemp EH, Waterman EA, et al. Detection of binding and blocking autoantibodies to the human sodium-iodide symporter in patients with autoimmune thyroid disease. *J Clin Endocrinol Metab.* 2000;85:2020-2027.
67. Chin HS, Chin DK, Morgenthaler NG, Vassart G, Costagliola S. Rarity of anti- Na+/I− symporter (NIS) antibody with iodide uptake inhibiting activity in autoimmune thyroid diseases (AITD). *J Clin Endocrinol Metab.* 2000;85:3937-3940.
68. Tonacchera M, Agretti P, Ceccarini G, et al. Autoantibodies from patients with autoimmune thyroid disease do not interfere with the activity of the human iodide symporter gene stably transfected in CHO cells. *Eur J Endocrinol.* 2001;144:611-618.
69. Ajjan RA, Weetman AP. Techniques to quantify TSH receptor antibodies. *Nat Clin Pract Endocrinol Metab.* 2008;4:461-468.
70. Lavard L, Perrild H, Jacobsen BB, Hoier-Madsen M, Bendinelli G, Vitti P. Prevalence of thyroid peroxidase, thyroglobulin and thyrotropin receptor antibodies in a long-term follow-up of juvenile Graves disease. *Autoimmunity.* 2000;32:167-172.
71. Vos XG, Smit N, Endert E, Tijssen JG, Wiersinga WM. Frequency and characteristics of TBII-seronegative patients in a population with untreated Graves' hyperthyroidism: a prospective study. *Clin Endocrinol (Oxford).* 2008;69:311-317.
72. Gerding MN, van der Meer JW, Broenink M, Bakker O, Wiersinga WM, Prummel MF. Association of thyrotrophin receptor antibodies with the clinical features of Graves' ophthalmopathy. *Clin Endocrinol (Oxford).* 2000;52:267-271.
73. Khoo TK, Bahn RS. Pathogenesis of Graves' ophthalmopathy: the role of autoantibodies. *Thyroid.* 2007;17:1013-1018.
74. Khoo DH, Eng PH, Ho SC, et al. Graves' ophthalmopathy in the absence of elevated free thyroxine and triiodothyronine levels: prevalence, natural history, and thyrotropin receptor antibody levels. *Thyroid.* 2000;10:1093-1100.
75. Eckstein AK, Plicht M, Lax H, et al. Thyrotropin receptor autoantibodies are independent risk factors for Graves' ophthalmopathy and help to predict severity and outcome of the disease. *J Clin Endocrinol Metab.* 2006;91:3464-3470.
76. Vanderpump MP, Tunbridge WM, French JM, et al. The incidence of thyroid disorders in the community: a twenty-year follow-up of the Whickham Survey. *Clin Endocrinol (Oxford).* 1995;43:55-68.
77. Fatourechi V. Subclinical hypothyroidism: how should it be managed? *Treat Endocrinol.* 2002;1:211-216.
78. Martino E, Bartalena L, Bogazzi F, Braverman LE. The effects of amiodarone on the thyroid. *Endocr Rev.* 2001;22:240-254.
79. Basaria S, Cooper DS. Amiodarone and the thyroid. *Am J Med.* 2005;118:706-714.
80. Evans C, Jordan NJ, Owens G, Bradley D, Ludgate M, John R. Potent thyrotropin receptor-blocking antibodies: a cause of transient congenital hypothyroidism and delayed thyroid development. *Eur J Endocrinol.* 2004;150:265-268.

81. Bryant WP, Bergert ER, Morris JC. Identification of thyroid blocking antibodies and receptor epitopes in autoimmune hypothyroidism by affinity purification using synthetic TSH receptor peptides. *Autoimmunity.* 1995;22:69-79.
82. Iitaka M, Kakinuma S, Yamanaka K, et al. Induction of autoimmune hypothyroidism and subsequent hyperthyroidism by TSH receptor antibodies following subacute thyroiditis: a case report. *Endocr J.* 2001;48:139-142.
83. Lazarus JH. Thyroid disorders associated with pregnancy: etiology, diagnosis, and management. *Treat Endocrinol.* 2005;4:31-41.
84. Lazarus JH, Premawardhana LD. Screening for thyroid disease in pregnancy. *J Clin Pathol.* 2005;58:449-452.
85. Chan GW, Mandel SJ. Therapy insight: management of Graves' disease during pregnancy. *Nat Clin Pract Endocrinol Metab.* 2007;3:470-478.
86. Nayak B, Hodak SP. Hyperthyroidism. *Endocrinol Metab Clin North Am.* 2007;36:617-56, v.
87. Klein RZ, Haddow JE, Faix JD, et al. Prevalence of thyroid deficiency in pregnant women. *Clin Endocrinol (Oxford).* 1991;35:41-46.
88. Pop VJ, de Vries E, van Baar AL, et al. Maternal thyroid peroxidase antibodies during pregnancy: a marker of impaired child development? *J Clin Endocrinol Metab.* 1995;80:3561-3566.
89. Wasserman EE, Nelson K, Rose NR, et al. Maternal thyroid autoantibodies during the third trimester and hearing deficits in children: an epidemiologic assessment. *Am J Epidemiol.* 2008;167:701-710.
90. Negro R, Formoso G, Mangieri T, Pezzarossa A, Dazzi D, Hassan H. Levothyroxine treatment in euthyroid pregnant women with autoimmune thyroid disease: effects on obstetrical complications. *J Clin Endocrinol Metab.* 2006;91:2587-2591.
91. Glinoer D. Miscarriage in women with positive anti-TPO antibodies: is thyroxine the answer? *J Clin Endocrinol Metab.* 2006;91:2500-2502.
92. Hara T, Tamai H, Mukuta T, Fukata S, Kuma K. The role of thyroid stimulating antibody (TSAb) in the thyroid function of patients with post-partum hypothyroidism. *Clin Endocrinol (Oxford).* 1992;36:69-74.
93. Hidaka Y, Tamaki H, Iwatani Y, Tada H, Mitsuda N, Amino N. Prediction of post-partum Graves' thyrotoxicosis by measurement of thyroid stimulating antibody in early pregnancy. *Clin Endocrinol (Oxford).* 1994;41:15-20.
94. Sarlis NJ, Brucker-Davis F, Swift JP, Tahara K, Kohn LD. Graves' disease following thyrotoxic painless thyroiditis. Analysis of antibody activities against the thyrotropin receptor in two cases. *Thyroid.* 1997;7:829-836.
95. Shorey S, Badenhoop K, Walfish PG. Graves' hyperthyroidism after postpartum thyroiditis. *Thyroid.* 1998;8:1117-1122.
96. Harish K. Thyroglobulin: current status in differentiated thyroid carcinoma (review). *Endocr Regul.* 2006;40:53-67.
97. Spencer CA, Lopresti JS. Measuring thyroglobulin and thyroglobulin autoantibody in patients with differentiated thyroid cancer. *Nat Clin Pract Endocrinol Metab.* 2008;4:223-233.

Chapter 7
Thyroglobulin Measurement

Carole Spencer and Ivana Petrovic

7.1 Tg Biosynthesis and Metabolic Clearance

The thyroglobulin (Tg) gene is encoded by human chromosome 8q24.2–8q24.3 in a 8.5 kb coding sequence covering 48 exons. As illustrated in Fig. 7.1, transcription of the 330 kDa Tg monomeric protein is regulated by a number of transcription factors that include TTF-1, TTF-2, and Pax-8 [1–3]. Posttranslational processing is complex and necessitates multiple molecular chaperones to control the glycosylation, appropriate folding, dimerization, and trafficking of the mature protein to the apical membrane where thyroid peroxidase catalyses the iodination of the hormonogenic sites [1, 3–6]. Comparisons between Tg derived from papillary cancers versus normal thyroid tissue show differences in carbohydrate, iodine content, sulfation, charge, and immunological properties [7–13]. These differences likely result from defective posttranslational processing of tumor-derived Tg leading to the secretion of Tg molecules with an abnormal tertiary structure. Because Tg epitopes are conformational, any alteration in the tertiary structure of the molecule has the potential to disrupt the immunological interaction(s) with the assay reagents [7, 10, 11, 14–16]. The half-life of Tg in serum approximates 3 days and is determined by the terminal sialic acid content of the molecule [17]. Both the sialic acid and iodine content of the Tg derived from papillary tumors tend to be lower than normal, suggesting the possibility for differences in the metabolic clearance of Tg protein secreted by different tumors [8, 17–19]. An accelerated metabolic clearance of tumor-derived Tg could be the reason why serum Tg can be paradoxically low or even undetectable in some patients with a significant tumor burden [11, 12, 20–24].

C. Spencer (✉)
Department of Medicine, Keck School of Medicine, University of Southern California, Los Angeles, CA 90032, USA
e-mail: cspencer@usc.edu

G. A. Brent (ed.), *Thyroid Function Testing,*
DOI 10.1007/978-1-4419-1485-9_7, © Springer Science+Business Media, LLC 2010

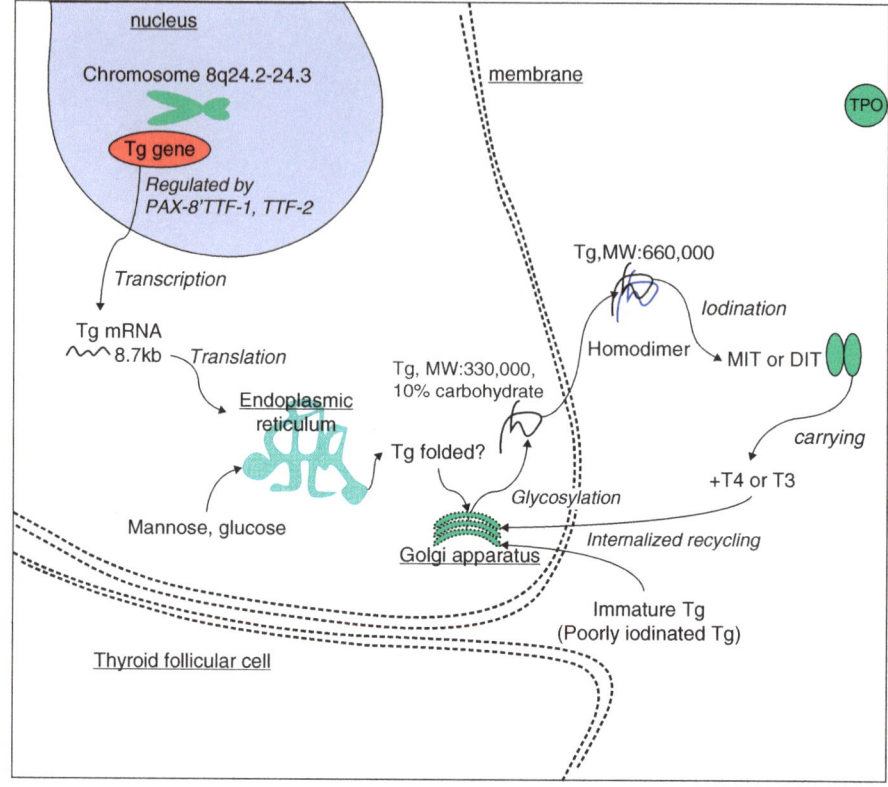

Fig. 7.1 Gene regulation and synthesis of thyroglobulin (*Tg*) in normal thyroid follicular epithelial cells. (Reproduced with permission from [3])

7.2   Tg Assay Methodology: Technical Issues

Tg measurement still remains technically challenging. Most laboratories favor automated immunometric assay (IMA) methods because they are nonisotopic, require shorter incubations than radioimmunoassay (RIA; hours vs. days), and can be automated. Manufacturers are beginning to use a two-step approach to overcome the "hook" problems that plague tumor-marker IMAs, wherein high antigen concentrations exceed the binding capacity of the capture antibody and cause inappropriately low results [25–28]. Unfortunately, Tg IMA methodology appears to have a greater propensity for interference, both from human anti-mouse antibodies (HAMA; see Sect. 7.2.3.1) and Tg autoantibodies (TgAb; see Sect. 7.2.3.2) as compared with RIA [16]. RIA is not influenced by HAMA; however TgAb has the potential to interfere and cause false low or high RIA values depending on the specificity of the RIA reagents employed [26, 29–33].

7.2.1 Standardization/Specificity

Despite the introduction of a Thyroglobulin Certified Reference Material (CRM-457) more than 10 years ago [34], some methods are still not CRM-457 standardized (Table 7.1), and the coefficient of variation between Tg methods approximates 30% (Fig. 7.2 panels (a) and (b))—twice the within-person biologic variability (~15%) [16, 35–39]. A recent study found that the variability among IMA methods was higher than among RIA methods, even when measuring Tg in normal euthyroid subjects (44% vs. 29%) [16]. This variability may, in part, result from standardization and assay matrix differences, but also likely reflects the use of monoclonal antibody (MAb) reagents with narrow epitope recognition for different Tg isoforms, as compared with the broad epitope recognition inherent to the polyclonal antibodies (PAb) used for RIA (Table 7.1) [7, 10, 11, 26, 40]. It is not surprising that IMA methods vary in their specificity for measuring abnormal tumor-derived Tg isoforms given the conformational nature of Tg epitopes and the potential for tumors to secrete immature Tg isoforms with compromised immunologic recognition and/or abnormal metabolic clearances (see Sect. 7.1) [11, 12, 14–16, 18, 24].

Changing Tg methods during long-term monitoring of patients with differentiated thyroid cancers (DTC) has the potential to disrupt patient care given the magnitude of bias between tests by different manufacturers [39, 41, 42]. As shown in Fig. 7.2, values reported by different Tg assays vary as much as threefold, even when TgAb is not detected. Differences of this magnitude would certainly be interpreted as clinically significant (>1.5 µg/L [ng/mL][1]) [41], and have the potential to either mask a rise in Tg due to recurrence, or prompt unnecessary concern for recurrence. Methodologic variability also compromises the current practice of using fixed Tg cutoff values to assess risk for persistent/recurrent disease. For example, the 72-hour post recombinant human TSH (rhTSH) serum Tg cutoff value of 2.0 µg/L (ng/mL) that has become the "gold standard" for rhTSH-stimulated Tg testing (see Sect. 7.6.4.2) has been universally adopted without compensating for differences in assay standardization [43–48]. Because assay 2 from Table 7.1 is only ~50% standardized against CRM-457, a Tg cutoff of 2.0 µg/L (ng/mL) reported by this assay would be equivalent to 4.0 µg/L (ng/mL) when using CRM-457 standardization. These standardization/specificity problems can be mitigated by evaluating trends in the serial Tg measurements used to follow patients with DTC (made with the same assay under the same TSH conditions) in preference to employing a fixed Tg cutoff [46, 48–50, 52–57]. When practical, the archiving of unused specimens allows the concurrent remeasurement of a past with a current specimen, thereby eliminating run-to-run variability and facilitating rebaselining, should a change in Tg method become necessary.

---

[1] Serum Tg values expressed in terms of 1:1 CRM-457 standardization.

Table 7.1 Comparison of nine current Tg assays (assay numbers relate to Fig. 7.2)

Assay no. (from Fig. 7.2)	1	2	3	4	5	6	7	8	9
Assay name	Access Tg	Tg-Plus	Tg IRMA	Immulite 2000	Tg	Tg RIA	Elecsys Tg	Tg	Wallac Delfia Tg
Manufacturer	Beckman Couter, USA	BRAHMS diagnostica, Germany	CIS bio-Schering, Germany	Siemens, USA	Genesis Diagnostics, UK	University Southern California, USA	Roche, Germany	Sanofi Pasteur, France	Perkin-Elmer, Finland
Assay type	Noncompetitive ICMA	Noncompetitive IRMA	Noncompetitive IRMA	Noncompetitive ICMA	Noncompetitive ELISA	Competitive RIA	Noncompetitive IECMA	Noncompetitive IRMA	Noncompetitive IFMA
Capture antibody	4x MAb	PAb (rabbit)	4x MAb	MAb	PAb (rabbit)	PAb (rabbit)	MAb	4x MAb	MAb
Tracer	AP-MAb	^{125}-I-MAb	^{125}-I-MAb	AP-PAb (sheep)	AP-PAb (rabbit)	^{125}-I-Tg	Ru complex-MAb	^{125}-I-MAb	Eu-MAb
Sample size (µL)	40	100	100	50	50	200	20	100	50
1:1 CRM-457 standardization	Yes	No (factor of 2)	Yes	Yes	No	Yes	Yes	No	No
Functional sensitivity (µg/L)*,#	0.1 [51]	0.4*	0.7	0.9	?	0.5	1.0	?	?
Reference range (µg/L)*	3–32 [16]	2–34 [16]	2.1–43 [16]	1.6–60	2.0–50	3.0–40	1.4–78	1.5–50 [115]	1.7–35

* expressed relative to 1:1 CRM-457 standardization
# defined by NACB guidelines [41]
[ ] literature citation, no manufacturer data

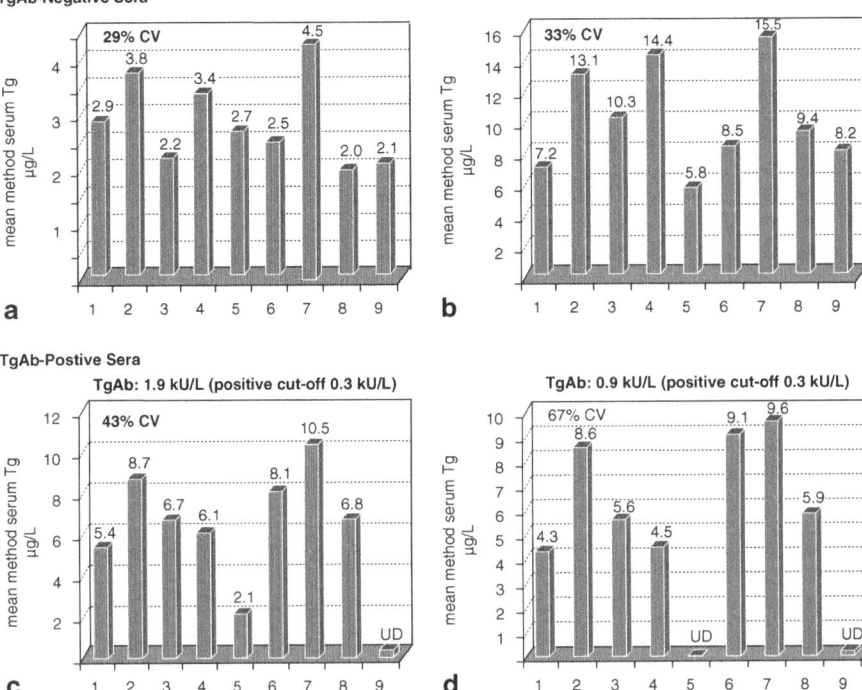

Fig. 7.2 Comparison of mean Tg values measured for sera from single donations measured by nine different Tg assays in 22 different laboratories (assays identified in Table 7.1). Sera **a** and **b** had no TgAb detected by any of three TgAb assays: Kronus/RSR, Siemens Immulite, and Beckman Access. Sera **c** and **d** had a low level of TgAb detected by Kronus/RSR; both were judged negative by the Access method and only **c** was judged marginally positive by Immulite TgAb. *UD* undetectable. (Data is taken from the UK NEQAS Thyroglobulin Surveys [www.birminghamquality. org.uk] and used with permission from Finlay MacKenzie [Program Director])

7.2.2 Methodologic Sensitivity

The adoption of IMA methodology for Tg measurement has not, in general, led to an improvement in assay sensitivity relative to RIA methodology. In fact, most current Tg assays (Table 7.1) are still only first generation in nature with functional sensitivities between 0.5 and 1.0 μg/L (ng/mL)—similar to that achieved with RIA methodology [16, 58]. Because first generation functional sensitivity is only marginally below the lower reference limit for euthyroid control subjects with intact thyroid glands (Table 7.1), such assays clearly have suboptimal sensitivity for detecting small amounts of persistent/recurrent tumor [16, 46]. The measurement of Tg following TSH (endogenous or rhTSH) stimulation has been used to overcome Tg assay insensitivity (see Sect. 7.6.4.2)—analogous to the use of TRH stimulation to overcome the insensitivity of the insensitive first generation TSH assays [44–46, 59]. Over the last decade, more sensitive second generation Tg IMA methods (functional sensitivities 0.05–0.1 µg/L [ng/mL]) have become available [39, 51, 57]. These more sensitive assays provide superior diagnostic potential for monitoring the trend in basal Tg measured without the need for expensive rhTSH stimulation (see Sect. 7.6.4.2) [42, 51, 57, 60–62].

Most laboratories adopt the manufacturer's information on assay sensitivity as the basis for setting the assay detection limit; however some manufacturers do not provide this data (Table 7.1) [40]. Generally assay information is presented in terms of analytical or functional sensitivity, or both [41]. Unfortunately, manufacturers tend to make exaggerated claims for the sensitivity of their products and fail to determine functional sensitivity according to established guidelines [41]. Furthermore, some manufacturers use descriptive terms such as "ultrasensitive" for marketing purposes, or only cite assay analytical sensitivity, a within-run precision that is clinically irrelevant [63].

Functional sensitivity is a clinically relevant parameter relating to the low-end between-run precision of the assay that is used to define the lower reporting limit [41]. Specifically, functional sensitivity is defined as the serum Tg value that can be measured with a between-run coefficient of variation of 20% with the following stipulations (http://www.aacc.org/members/nacb/LMPG/OnlineGuide/PublishedGuidelines/ThyroidDisease/Pages/default.aspx):

- Precision should be determined in TgAb-free human serum to eliminate matrix effects [40].
- The precision assessment should be made over a 6–12 month period to represent the clinical interval used for monitoring patients with DTC.
- At least two different lots of reagents and two instrument calibrators should be used when evaluating precision, because long-term precision is dependent on the consistency of the manufacturers's reagents.

Current American Thyroid Association and European Thyroid Association guidelines for managing patients with DTC suggest that an "undetectable" basal and rhTSH-stimulated Tg should be used as a parameter for assigning a disease-free status [45, 46]. However, the use of the term "undetectable" is problematic given the tenfold difference in functional sensitivity among current assays (Table 7.1). Specifically, patients with an "undetectable" Tg status using a first generation assay often have a low but detectable Tg when measured by a second generation assay [39, 42, 51].

7.2.3   Interferences

An unintended consequence of adopting IMA methodology for Tg measurement has been an exacerbation of the problem of both HAMA and TgAb interferences.

7.2.3.1 HAMA Interference with Serum Tg Measurement

Heterophile antibodies are human antibodies with specificities for animal immu-noglobulins. HAMA interference is caused by mouse antibodies in the specimen and is especially problematic for IMA methods that employ monoclonal antibodies (MAb) of murine origin [64, 65]. Patients who handle animals or receive mouse MAb for diagnostic imaging or medical therapy for malignancies are especially prone to develop HAMA [65, 66]. IMA methodology is based on noncompetitive binding of antigen by two antibody reagents (a capture and tracer antibody) tar-geted against different epitopes. Combinations of mono- and polyclonal antibodies are usually employed (Table 7.1). HAMA prevalences between 0.05 and 3.0% in patient blood samples have been reported [66, 67]. Manufacturers reduce the risk of HAMA interference by adding nonimmune mouse serum to their assay reagents, but this practice does not eliminate all HAMA interferences. When a serum Tg value appears inappropriately high or fails to respond appropriately to TSH changes (ris-ing with TSH stimulation and falling with TSH suppression), the physician should ask the laboratory to remeasure that specimen using a different manufacturer's method or rerun the specimen in a blocker tube (Scantibodies, Santee, CA, USA) [68]. Unfortunately, these approaches do not detect or eliminate all HAMA interfer-ences [70, 71].

Interference typically results when HAMA in the specimen interacts with both antibody reagents to create a false signal that simulates the presence of antigen (Tg) [67]. Rarely, HAMA can cause a false low result by blocking Tg from par-ticipating in antibody binding [67, 72]. In contrast, the competitive RIA format that uses high affinity polyclonal antibodies (often rabbit) is not influenced by HAMA [73]. Unrecognized HAMA interference has the potential to negatively impact patient care by prompting unnecessary imaging or radioiodine (RAI) treat-ment, or in the case of a falsely low Tg, mask the presence of persistent/recurrent disease [74].

7.2.3.2 TgAb Interference with Serum Tg Measurement

Because TgAb interference is the most common type of interference affecting serum Tg measurement, guidelines state that it is mandatory to measure TgAb in every specimen sent for Tg testing [41]. Although the propensity for interference is related to the TgAb concentration, high TgAb levels do not necessarily produce interfer-ence [26, 75]. Conversely, interference can result from low levels of TgAb that may be detected by one method but not another [16]. This is seen in panels (c) and (d) of Fig. 7.2 in which extreme between-method variability was observed (43% and 67% CV, respectively). Both specimens (c) and (d) had TgAb measured by three different methods (Kronus/RSR, Beckman Access, and Siemens Immulite). Both displayed a low level of TgAb when measured by Kronus/RSR, but both were nega-tive by Access. Immulite only detected a marginal level of TgAb in specimen (c). This emphasizes the method dependence of TgAb detection and that the potential for TgAb interference is multifactorial relating to the format of Tg assay used (IMA or RIA), the concentration of TgAb, and the affinity and specificity of that TgAb for both endogenous Tg and the assay reagent(s) [16, 76]. Conversely, some TgAb methodologies may report false low TgAb values because of interference by high concentrations of endogenous Tg in the specimen [77, 78].

When TgAb is present in a serum specimen, equilibria will develop between the endogenous entities (free Tg, TgAb, and Tg/TgAb immune complexes). During Tg measurement (either by IMA or RIA), these entities can interact with added Tg (i.e., tracer) and the antibody reagent(s) in an unpredictable way. The measurement of any single entity may be influenced by the presence of the other two in various ways: (1) immunobinding of an "irrelevant" entity by added reagents (e.g., ^{125}I-Tg tracer binding to endogenous TgAb), (2) displacement of binding of an added reagent (e.g., ^{125}I-Tg tracer) because of competition from the endogenous component already present (e.g., endogenous Tg), and (3) depending on the ability of the method to detect various epitopes, only free Tg, TgAb-complexed Tg, or TgAb may participate in the reaction [79].

The exogenous Tg recovery test approach has often been used to screen for TgAb. Although there is some correlation between the TgAb concentration and the potential for a low Tg recovery, many studies have now shown that recoveries are an unreliable way to detect TgAb [16, 26, 30, 41, 69, 80–82]. Three variables limit the validity of using the recovery of an exogenous Tg spike to detect TgAb [26]. First, there may be differences in the immunologic recognition of the Tg isoforms in the exogenous Tg (typically derived from nonneoplastic tissue) and endogenous Tg isoforms (secreted by tumor) [7, 11, 10]. Different Tg–TgAb complexes could result if the affinity of the exogenous versus endogenous Tg for the TgAb in that specimen differs. Second, recoveries are influenced by the relative concentrations of the endogenous Tg versus the exogenous Tg added to the specimen [26]. Often the concentration of the exogenous Tg spike is much higher than the concentration of the endogenous Tg, giving rise to a high concentration of free Tg and an overestimation of recovery. Third, it takes time for immune complexes involving large molecules like Tg to reach equilibrium [83]. Typically, recovery protocols add the exogenous Tg to the serum specimen immediately before the addition of assay reagents. Failure to allow the exogenous Tg to equilibrate with the endogenous Tg and TgAb has the potential to create a falsely high recovery [26]. Current guidelines recommend that Tg recoveries be discouraged and eliminated [41].

7.3   TgAb Measurements Used as a Surrogate Tumor Marker

Tg autoantibodies predominantly belong to the immunoglobulin G (IgG) subclass, are not complement fixing, and are generally conformational [14]. Over 20% of DTC patients have TgAb detected in their circulation as compared with ~11% of the general population [75, 80, 84–86]. All sera sent for Tg measurement require adjunctive

TgAb testing because a patient's TgAb status can change over time and even very low TgAb concentrations can interfere with Tg measurements [16, 41, 75, 80, 85, 87].

There has been growing recognition that serial TgAb levels can be monitored as a surrogate tumor marker, because TgAb concentrations respond to changes in circulating Tg antigen [14, 41, 75, 86, 88–90]. Specifically, patients who have TgAb detected at the time of their thyroidectomy and are rendered disease-free show declining TgAb levels that become undetectable over a median period of 3 years [89–91]. In contrast, patients with persistent/recurrent disease typically maintain detectable, and often exhibit rising, TgAb concentrations [75, 80, 85, 91]. Serial TgAb measurements can only be monitored if the same method is used (Fig. 7.2 panels (c) and (d)). This is because current TgAb tests differ in sensitivity and specificity and report qualitatively and quantitatively different values despite claiming standardization against the same International Reference Preparation (WHO 65/93) [16, 75, 92].

7.4   Tg mRNA as a Tumor Marker

Reverse transcription-polymerase chain reaction (RT-PCR) has been used to detect Tg mRNA in peripheral blood. The goal was to use Tg mRNA as a post-operative tumor marker that would not be subject to TgAb interference [93–101]. No correlation between Tg mRNA and serum Tg concentrations has been shown. Despite early reports of promise, subsequent studies have shown that Tg mRNA measurements lack optimal specificity and practicality to be clinically useful [95–97, 99, 102–108]. Specifically, Tg mRNA has been detected in a number of nonthyroidal tissues such as lymphocytes, leukocytes, and kidney and is no longer considered thyroid-specific [93, 98, 101, 109]. Additional problems include the use of primers that detect Tg splice variants, sample-handling techniques that introduce variability, and difficulties in quantifying the Tg mRNA detected [99, 110]. Whereas rhTSH administration has been shown to stimulate Tg mRNA, it is doubtful whether even this maneuver will increase the diagnostic utility of this test as compared with less expensive serum Tg measurements [111, 112]. The current consensus is that Tg mRNA testing is not clinically useful, even for patients with TgAb in whom Tg IMA measurements are compromised by interference.

7.5   The Clinical Utility of Tg Measurement when TgAb
Is Present

Circulating TgAb interferes with serum Tg measurements in a qualitative, quantitative, and method-dependent manner [30, 33, 75]. Interference with IMA methodology is always unidirectional (underestimation), whereas RIA methods have the potential to either under- or overestimate Tg depending on the affinity and specificity of the antibody reagents [16, 26, 29, 30, 32, 33, 75, 113, 114]. It appears that RIA methods quantify total Tg (free Tg + TgAb-complexed Tg), whereas IMA methods mainly detect the free Tg moeity. Unsuccessful attempts to overcome this interference have involved the development of multisite IMAs using selected MAbs having specificities for Tg epitopic domains different from those commonly involved in thyroid autoimmunity [90, 114, 115]. The failure of this approach suggests that steric inhibition might prevent the Tg that is complexed with TgAb from participating in the two-site, noncompetitive IMA reaction. Even if TgAb interference could be technically overcome, there is some evidence that Tg/TgAb complexes may have enhanced clearance relative to free Tg, resulting in lower total (free + TgAb-complexed) Tg levels in the presence of TgAb [114, 116, 117]. This might explain why the Tg response to TSH stimulation is typically blunted or absent in the presence of TgAb, irrespective of the class of Tg assay used [42]. Current guidelines recommend that IMA methodology not be used when TgAb is present, because falsely low/paradoxically undetectable Tg values can mask the presence of disease [16, 29, 41, 82, 114]. This interference is a serious flaw of IMA methodology because patients with persistent TgAb have an increased risk of having persistent/recurrent disease [82, 118].

When Tg is measured by both an IMA and RIA method, discordance between the values (low/undetectable Tg by IMA versus a detectable Tg by RIA) appears to indicate the presence of TgAb interference [62, 75, 119]. RIA methodology appears to be less prone to TgAb interference than IMA, but retains a propensity for TgAb to interfere if the first antibody reagent (usually a rabbit PAb) has low affinity and/or the specificity of second antibody fails to exclusively target rabbit in preference to human immunoglobulins [33, 120, 121]. Indications that some RIA methods report valid total Tg (free + TgAb-complexed) measurements are threefold. First, euthyroid subjects with intact thyroid glands and circulating TgAb have serum Tg values that fall appropriately within the assay reference range for TgAb-negative controls. In contrast, low/undetectable Tg values are reported for many of these same sera when measured by IMA methodology [16]. Second, appropriately high Tg RIA values have been reported for Graves' hyperthyroid patients [122]. In contrast, low or paradoxically undetectable Tg IMA values have been reported for Graves' patients with TgAb [114, 120]. Thirdly, DTC patients with documented disease and circulating TgAb often have a detectable Tg level measured by RIA, but a paradoxically undetectable Tg measured by IMA [75, 82].

Most laboratories favor the convenience of using IMA methodology. However, concerns for TgAb interference have prompted some laboratories to adopt a dual strategy for serum Tg measurement. Specifically, the TgAb status is first measured by a sensitive TgAb immunoassay. If TgAb is absent, serum Tg is measured by IMA, but if TgAb is present, serum Tg is measured by an RIA method. When no Tg RIA method is available, serial TgAb concentrations (measured by the same method) can be used as a surrogate tumor marker in preference to Tg IMA determinations [see Sect. 7.3].

7.6 The Clinical Utility of Tg Measurement when TgAb Is Absent

Tg measurement is primarily used as a post-operative tumor marker for managing patients with DTC (see Sect. 7.6.4). In addition, serum Tg measurement is sometimes useful for investigating certain nonneoplastic conditions (see Sect. 7.6.3).

7.6.1 Factors Influencing Circulating Tg Concentrations

Serum Tg concentrations reflect the net sum of three factors: (1) the mass of thyroid tissue present (normal, remnant, and/or tumor); (2) any inflammation of, or injury to, thyroid tissue, secondary to fine needle aspiration biopsy (FNAB), surgery, RAI therapy, or thyroiditis; and (3) the degree of TSH receptor stimulation (by endogenous or rhTSH, high levels of human chorionic gonadotropin (hCG), or the thyroid stimulating immunoglobulins of Graves' disease). These factors should all be considered when interpreting serum Tg concentrations.

1. *Thyroid mass*
   Serum Tg concentrations are increased in both simple and nodular goiter and many cases of thyroid neoplasia [123–126]. Conversely, a low or undetectable serum Tg is expected with thyroid agenesis, thyroid atrophy, and thyroidectomy. When thyroidectomized DTC patients have lymph node metastases, serum Tg concentrations correlate with lymph node mass and number [127]. However, lymph nodes are not very efficient Tg secretors and patients with a small lymph node burden may have a serum Tg below the detection limit of the first generation assays, even when rhTSH stimulation is used [128].

2. *Thyroid injury*
   Any source of thyroid injury—FNAB, thyroid surgery, RAI treatment, or thyroiditis—increases serum Tg concentrations. However, the temporal pattern of the Tg elevation and recovery to baseline will depend on the type of injury. Both thyroidectomy and FNAB produce an acute rise (hours) in Tg followed by a fairly rapid decline related to the half-life of circulating Tg (~3 days) and the healing of surgical margins [129, 130]. RAI produces a slower (days–weeks) rise in Tg secondary to radiolytic tissue damage with a slower resolution (months) [131]. The rise in serum Tg secondary to the inflammation associated with thyroiditis lasts the longest (~2 years) [132].

3. *TSH stimulation*
   The degree and chronicity of TSH receptor stimulation by TSH (endogenous and rhTSH), thyroid stimulating immunoglobulins (Graves' hyperthyroidism), and high hCG concentrations (first trimester pregnancy) increases Tg secretion. The magnitude of the change in serum Tg relates to the type and chronicity of the stimulus. TSH stimulation produces a 10–20-fold rise in serum Tg concentrations relative to baseline (see Sect. 7.6.4.2). In contrast, chronic thyroid

hormone suppression of TSH induces an ~50% reduction in serum Tg concentrations [133, 134]. As would be expected, the stimulating TSH receptor antibodies of Graves' hyperthyroidism result in high serum Tg concentrations (although TgAb interference can mask this elevation if an IMA method is used) [114, 122]. Because hCG shares some homology with TSH, the high hCG concentrations characteristic of first trimester pregnancy stimulate thyroid tissue and have the potential to raise serum Tg. Whereas the pregnancy-associated Tg rise is minimal for patients without DTC, a small Tg increase may be seen when monitoring pregnant DTC patients with a low serum Tg [135, 136]. Tg typically returns to baseline postpartum [137].

7.6.2   Serum Tg Reference Range

Tg assay reference ranges are typically established from a cohort of euthyroid TgAb-negative subjects. This range is only relevant to patients with an intact thyroid gland and does not apply to postoperative DTC management [41]. The average serum Tg reported for euthyroid subjects averages 10–13 µg/L (ng/mL) [42]. Given that such subjects have a thyroid volume approximating 10–15 g when iodine is sufficient, it is logical to predict that 1 g of normal thyroid tissue normally gives rises to approximately 1.0 µg/L (ng/mL) Tg in the circulation when TSH is not stimulated [137, 138]. Along these lines, the 1–2 g thyroid remnant typically left following near-total thyroidectomy would be expected to produce a serum Tg below 2.0 µg/L (ng/mL) in the absence of TSH stimulation, and below 10 µg/L (ng/mL) if endogenous TSH were high [46, 139]. The assay reference range only provides a useful benchmark if an adjustment is made for the influence of TSH (Sect. 7.6.1) and the degree of thyroid surgery. For example, the reference range should be reduced by 50% for patients who have had a lobectomy and have TSH within the reference range and a further 50% if such patients have chronic TSH suppression (Sect. 7.6.1) [41].

As seen in Table 7.1, Tg reference ranges differ among methods. CRM-457 standardization has not been universally adopted, and most assays have a functional sensitivity limit that is close to the lower reference limit. The broad variability in upper reference limits likely reflects assay specificity differences (see Sect. 7.2.1) and the rigor for selecting subjects without thyroid pathology.

As with other thyroid tests, serum Tg has a high index of individuality (IoI) [36, 140]. Broad between-method biases (Fig. 7.2 panels (a) and (b)) resulting from specificity differences exacerbated by standardization biases far exceed the narrow within-person biologic variability of serum Tg (~15%) [16, 36, 37]. Disruption of serial monitoring resulting from a change in Tg method can be ameliorated by archiving specimens for rebaselining Tg concentrations, should a change in method become necessary [41].

7.6.3   Serum Tg Measurements for Nonmalignant Thyroid Conditions

Although Tg measurement is primarily used as a tumor marker for DTC, serum Tg testing can sometimes be useful for evaluating nonmalignant thyroidal conditions.

7.6.3.1   Assessment of Population Iodine Status

Serum Tg concentrations are higher in areas of iodine deficiency as a reflection of endemic goiter [141]. Iodine deficiency is a worldwide problem responsible for goiter, intellectual deficiency, and in severe cases, hearing loss, neurological dysfunction, and cretinism [142] (discussed in depth in Chap. 3). Tg is conserved throughout vertebrates as the matrix for iodine storage because an adequate iodine supply is essential for thyroid hormone biosynthesis [143]. Given the interdependence between Tg, dietary iodine supply, and thyroid hormone biosynthesis, it is not surprising that the circulating Tg concentration provides a good marker of iodine status [143–145]. Measurements of urinary iodine are a relatively short-term indicator of dietary iodine intake, while the large reservoir of iodine stored in thyroid follicles as iodinated Tg acts as a buffer against short-term reductions in dietary iodine [146]. As a result, the within-person variability in serum Tg concentrations remains relatively narrow (~15%), facilitating the use of serum Tg as an integrated, biochemical readout of iodine sufficiency for population studies [36, 37, 145]. A recent technique to measure Tg in dried blood spots appears to hold promise as a way to monitor iodine intake in children [147].

7.6.3.2   Congenital Hypothyroidism

Congenital hypothyroidism is detected by neonatal screening in 1 in 3,000–4,000 neonates [2, 148] (discussed in Chap. 9). The prevalence is higher in some ethnic groups and is increased in iodine deficient regions of the world [149]. The majority of cases (80–85%) are thyroid developmental defects (thyroid dysgeneis), whereas 10–15% of cases arise from a spectrum of genetic defects that cause thyroid dyshormonogenesis [148]. Many of these defects result from autosomal recessive Tg gene mutations. Serum Tg measurement has become an important parameter for establishing the etiology of congenital hypothyroidism and, recently, rhTSH stimulated Tg testing has been used to confirm the diagnosis without thyroid hormone withdrawal [111, 150]. A low or undetectable Tg is characteristic of thyroid dysgenesis, whereas a high serum Tg suggests thyroid dyshormonogenesis [150, 151]. Thirty-five loss-of-function Tg mutations have been identified and associated with a range of phenotypes from mild to severe hypothyroidism [124, 152–154]. These mutations typically give rise to goiters that grow continuously, often to a remarkable size. Most commonly, individuals are homozygous for the mutation, although loss of function in both alleles can result from compound heterozygous mutations.

7.6.3.3 Thyrotoxicosis Factitia

Thyrotoxicosis factitia results from the intentional, unintentional, or accidental ingestion of excess thyroid hormone [155, 156]. Serum Tg measurement is the most useful biochemical test for distinguishing thyrotoxicosis factitia from endogenous causes of hyperthyroidism (Graves' disease, toxic multinodular goiter, or subacute thyroiditis). TSH is universally low in both exogenous and endogenous causes of thyrotoxicosis, whereas the low serum Tg characteristic of thyrotoxicosis factitia is in sharp contrast to the high Tg state seen with excess thyroid hormone secretion [157]. RAI uptakes have limited diagnostic value because low uptakes are characteristic of both thyrotoxicosis factitia and subacute thyroiditis [156, 158]. The degree of thyroid hormone(s) elevation relates to the source of the thyroid hormone ingested. Thyroid extract preparations or the unintentional ingestion of bovine thyroid tissue inadvertently included in neck trimmings ("hamburger thyrotoxicosis") can result in elevations in both thyroid hormones [156, 159]. Some dietary supplements contain triiodothyronine (T3) or triiodothyroacetic acid (Triac). These hormones have shorter half-lives than thyroxine and may be difficult to detect unless the specimen is drawn within hours of ingestion.

7.6.3.4 Subacute Thyroiditis

Tg is released into the circulation following thyroid injury caused by both acute and chronic thyroid inflammation. Serum Tg concentrations are elevated in patients with thyrotoxicosis caused by either subacute or silent (painless) thyroiditis, including postpartum thyroiditis and radiation thyroiditis [160, 161]. In both subacute and silent thyroiditis the duration of clinical symptoms is typically limited to several weeks, whereas it can take between 1 and 2 years for thyroid iodine stores and serum Tg concentrations to normalize [132, 161–163]. Most episodes of subacute thyroiditis are not associated with the development of thyroid autoantibodies, however, TgAb is commonly present in most cases of Hashimoto's or postpartum thyroiditis and these limit the clinical utility of Tg testing by IMA methodology (see Sect. 7.2.3.2).

7.6.3.5 Goiter

Patients with goiter of any etiology have high serum Tg concentrations that result from increased thyroid mass [123, 164–166]. In cases of multinodular goiter, serum Tg is inversely related to TSH and generally correlates with goiter size [126]. Because most cases of goiter result from iodine deficiency (see Sect. 7.6.3.1), the elevated Tg concentrations correlate with reduced iodine content and low intrathyroidal iodine stores and fall in response to iodine repletion [146, 167, 168]. Tg measurement can be used to assess the efficacy of surgical treatment for goiter. Conversely, serial Tg measurements can be used to monitor regrowth of the remnant over time [169].

7.6.4 Tg Measurement for Differentiated Thyroid Cancer

The thyroid-specific origin of Tg has led to its use as a tumor marker for the postoperative management of DTC [45, 46]. The expression of Tg and other thyroid-specific proteins correlate with the degree of differentiation of the tumor [170]. Patients with thyroid cancers frequently have a preoperative serum Tg concentration that is elevated above the reference range, the highest levels being observed with follicular > Hurthle > papillary > medullary cancers [125]. Despite this, the diagnostic work-up of a thyroid nodule does not include a serum Tg measurement because Tg elevations are not diagnostic for tumor and do not distinguish between patients with and without metastases [46, 125]. In contrast, recent retrospective studies suggest that the preoperative TSH is a biochemical marker for the risk of malignancy in a thyroid nodule, even across TSH concentrations within the reference range [171–173]. Thus, following a cytological diagnosis of DTC, a preoperative ultrasound, but not serum Tg measurement, is currently recommended by guidelines [46]. Despite this, some contend that the preoperative serum Tg may indicate the tumor's capacity for Tg secretion, provided that the preoperative specimen is drawn more than 2 weeks after the FNAB (see Sect. 7.6.1) [46, 130]. Specifically, preoperative Tg will be a sensitive tumor marker when the tumor is small and the preoperative Tg high, as contrasted with a large tumor but a low preoperative serum Tg, in which case there is a lack of evidence that the tumor has the capability for Tg secretion [170].

Early (2–6 months) postoperative Tg measurements are reported to have prognostic value—the higher the Tg, the greater the likelihood that persistent disease is present [48, 174–182]. However, the mere detection of Tg postoperatively does not distinguish between neoplastic and normal thyroid remnant as the source of Tg. When thyroid hormone therapy is initiated immediately following thyroidectomy to prevent the expected rise in TSH, the 1–2 g surgical remnant would be expected to give rise to a serum Tg ≤ 2.0 μg/L (ng/mL) (see Sect. 7.6.2 for rationale) [41, 139]. It is important to recognize that serum Tg may remain detectable even after RAI treatment, because RAI does not always completely eradicate all normal remnant tissue [183, 184]. Whether Tg is detected postoperatively will depend on the sensitivity and specificity of the Tg assay used (see Sect. 7.2.2). When the origin of the circulating Tg is normal tissue, the serum Tg concentration reflects the size of the surgical remnant and the degree of TSH stimulation. When persistent/recurrent tumor is present, the neoplastic Tg contribution will relate to the mass of tumor, the ability of that tumor to secrete Tg, the TSH sensitivity of that tumor tissue, and the ability of the assay to detect the neoplastic Tg isoforms secreted. These patient-specific variables together with differences in assay sensitivity and specificity (see Sects. 7.2.1 and 7.2.2) prevent the adoption of a universal serum Tg cutoff value with a high positive predictive value (PPV) for disease [181]. In contrast, studies have shown that the use of a rising Tg trend (measured with the same assay and under the same TSH conditions) has a higher PPV than that associated with the use of a fixed Tg cutoff [46, 48–50, 52, 55, 128, 185–187]. Ultrasound used in conjunction with Tg testing further improves PPV, whereas diagnostic RAI scanning (DxWBS) is now recognized as having low diagnostic sensitivity [46, 48, 49, 52, 128, 185–188].

7.6.4.1 Clinical Utility of Basal Tg Measured Without TSH Stimulation

Although the incidence of DTC has been increasing over the last two decades [189], tumor-related mortality, especially for papillary cancers diagnosed before age 40, remains low with only a minority of patients having persistent/recurrent disease detected during long-term follow-up [190, 191]. This necessitates that protocols used for postoperative DTC management have a high negative predictive value (NPV) in order to limit unnecessary testing and focus investigations on the minority of individuals at risk for disease. Patients with DTC are typically maintained on high doses of levothyroxine to suppress the trophic influence of TSH [46, 192–195]. Serum Tg shows a 5–20-fold rise above basal with either endogenous TSH stimulation or rhTSH administration [43]. In the absence of TSH stimulation, an "undetectable" Tg has a lower NPV than a comparable TSH-stimulated Tg measured by the same assay. Conversely, a "detectable" basal Tg has a higher PPV than a comparable Tg level measured under high TSH conditions [39, 43, 44]. When adopting "detectability" as a risk factor for disease, the use of a more sensitive second generation assay (Sect. 7.2.2) will obviously improve NPV at the expense of lowering the PPV (i.e., fewer false negatives and more false positives) [39, 51, 60, 61]. An increasing number of studies of second generation assay performance report that a basal Tg below 0.1 μg/L (ng/mL) obviates the need for rhTSH stimulation [39, 42, 51, 61, 62]. A current controversy relates to the interpretation of low but detectable basal Tg values (in the 0.1–1.0 μg/L (ng/mL) range) [60]. This dilemma can be overcome by evaluating the trend in basal Tg concentrations [46, 48–50, 52–57]. Because the efficacy of RAI treatment of low-risk patients has become controversial, there will be a growing number of patients in whom a nonneoplastic source of Tg would be expected to give rise to a low (usually clinically inconsequential) serum Tg detectable by second generation assay [46, 49, 50, 52, 57, 193, 196–202]. Such patients should be monitored using Tg trends and not Tg "detectability" [48, 49, 52, 57].

7.6.4.2 Clinical Utility of TSH-Stimulated Tg Measurements

The degree of differentiation of the tumor determines the presence of TSH receptors and the magnitude of the response to TSH stimulation [170, 203]. Most tumors respond to TSH by elevating serum Tg 5–20-fold above baseline [42, 43, 51]. This is why serum Tg is frequently measured under high TSH conditions (either following thyroid hormone withdrawal or after rhTSH administration) as a way to overcome first generation Tg assay insensitivity [43, 44, 46, 204]. Typically, chronic endogenous TSH stimulation increases serum Tg twofold higher than rhTSH stimulation [43, 46]. Studies report that a serum Tg below 2.0 µg/L (ng/mL) measured 72 hours after rhTSH has a high NPV (>95%) although an rhTSH-stimulated serum Tg below this cutoff does not guarantee the absence of tumor [43, 44, 46–48, 50, 51, 53, 55, 60, 178, 127, 128, 175, 178, 180, 205–207]. In contrast, the PPV of rhTSH-stimulated Tg values above 2.0 µg/L (ng/mL) only approximates 50%. This is in part because DTC has a low recurrence rate, but also reflects patient-specific variables, such as the size of the surgical remnant, and differences in tumor sensitivity to TSH compounded by assay sensitivity/standardization differences (Sects. 7.2.1 ad 7.2.2). In a metaanalysis of 784 DTC patients with rhTSH-stimulated Tg below 1.0 µg/L (ng/mL), 8.7% were found to have disease [44]. In most cases (5.4%) disease was local and would have likely been detected by ultrasound [44, 46, 128].

The low PPV and expense of rhTSH stimulation testing has prompted a debate concerning the necessity of using rhTSH-stimulated Tg measured by second generation assay [42, 51, 60–62]. Both bovine TSH and more recently rhTSH administration have demonstrated strong correlations (an approximate tenfold relationship) between basal and TSH-stimulated Tg (Fig. 7.3a) [42 ,51, 208, 209]. This relationship dictates that a basal Tg below 0.1 µg/L (ng/mL) will be highly predictive of a negative rhTSH-stimulated Tg response (below 2.0 µg/L [ng/mL] cutoff) (Fig. 7.3b) [39, 42, 43, 51, 57, 61, 62].

Current guidelines acknowledge that TSH-stimulated Tg testing is less sensitive than ultrasound for detecting small lymph node metastases [46, 53, 127, 128, 176,

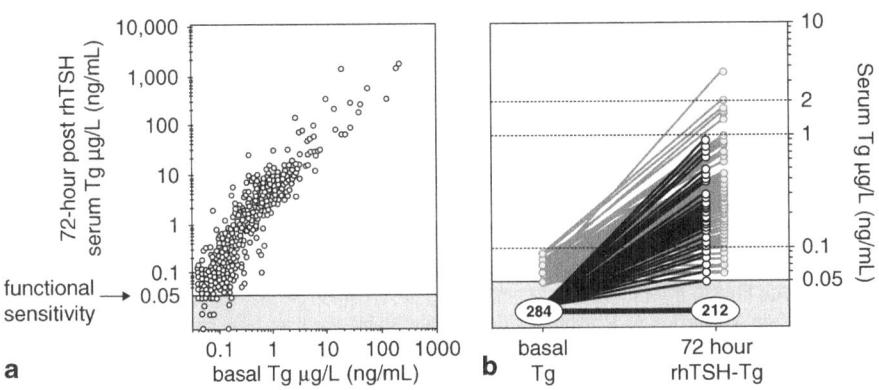

Fig. 7.3 a Correlation between basal Tg and 72-hour post rhTSH-stimulated Tg concentrations measured by a second generation Tg assay (Beckman Access) in sera from 950 DTC patients without TgAb detected (rhTSH − Tg = 17.6 × basal Tg − 12.9, r = 0.72, p < 0.0001). **b** Individual basal Tg and rhTSH-stimulated responses for the 384 patients with basal Tg below 0.1 µg/L (ng/mL). (Reproduced with permission from [42])

186]. In fact, TSH-stimulated Tg may fail to rise above 1.0 μg/L (ng/mL) when neoplastic foci are small, or even with some cases of distant metastases [53, 127, 128, 210]. Impaired TSH-stimulation could reflect either tumor dedifferentiation, a Tg method that did not have adequate specificity for the tumor-derived Tg isoforms (see Sect. 7.2.1), or interference by HAMA or TgAb (see Sects. 7.2.3.1 and 7.2.3.2) [72, 170]. In fact, when a serum Tg level appears inappropriate, or a detectable basal Tg fails to respond appropriately to TSH stimulation, the possibility of HAMA and/or TgAb (see Sects. 7.2.3.1 and 7.2.3.2) interference should be investigated.

7.6.4.3 Tg Measured in Cyst Fluid and FNAB Needle Washouts

Because Tg protein is tissue-specific, the detection of Tg in nonthyroidal tissues or fluids (such as pleural fluid) indicates metastatic thyroid cancer [211]. Struma ovarii is the only (rare) condition in which the source of Tg in the circulation is not from the thyroid [212]. Cystic thyroid nodules are commonly encountered in clinical practice, the large majority arising from follicular epithelium and the minority from parathyroid epithelium. A high concentration of Tg or parathyroid hormone (PTH) measured in the cyst fluid provides a reliable indicator of the tissue origin of the cyst that can often aid the decision for surgery [211]. Lymph node metastases are found in approximately 50% of patients with papillary cancers and 20% of follicular cancers [213, 214]. High-resolution ultrasound has now become an important component of protocols used for postoperative surveillance for recurrence [46]. Although ultrasound characteristics are helpful for distinguishing benign reactive lymph nodes from those suspected for malignancy, the finding of Tg in the needle washout of a lymph node biopsy has higher diagnostic accuracy than the ultrasound appearance [215–219]. The current protocol recommends rinsing the needle in 1.0 mL of saline and sending this specimen to the laboratory for Tg analysis. This procedure is now widely accepted as a useful adjunctive test for improving the diagnostic sensitivity of the cytological evaluation of a suspicious lymph node or thyroid mass [216–219].

References

1. van de Graaf SA, Ris-Stalpers C, Pauws E, Mendive FM, Targovnik HM, de Vijlder JJ. Up to date with human thyroglobulin. *J Endocrinol.* 2001;170:307-321.
2. De Felice M, Di Lauro R. Thyroid development and its disorders: genetics and molecular mechanisms. *Endocr Rev.* 2004;25:722-746.
3. Lin JD. Thyroglobulin and human thyroid cancer. *Clin Chim Acta.* 2008;338:15-21.
4. Lee J, Di Jeso B, Arvan P. The cholinesterase-like domain of thyroglobulin functions as an intramolecular chaperone. *J Clin Invest.* 2008;118:2950-2958.
5. Arvan P, Kim PS, Kuliawat R, et al. Intracellular protein transport to the thyrocyte plasma membrane: potential implications for thyroid physiology. *Thyroid.* 1997;7:89-105.
6. Di Jeso B, Ulianich L, Pacifico F, et al. Folding of thyroglobulin in the calnexin/calreticulin pathway and its alteration by loss of Ca2+ from the endoplasmic reticulum. *Biochem J.* 2003;370:449-458.

7. Kim PS, Dunn AD, Dunn JT. Altered immunoreactivity of thyroglobulin in thyroid disease. *J Clin Endocrinol Metab.* 1988;67:161-168.

8. Schneider A, Ikekubo K, Kuma K. Iodine content of serum thyroglobulin in normal individuals and patients with thyroid tumors. *J Clin Endocrinol Metab.* 1983;57:1251-1256.

9. Gérard AC, Daumerie C, Mestdagh C, et al. Correlation between the loss of thyroglobulin iodination and the expression of thyroid-specific proteins involved in iodine metabolism in thyroid carcinomas. *J Clin Endocrinol Metab.* 2003;88:4977-4983.

10. de Micco C, Ruf J, Carayon P, Christian MA, Henry JF, Toga M. Immunohistochemical study of thyroglobulin in thyroid carcinomas with monoclonal antibodies. *Cancer.* 1987;59:471-476.

11. Schulz R, Bethauser H, Stempka L, Heilig B, Moll A, Hufner M. Evidence for immunological differences between circulating and tissue-derived thyroglobulin in men. *Eur J Clin Invest.* 1989;19:459-463.

12. Shimizu K, Nakamura K, Kobatake S, et al. The clinical utility of Lens culinaris agglutinin-reactive thyroglobulin ratio in serum for distinguishing benign from malignant conditions of the thyroid. *Clin Chim Acta.* 2007;379:101-104.

13. Emoto N, Kunii YK, Ashizawa M, et al. Reduced sulfation of chondroitin sulfate in thyroglobulin derived from human papillary thyroid carcinomas. *Cancer Sci.* 2007;98:1577-1581.

14. McLachlan SM, Rapoport B. Why measure thyroglobulin autoantibodies rather than thyroid peroxidase autoantibodies. *Thyroid.* 2004;14:510-520.

15. Prentice L, Kiso Y, Fukuma N, et al. Monoclonal thyroglobulin autoantibodies: variable region analysis and epitope recognition. *J Clin Endocrinol Metab.* 1995;80:977-986.

16. Spencer CA, Bergoglio LM, Kazarosyan M, Fatemi S, LoPresti JS. Clinical impact of thyroglobulin (Tg) and Tg autoantibody method differences on the management of patients with differentiated thyroid carcinomas. *J Clin Endocrinol Metab.* 2005;90:5566-5575.

17. Morell AG, Gregoriadis G, Scheinberg IH, Hickman J, Ashwell G. The role of sialic acid in determining the survival of glycoproteins in the circulation. *J Biol Chem.* 1971;246:1461-1467.

18. Sinadinovic J, Cvejic D, Savin S, Jancic-Zuguricas M, Micic JV. Altered terminal glycosylation of thyroglobulin in papillary thyroid carcinoma. *Exp Clin Endocrinol.* 1992;100:124-128.

19. Bastiani P, Papandreou MJ, Blanck O, Fenouillet E, Thibault V, Miquelis R. On the relationship between completion of N-acetyllactosamine oligosaccharide units and iodine content of thyroglobulin: a reinvestigation. *Endocrinology.* 1995;136:4204-4209.

20. Feldt-Rasmussen U. Serum thyroglobulin and thyroglobulin autoantibodies in thyroid diseases. Pathogenic and diagnostic aspects. *Allergy.* 1983;38:369-387.

21. Jeevanram RK, Shah DH, Sharma SM, Ganatra RD. Disappearance rate of endogenously radioiodinated thyroglobulin and thyroxine after radioiodine treatment. *Cancer.* 1982;49:2281-2284.

22. Hocevar M, Auersperg M, Stanovnik L. The dynamics of serum thyroglobulin elimination from the body after thyroid surgery. *Eur J Surg Oncol.* 1997;23:208-210.

23. Ikekubo K, Pervos R, Schneider AB. Clearance of normal and tumor-related thyroglobulin from the circulation of rats: role of the terminal sialic acid residues. *Metabolism.* 1980;29:673-681.

24. Magro G, Perissinotto D, Schiappacassi M, et al. Proteomic and postproteomic characterization of keratan sulfate-glycanated isoforms of thyroglobulin and transferrin uniquely elaborated by papillary thyroid carcinomas. *Am J Pathol.* 2003;163:183-196.

25. Cole TG, Johnson D, Eveland BJ, Nahm MH. Cost-effective method for detection of "hook effect" in tumor marker immunometric assays. *Clin Chem.* 1993;39:695-696.

26. Spencer CA, Takeuchi M, Kazarosyan M. Current status and performance goals for serum thyroglobulin assays. *Clin Chem.* 1996;42:164-173.

27. Schofl C, Schofl-Siegert B, Karstens JH, et al. Falsely low serum prolactin in two cases of invasive macroprolactinoma. *Pituitary.* 2002;5:261-265.

28. Morgenthaler NG, Froehlich J, Rendl J, et al. Technical evaluation of a new immunoradiometric and a new immunoluminometric assay for thyroglobulin. *Clin Chem.* 2002;48:1077-1083.

29. Feldt-Rasmussen U, Schlumberger M. European interlaboratory comparison of serum thyroglobulin measurement. *J Endocrinol Invest.* 1988;11:175-181.

30. Schaadt B, Feldt-Rasmussen U, Rasmussen B, et al. Assessment of the influence of thyroglobulin (Tg) autoantibodies and other interfering factors on the use of serum Tg as tumor marker in differentiated thyroid carcinoma. *Thyroid.* 1995;5:165-170.

31. Kato R, Maruyama M, Sekino T, Kasuga Y. A new assay for thyroglobulin concentration in serum using monoclonal antibodies against synthetic peptides. *Clin Chim Acta.* 2000;298: 69-84.

32. Weightman DR, Mallick UK, Fenwick JD, et al. Discordant serum thyroglobulin results generated by two classes of assay in patients with thyroid carcinoma: correlation with clinical outcome after 3 years of follow-up. *Cancer.* 2003;98:41-47.

33. Schneider AB, Pervos R. Radioimmunoassay of human thyroglobulin: effect of antithyroglobulin autoantibodies. *J Clin Endocrinol Metab.* 1978;47:126-137.

34. Feldt-Rasmussen U, Profilis C, Colinet E, et al. Human thyroglobulin reference material (CRM 457) 1st part: assessment of homogeneity, stability and immunoreactivity. *Ann Biol Clin (Paris).* 1996;54:337-342.

35. Iervasi A, Iervasi G, Carpi A, Zucchelli GC. Serum thyroglobulin measurement: clinical background and main methodological aspects with clinical impact. *Biomed Pharmacother.* 2006;60:414-424.

36. Jensen E, Petersen PH, Blaabjerg O, Hegedus L. Biological variation of thyroid autoantibodies and thyroglobulin. *Clin Chem Lab Med.* 2007;45:1058-1064.

37. Feldt-Rasmussen U, Petersen PH, Blaabjerg O, Horder M. Long-term variability in serum thyroglobulin and thyroid related hormones in healthy subjects. *Acta Endocrinol (Copenhagen).* 1980;95:328-334.

38. Ferrari L, Biancolini D, Seregni E, et al. Critical aspects of immunoradiometric thyroglobulin assays. *Tumori.* 2003;89:537-539.

39. Schlumberger M, Hitzel A, Toubert ME, et al. Comparison of seven serum thyroglobulin assays in the follow-up of papillary and follicular thyroid cancer patients. *J Clin Endocrinol Metab.* 2007;92:2487-2495.

40. Ross HA, Netea-Maier RT, Schakenraad E, Bravenboer B, Hermus AR, Sweep FC. Assay bias may invalidate decision limits and affect comparability of serum thyroglobulin assay methods: an approach to reduce interpretation differences. *Clin Chim Acta.* 2008;394:104-109.

41. Baloch Z, Carayon P, Conte-Devolx B, et al. Laboratory medicine practice guidelines: laboratory support for the diagnosis and monitoring of thyroid disease. *Thyroid.* 2003;13:57-67.

42. Spencer CA, Lopresti JS. Measuring thyroglobulin and thyroglobulin autoantibody in patients with differentiated thyroid cancer. *Nat Clin Pract Endocrinol Metab.* 2008;4:223-233.

43. Haugen BR, Ladenson PW, Cooper DS, et al. A comparison of recombinant human thyrotropin and thyroid hormone withdrawal for the detection of thyroid remnant or cancer. *J Clin Endocrinol Metab.* 1999;84:3877-3885.

44. Mazzaferri EL, Robbins RJ, Spencer CA, et al. A consensus report of the role of serum thyroglobulin as a monitoring method for low-risk patients with papillary thyroid carcinoma. *J Clin Endocrinol Metab.* 2003;88:1433-1441.

45. Pacini F, Schlumberger M, Dralle H, et al. European consensus for the management of patients with differentiated thyroid carcinoma of the follicular epithelium. *Eur J Endocrinol.* 2006;154:787-803.

46. Cooper DS, Doherty GM, Haugen BR, et al. Management guidelines for patients with thyroid nodules and differentiated thyroid cancer. The American Thyroid Association Guidelines Taskforce. *Thyroid.* 2006;16:109-142.

47. Giovanella L, Ceriani L, Ghelfo A, et al. Thyroglobulin assay during thyroxine treatment in low-risk differentiated thyroid cancer management: comparison with recombinant human thyrotropin-stimulated assay and imaging procedures. *Clin Chem Lab Med.* 2006;44:648-652.

48. Giovanella L, Ceriani L, Suriano S, Ghelfo A, Maffioli M. Thyroglobulin measurement before rhTSH-aided 131-I ablation in detecting metastases from differentiated thyroid carcinoma. *Clin Endocrinol (Oxford).* 2008;68:659-663.

49. Baudin E, Do Cao C, Cailleux AF, Leboulleux S, Travagli JP, Schlumberger M. Positive predictive value of serum thyroglobulin levels, measured during the first year of follow-

up after thyroid hormone withdrawal, in thyroid cancer patients. *J Clin Endocrinol Metab.* 2003;88:1107-1111.

50. Schaap J, Eustatia-Rutten CF, Stokkel M, et al. Does radioiodine therapy have disadvantageous effects in non-iodine accumulating differentiated thyroid carcinoma. *Clin Endocrinol (Oxford).* 2002;57:117-124.

51. Iervasi A, Iervasi G, Ferdeghini M, et al. Clinical relevance of highly sensitive Tg assay in monitoring patients treated for differentiated thyroid cancer. *Clin Endocrinol (Oxford).* 2007;67:434-441.

52. Tuttle RM, Leboeuf R. Follow up approaches in thyroid cancer: a risk adapted paradigm. *Endocrinol Metab Clin North Am.* 2008;37:419-435.

53. Huang SH, Wang PW, Huang YE, et al. Sequential follow-up of serum thyroglobulin and whole body scan in thyroid cancer patients without initial metastasis. *Thyroid.* 2006;16:1273-1278.

54. Pacini F, Agate L, Elisei R, et al. Outcome of differentiated thyroid cancer with detectable serum Tg and negative diagnostic 131-I whole body scan: comparison of patients treated with high 131-I activities versus untreated patients. *J Clin Endocrinol Metab.* 2001;86:4092-4097.

55. Valadão MM, Rosário PW, Borges MA, et al. Positive predictive value of detectable stimulated tg during the first year after therapy of thyroid cancer and the value of comparison with Tg-ablation and Tg measured after 24 months. *Thyroid.* 2006;16:1145-1149.

56. Rosario P, Borges M, Reis J, Alves MF. Effect of suppressive therapy with levothyroxine on the reduction of serum thyroglobulin after total thyroidectomy. *Thyroid.* 2006;16:199-200.

57. Zophel K, Wunderlich G, Smith BR. Serum thyroglobulin measurements with a high sensitivity enzyme-linked immunosorbent assay: is there a clinical benefit in patients with differentiated thyroid carcinoma? *Thyroid.* 2003;13:861-865.

58. Van Herle AJ, Uller RP, Matthews NI, Brown J. Radioimmunoassay for measurement of thyroglobulin in human serum. *J Clin Invest.* 1973;52:1320-1327.

59. Spencer CA, LoPresti JS, Patel A, et al. Applications of a new chemiluminometric thyrotropin assay to subnormal measurement. *J Clin Endocrinol Metab.* 1990;70:453-460.

60. Mazzaferri EL. Will highly sensitive thyroglobulin assays change the management of thyroid cancer? *Clin Endocrinol (Oxford).* 2007;67:321-323.

61. Smallridge RC, Meek SE, Morgan MA, et al. Monitoring thyroglobulin in a sensitive immunoassay has comparable sensitivity to recombinant human tsh-stimulated thyroglobulin in follow-up of thyroid cancer patients. *J Clin Endocrinol Metab.* 2007;92:82-87.

62. Rosario PW, Purisch S. Does a highly sensitive thyroglobulin (Tg) assay change the clinical management of low-risk patients with thyroid cancer with Tg on T4 < 1 ng/ml determined by traditional assays? *Clin Endocrinol (Oxford).* 2008;68:338-342.

63. Rodbard D. Statistical estimation of the minimal detectable concentration ("sensitivity") for radioligand assays. *Anal Biochem.* 1978;90:1-12.

64. Després N, Grant AM. Antibody interference in thyroid assays: a potential for clinical misinformation. *Clin Chem.* 1998;44:440-454.

65. Kricka LJ. Human anti-animal antibody interferences in immunological assays. *Clin Chem.* 1999;45:942-956.

66. Choi WW, Srivatsa S, Ritchie JC. Aberrant thyroid testing results in a clinically euthyroid patient who had received a tumor vaccine. *Clin Chem.* 2005;51:673-675.

67. Ismail AAA, Walker PL, Cawood ML, Barth JH. Interference in immunoassay is an underestimated problem. *Ann Clin Biochem.* 2002;39:366-373.

68. Preissner CM, O'Kane DJ, Singh RJ, Morris JC, Grebe SK. Phantoms in the assay tube: heterophile antibody interferences in serum thyroglobulin assays. *J Clin Endocrinol Metab.* 2003;88:3069-3074.

69. Massart C, Corcuff JB, Bordenave L. False-positive results corrected by the use of heterophilic antibody-blocking reagent in thyroglobulin immunoassays. *Clin Chim Acta.* 2008;388:211-213.

70. Boscato LM, Stuart MC. Incidence and specificity of interference in two-site immunoassays. *Clin Chem.* 1986;32:1491-1495.

71. Tan MJ, Tan F, Hawkins R, Mukherjee JJ. A hyperthyroid patient with measurable thyroid-stimulating hormone concentration—a trap for the unwary. *Ann Acad Med Singapore.* 2006;35:500-503.

72. Giovanella L, Ghelfo A. Undetectable serum thyroglobulin due to negative interference of heterophile antibodies in relapsing thyroid carcinoma. *Clin Chem.* 2007;53:1871-1872.

73. Levinson SS, Miller JJ. Towards a better understanding of heterophile (and the like) antibody interference with modern immunoassays. *Clin Chim Acta.* 2002;325:1-15.

74. Rotmensch S, Cole LA. False diagnosis and needless therapy of presumed malignant disease in women with false-positive human chorionic gonadotropin concentrations. *Lancet.* 2000;355:712-715.

75. Spencer CA, Takeuchi M, Kazarosyan M, et al. Serum thyroglobulin autoantibodies: prevalence, influence on serum thyroglobulin measurement and prognostic significance in patients with differentiated thyroid carcinoma. *J Clin Endocrinol Metab.* 1998;83:1121-1127.

76. Benvenga S, Burek CL, Talor M, Rose NR, Trimarchi F. Heterogeneity of the thyroglobulin epitopes associated with circulating thyroid hormone autoantibodies in hashimoto's thyroiditis and non-autoimmune thyroid diseases. *J Endocrinol Invest.* 2002;25:977-982.

77. Pinchera A, Mariotti S, Vitti P, et al. Interference of serum thyroglobulin in the radioassay for serum antithyroglobulin antibodies. *J Clin Endocrinol Metab.* 1977;45:1077-1088.

78. Feldt-Rasmussen U, Høier-Madsen M, Hansen HS, Blichert-Toft M. Comparison between homogeneous phase radioassay and enzyme-linked immunosorbent assay for measurement of antithyroglobulin antibody content in serum. *Acta Pathol Microbiol Immunol Scand.* 1986;94:33-38.

79. Feldt-Rasmussen U. Serum thyroglobulin and thyroglobulin autoantibodies in thyroid diseases. pathogenetic and diagnostic aspects. *Allergy.* 1983;38:369-387.

80. Görges R, Maniecki M, Jentzen W, et al. Development and clinical impact of thyroglobulin antibodies in patients with differentiated thyroid carcinoma during the first 3 years after thyroidectomy. *Eur J Endocrinol.* 2005;153:49-55.

81. Sapin R, Gasser F, Chambron J. Recovery determination in 600 sera analyzed for thyroglobulin with a recently commercialized IRMA kit. *Clin Chem.* 1992;38:1920-1921.

82. Okosieme OE, Evans C, Moss L, Parkes AB, Premawardhana LD, Lazarus JH. Thyroglobulin antibodies in serum of patients with differentiated thyroid cancer: relationship between epitope specificities and thyroglobulin recovery. *Clin Chem.* 2005;51:729-734.

83. Ratcliffe JG, Ayoub LA, Pearson D. The measurement of serum thyroglobulin in the presence of thyroglobulin antibodies. *Clin Endocrinol (Oxford).* 1981;15:507-518.

84. Hollowell JG, Staehling NW, Hannon WH, et al. Serum thyrotropin, thyroxine, and thyroid antibodies in the United States population (1988 to 1994): NHANES III. *J Clin Endocrinol Metab.* 2002;87:489-499.

85. Chung JK, Park YJ, Kim TY, et al. Clinical significance of elevated level of serum antithyroglobulin antibody in patients with differentiated thyroid cancer after thyroid ablation. *Clin Endocrinol (Oxford).* 2002;57:215-221.

86. Pacini F, Mariotti S, Formica N, et al. Thyroid autoantibodies in thyroid cancer: incidence and relationship with tumour outcome. *Acta Endocrinol (Copenhagen).* 1988;119:373-380.

87. Cubero JM, Rodríguez-Espinosa J, Gelpi C, Estorch M, Corcoy R. Thyroglobulin autoantibody levels below the cut-off for positivity can interfere with thyroglobulin measurement. *Thyroid.* 2003;13:659-661.

88. Küçük ON, Aras G, Kulak HA, et al. Clinical importance of anti-thyroglobulin auto-antibodies in patients with differentiated thyroid carcinoma: comparison with 99mTc-MIBI scans. *Nucl Med Commun.* 2006;27:873-876.

89. Chiovato L, Latrofa F, Braverman LE, et al. Disappearance of humoral thyroid autoimmunity after complete removal of thyroid antigens. *Ann Intern Med.* 2003;139:346-351.

90. Thomas D, Liakos V, Vassiliou E, Hatzimarkou F, Tsatsoulis A, Kaldrimides P. Possible reasons for different pattern disappearance of thyroglobulin and thyroid peroxidase autoantibodies in patients with differentiated thyroid carcinoma following total thyroidectomy and iodine-131 ablation. *J Endocrinol Invest.* 2007;30:173-180.

91. Rubello D, Casara D, Girelli ME, Piccolo M, Busnardo B. Clinical meaning of circulating antithyroglobulin antibodies in differentiated thyroid cancer: a prospective study. *J Nucl Med.* 1992;33:1478-1480.

92. Sapin R, d'Herbomez M, Gasser F, Meyer L, Schlienger JL. Increased sensitivity of a new assay for anti-thyroglobulin antibody detection in patients with autoimmune thyroid disease. *Clin Biochem.* 2003;36:611-616.

93. Sellitti DF, Akamizu T, Doi SQ, et al. Renal expression of two 'thyroid-specific' genes: thyrotropin receptor and thyroglobulin. *Exp Nephrol.* 2000;8:235-243.

94. Barzon L, Boscaro M, Pacenti M, Taccaliti A, Palu G. Evaluation of circulating thyroid-specific transcripts as markers of thyroid cancer relapse. *Int J Cancer.* 2004;110:914-920.

95. Eszlinger M, Neumann S, Otto L, Paschke R. Thyroglobulin mRNA quantification in the peripheral blood is not a reliable marker for the follow-up of patients with differentiated thyroid cancer. *Eur J Endocrinol.* 2002;147:575-582.

96. Grammatopoulos D, Elliott Y, Smith SC, et al. Measurement of thyroglobulin mRNA in peripheral blood as an adjunctive test for monitoring thyroid cancer. *Mol Pathol.* 2003;56:162-166.

97. Elisei R, Vivaldi A, Agate L, et al. Low specificity of blood thyroglobulin messenger ribonucleic acid assay prevents its use in the follow-up of differentiated thyroid cancer patients. *J Clin Endocrinol Metab.* 2004;89:33-39.

98. Kaufmann S, Schmutzler C, Schomburg L, et al. Real time RT-PCR analysis of thyroglobulin mRNA in peripheral blood in patients with congenital athyreosis and with differentiated thyroid carcinoma after stimulation with recombinant human thyrotropin. *Endocr Regul.* 2004;38:41-49.

99. Ringel MD. Editorial: molecular detection of thyroid cancer: differentiating "signal" and "noise" in clinical assays. *J Clin Endocrinol Metab.* 2004;89:29-32.

100. Verburg FA, Lips CJ, Lentjes EG, de Klerk JM. Detection of circulating Tg-mRNA in the follow-up of papillary and follicular thyroid cancer: how useful is it? *Br J Cancer.* 2004;91:200-204.

101. Amakawa M, Kato R, Kameko F, Maruyama M,Tajiri J. Thyroglobulin mRNA expression in peripheral blood lymphocytes of healthy subjects and patients with thyroid disease. *Clin Chim Acta.* 2008;390:97-103.

102. Tallini G, Ghossein RA, Emanuel J, et al. Detection of thyroglobulin, thyroid peroxidase, and RET/PTC1 mRNA transcripts in the peripheral blood of patients with thyroid disease. *J Clin Oncol.* 1998;16:1158-1166.

103. Ringel MD, Balducci-Silano PL, Anderson JS, et al. Quantitative reverse transcription-polymerase chain reaction of circulating thyroglobulin messenger ribonucleic acid for monitoring patients with thyroid carcinoma. *J Clin Endocrinol Metab.* 1999;84:4037-4042.

104. Bellantone R, Lombardi CP, Bossola M, et al. Validity of thyroglobulin mRNA assay in peripheral blood of postoperative thyroid carcinoma patients in predicting tumor recurrences varies according to the histologic type: results of a prospective study. *Cancer.* 2001;92:2273-2279.

105. Chinnappa P, Taguba L, Arciaga R, et al. Detection of thyrotropin-receptor messenger ribonucleic acid (mRNA) and thyroglobulin mRNA transcripts in peripheral blood of patients with thyroid disease: sensitive and specific markers for thyroid cancer. *J Clin Endocrinol Metab.* 2004;89:3705-3709.

106. Lombardi CP, Bossola M, Princi P, et al. Circulating thyroglobulin mRNA does not predict early and midterm recurrences in patients undergoing thyroidectomy for cancer. *Am J Surg.* 2008;196:326-332.

107. Takano T, Miyauchi A, Yoshida H, Hasegawa Y, Kuma K, Amino N. Quantitative measurement of thyroglobulin mRNA in peripheral blood of patients after total thyroidectomy. *Br J Cancer.* 2001;85:102-106.

108. Span PN, Sleegers MJ, van den Broek WJ, et al. Quantitative detection of peripheral thyroglobulin mRNA has limited clinical value in the follow-up of thyroid cancer patients. *Ann Clin Biochem.* 2003;40:94-99.

109. Bojunga J, Röddiger S, Stanisch M, et al. Molecular detection of thyroglobulin mRNA transcripts in peripheral blood of patients with thyroid disease by RT-PCR. *Br J Cancer.* 2000;82:1650-1655.

110. Savagner F, Rodien P, Reynier P, Rohmer V, Bigorgne JC, Malthiery Y. Analysis of Tg transcripts by real-time RT-PCR in the blood of thyroid cancer patients. *J Clin Endocrinol Metab.* 2002;87:635-639.

111. Fugazzola L, Persani L, Mannavola D, et al. Recombinant human TSH testing is a valuable tool for differential diagnosis of congenital hypothyroidism during L-thyroxine replacement. *Clin Endocrinol (Oxford).* 2003;59:230-236.

112. Rubio IG, Silva MN, Knobel M, et al. Peripheral blood levels of thyroglobulin mRNA and serum thyroglobulin concentrations after radioiodine ablation of multinodular goiter with or without pre-treatment with recombinant human thyrotropin. *J Endocrinol Invest.* 2007;30:535-540.

113. Jahagirdar VR, Strouhal P, Holder G, Gama R, Singh BM. Thyrotoxicosis factitia masquerading as recurrent Graves' disease: endogenous antibody immunoassay interference, a pitfall for the unwary. *Ann Clin Biochem.* 2008;45:325-327.

114. Mariotti S, Barbesino G, Caturegli P, et al. Assay of thyroglobulin in serum with thyroglobulin autoantibodies: an unobtainable goal? *J Clin Endocrinol Metab.* 1995;80:468-472.

115. Marquet PY, Daver A, Sapin R, et al. Highly sensitive immunoradiometric assay for serum thyroglobulin with minimal interference from autoantibodies. *Clin Chem.* 1996;42:258-262.

116. Weigle WO, High GJ. The behaviour of autologous thyroglobulin in the circulation of rabbits immunized with either heterologous or altered homologous thyroglobulin. *J Immunol.* 1967;98:1105-1114.

117. Feldt-Rasmussen U, Petersen PH, Date J, Madse CM. Sequential changes in serum thyroglobulin (Tg) and its autoantibodies (TgAb) following subtotal thyroidectomy of patients with preoperatively detectable TgAb. *Clin Endocrinol (Oxford).* 1980;12:29-38.

118. Hjiyiannakis P, Mundy J, Harmer C. Thyroglobulin antibodies in differentiated thyroid cancer. *Clin Oncol.* 1999;11:240-244.

119. Clark PM, Beckett G. Can we measure serum thyroglobulin? *Ann Clin Biochem.* 2002;39: 196-202.

120. Black EG, Hoffenberg R. Should one measure serum thyroglobulin in the presence of antithyroglobulin antibodies? *Clin Endocrinol (Oxford).* 1983;19:597-601.

121. Feldt-Rasmussen U, Rasmussen AK. Serum thyroglobulin (Tg) in presence of thyroglobulin autoantibodies (TgAb). Clinical and methodological relevance of the interaction between Tg and TgAb in vitro and in vivo. *J Endocrinol Invest.* 1985;8:571-576.

122. Uller RP, Van Herle AJ. Effect of therapy on serum thyroglobulin levels in patients with Graves' disease. *J Clin Endocrinol Metab.* 1978;46:747-755.

123. Fenzi GF, Ceccarelli C, Macchia E, et al. Reciprocal changes of serum thyroglobulin and TSH in residents of a moderate endemic goitre area. *Clin Endocrinol (Oxford).* 1985;23:115-122.

124. Pardo V, Rubio IG, Knobel M, et al. Phenotypic variation among four family members with congenital hypothyroidism caused by two distinct thyroglobulin gene mutations. *Thyroid.* 2008;18:783-786.

125. Ericsson UB, Tegler L, Lennquist S, Borup Christensen S, Stahl E, Thorell JI. Serum thyroglobulin in differentiated thyroid carcinoma. *Acta Chir Scand.* 1984;150:367-375.

126. Berghout A, Wiersinga WM, Smits NJ, Touber JL. Interrelationships between age, thyroid volume, thyroid nodularity, and thyroid function in patients with sporadic nontoxic goiter. *Am J Med.* 1990;89:602-608.

127. Bachelot A, Cailleux AF, Klain M, et al. Relationship between tumor burden and serum thyroglobulin level in patients with papillary and follicular thyroid carcinoma. *Thyroid.* 2002;12:707-711.

128. Pacini F, Molinaro E, Castagna MG, et al. Recombinant human thyrotropin-stimulated serum thyroglobulin combined with neck ultrasonography has the highest sensitivity in monitoring differentiated thyroid carcinoma. *J Clin Endocrinol Metab.* 2003;88:3668-3673.

129. Feldt-Rasmussen U, Petersen PH, Date J, Madsen CM. Serum thyroglobulin in patients undergoing subtotal thyroidectomy for toxic and nontoxic goiter. *J Endorinol Invest.* 1982;5:161-164.

130. Luboshitzky R, Lavi I, Ishay A. Serum thyroglobulin levels after fine-needle aspiration of thyroid nodules. *Endocr Pract.* 2006;12:264-269.

131. Feldt-Rasmussen U, Bech K, Date J, Johansen K. A prospective study of the differential changes in serum thyroglobulin and its autoantibodies during propylthiouracil or radioiodine therapy of patients with Graves' disease. *Acta Endocrinol (Copenhagen).* 1982;99:379-385.

132. Smallridge RC, De Keyser FM, Van Herle AJ, Butkus NE, Wartofsky L. Thyroid iodine content and serum thyroglobulin: cues to the natural history of destruction-induced thyroiditis. *J Clin Endocrinol Metab.* 1986;62:1213-1219.

133. Duick DS, Stein RB, Warren DW, Nicoloff JT. The significance of partial suppressibility of serum thyroxine by triiodothyronine administration in euthyroid man. *J Clin Endocrinol Metab.* 1975;41:229-234.

134. Gardner DF, Rothman J, Utiger RD. Serum thyroglobulin in normal subjects and patients with hyperthyroidism due to Graves' disease: effects of T3, iodide, 131I and antithyroid drugs. *Clin Endocrinol (Oxford).* 1979;11:585-594.

135. Glinoer D, De Nayer P, Bourdoux P, et al. Regulation of maternal thyroid during pregnancy. *J Clin Endocrinol Metab.* 1990;71:276-287.

136. Berghout A, Endert E, Ross A, Hogerzeil HV, Smits NJ, Wiersinga WM. Thyroid function and thyroid size in normal pregnant women living in an iodine replete area. *Clin Endocrinol (Oxford).* 1994;41:375-379.

137. Leboeuf R, Emerick LE, Martorella AJ, Tuttle RM. Impact of pregnancy on serum thyroglobulin and detection of recurrent disease shortly after delivery in thyroid cancer survivors. *Thyroid.* 2007;17:543-547.

138. Derumeaux H, Valeix P, Castetbon K, et al. Association of selenium with thyroid volume and echostructure in 35- to 60-year-old French adults. *Eur J Endocrinol.* 2003;148:309-315.

139. Shih ML, Lee JA, Hsieh CB, et al. Thyroidectomy for Hashimoto's thyroiditis: complications and associated cancers. *Thyroid.* 2008;18:729-734.

140. Fraser CG. Generation and application of data on biological variation in clinical chemistry. *Crit Rev Clin Lab Sci.* 1989;27:409-437.

141. Buchinger W, Lorenz-Wawschinek O, Semlitsch G, et al. Thyrotropin and thyroglobulin as an index of optimal iodine intake: correlation with iodine excretion of 39,913 euthyroid patients. *Thyroid.* 1997;7:593-597.

142. WHO/ICCIDD/UNICEF. Indicators for assessing iodine deficiency disorders and their control through salt iodization. *Document WHO/NUT.* 1994;6:36.

143. Rasmussen LB, Ovesen L, Bülow I, et al. Relations between various measures of iodine intake and thyroid volume, thyroid nodularity, and serum thyroglobulin. *Am J Clin Nutr.* 2002;76:1069-1076.

144. van den Briel T, West CE, Hautvast JG, Vulsma T, de Vijlder JJ, Ategbo EA. Serum thyroglobulin and urinary iodine concentration are the most appropriate indicators of iodine status and thyroid function under conditions of increasing iodine supply in schoolchildren in Benin. *J Nutr.* 2001;131:2701-2706.

145. Knudsen N, Bülow I, Jørgensen T, Perrild H, Ovesen L, Laurberg P. Serum Tg—a sensitive marker of thyroid abnormalities and iodine deficiency in epidemiological studies. *J Clin Endocrinol Metab.* 2001;86:2599-2603.

146. Rasmussen LB, Ovesen L, Christiansen E. Day-to-day and within-day variation in urinary iodine excretion. *Eur J Clin Nutr.* 1999;53:401-407.

147. Zimmermann MB, de Benoist B, Corigliano S, et al. Assessment of iodine status using dried blood spot thyroglobulin: development of reference material and establishment of an international reference range in iodine-sufficient children. *J Clin Endocrinol Metab.* 2006;91:4881-4887.

148. Brown RS, Demmer LA. The etiology of thyroid dysgenesis-still an enigma after all these years. *J Clin Endocrinol Metab.* 2002;87:4069-4071.

149. Brown AL, Fernhoff PM, Milner J, McEwen C, Elsas LS. Racial differences in the incidence of congenital hypothyroidism. *J Pediatr.* 1981;99:934-936.

150. Djemli A, Fillion M, Belgoudi J, et al. Twenty years later: a reevaluation of the contribution of plasma thyroglobulin to the diagnosis of thyroid dysgenesis in infants with congenital hypothyroidism. *Clin Biochem.* 2004;37:818-822.

151. Simsek E, Karabay M, Kocabay K. Neonatal screening for congenital hypothyroidism in West Black Sea area, Turkey. *Int J Clin Pract.* 2005;59:336-341.

152. Caputo M, Rivolta CM, Esperante SA, et al. Congenital hypothyroidism with goitre caused by new mutations in the thyroglobulin gene. *Clin Endocrinol (Oxford).* 2007;67:351-357.

153. Vono-Toniolo J, Rivolta CM, Targovnik HM, Medeiros-Neto G, Kopp P. Naturally occurring mutations in the thyroglobulin gene. *Thyroid.* 2005;15:1021-1033.

154. Rivolta CM, Targovnik HM. Molecular advances in thyroglobulin disorders. *Clin Chim Acta.* 2006;374:8-24.

155. Cohen JH, Ingbar SH, Braverman LE. Thyrotoxicosis due to ingestion of excess thyroid hormone. *Endocr Rev.* 1989;10:113-124.

156. Matsubara S, Inoh M, Tarumi Y, Sato M, Takahara J. An outbreak (159 cases) of transient thyrotoxicosis without hyperthyroidism in Japan. *Intern Med.* 1995;34:514-519.

157. Mariotti S, Martino E, Cupini C, et al. Low serum thyroglobulin as a clue to the diagnosis of thyrotoxicosis factitia. *N Engl J Med.* 1982;307:410-412.

158. Chow E, Siddique F, Gama R. Thyrotoxicosis factitia: role of thyroglobulin. *Ann Clin Biochem.* 2008;45:447-448.

159. Parmar MS, Sturge C. Recurrent hamburger thyrotoxicosis. *CMAJ.* 2003;169:45-47.

160. Fatourechi V, Aniszewski JP, Fatourechi GZ, et al. Clinical features and outcome of subacute thyroiditis in an incidence cohort: Olmsted County, Minnesota, study. *J Clin Endocrinol Metab.* 2003;88:2100-2105.

161. Parkes AB, Black EG, Adams H, et al. Serum thyroglobulin: an early indicator of autoimmune post-partum thyroiditis. *Clin Endocrinol.* 1994;41:9-14.

162. Fragu P, Rougier P, Schlumberger M, Tubiana M. Evolution of thyroid 127-I stores measured by X-ray fluorescence in subacute thyroiditis. *J Clin Endocrinol Metab.* 1982;54:162-166.

163. Madeddu G, Casu AR, Costanza C, et al. Serum thyroglobulin levels in the diagnosis and follow-up of subacute 'painful' thyroiditis. *Arch Intern Med.* 1985;145:243-247.

164. Feldt-Rasmussen U. Relationship between serum thyroglobulin, thyroid volume and serum TSH in healthy non-goitrous subjects and the relationship to seasonal variations in iodine intake. *Thyroidol Clin Exp.* 1989;1:115-118.

165. Hershman JM, Due DT, Sharp B, et al. Endemic goiter in Vietnam. *J Clin Endocrinol Metab.* 1983;57:243-249.

166. Feldt-Rasmussen U, Hegedus L, Hansen JM, Perrild H. Relationship between thyroid volume and serum thyroglobulin during long-term suppression with triiodothyronine in patients with diffuse non-toxic goitre. *Acta Endocrinol.* 1984;105:184-189.

167. Unger J, De Maertelaer V, Golstein J, Decoster C, Jonckheer MH. Relationship between serum thyroglobulin and intrathyroidal stable iodine in human simple goiter. *Clin Endocrinol.* 1985;23:1-6.

168. Glinoer D, De Nayer P, Delange F, et al. A randomized trial for the treatment of mild iodine deficiency during pregnancy: maternal and neonatal effects. *J Clin Endocrinol Metab.* 1995;80:258-269.

169. Date J, Feldt-Rasmussen U, Blichert-Toft M, Hegedus L, Graversen HP. Long-term observation of serum thyroglobulin after resection of nontoxic goiter and relation to ultrasonographically demonstrated relapse. *World J Surg.* 1996;20:351-356.

170. Lazar V, Bidart JM, Caillou B, et al. Expression of the Na+/I- symporter gene in human thyroid tumors: a comparison study with other thyroid-specific genes. *J Clin Endocrinol Metab.* 1999;84:3228-3234.

171. Boelaert K, Horacek J, Holder RL, Watkinson JC, Sheppard MC, Franklyn JA. Serum thyrotropin concentration as a novel predictor of malignancy in thyroid nodules investigated by fine-needle aspiration. *J Clin Endocrinol Metab.* 2006;91:4295-4301.

172. Haymart MR, Repplinger DJ, Leverson GE, et al. Higher serum thyroid stimulating hormone level in thyroid nodule patients is associated with greater risks of differentiated thyroid cancer and advanced tumor stage. *J Clin Endocrinol Metab.* 2008;93:809-814.

173. Jonklaas J, Nsouli-Maktabi H, Soldin S. Endogenous thyrotropin and triiodothyronine concentrations in individuals with thyroid cancer. *Thyroid.* 2008;18:943-952.

174. Ronga G, Filesi M, Ventroni G, Signore A. Value of the first serum thyroglobulin level after total thyroidectomy for the diagnosis of metastases from differentiated thyroid carcinoma. *Eur J Nucl Med.* 1999;26:1448-1452.

175. Lima N, Cavaliere H, Tomimori E, Knobel M, Medeiros-Neto G. Prognostic value of serial serum thyroglobulin determinations after total thyroidectomy for differentiated thyroid cancer. *J Endocrinol Invest.* 2002;25:110-115.

176. Lin JD, Huang MJ, Hsu BR, et al. Significance of postoperative serum thyroglobulin levels in patients with papillary and follicular thyroid carcinomas. *J Surg Oncol.* 2002;80:45-51.

177. Toubeau M, Touzery C, Arveux P, et al. Predictive value for disease progression of serum thyroglobulin levels measured in the postoperative period and after [131]-I ablation therapy in patients with differentiated thyroid cancer. *J Nucl Med.* 2004;45:988-994.

178. Kloos RT, Mazzaferri EL. A single recombinant human thyrotropin-stimulated serum thyroglobulin measurement predicts differentiated thyroid carcinoma metastases three to five years later. *J Clin Endocrinol Metab.* 2005;90:5047-5057.

179. Makarewicz J, Adamczewski Z, Knapska-Kucharska M, Lewinski A. Evaluation of the diagnostic value of the first thyroglobulin determination in detecting metastases after differentiated thyroid carcinoma surgery. *Exp Clin Endocrinol Diabetes.* 2006;114:485-489.

180. Kim TY, Kim WB, Kim ES, et al. Serum thyroglobulin levels at the time of 131I remnant ablation just after thyroidectomy are useful for early prediction of clinical recurrence in low-risk patients with differentiated thyroid carcinoma. *J Clin Endocrinol Metab.* 2005;90: 1440-1445.

181. Heemstra KA, Liu YY, Stokkel M, et al. Serum thyroglobulin concentrations predict disease-free remission and death in differentiated thyroid carcinoma. *Clin Endocrinol (Oxford).* 2007;66:58-64.

182. Hall FT, Beasley NJ, Eski SJ, Witterick IJ, Walfish PG, Freeman JL. Predictive value of serum thyroglobulin after surgery for thyroid carcinoma. *Laryngoscope.* 2003;113:77-81.

183. Pacini F, Schlumberger M, Harmer C, et al. Post-surgical use of radioiodine (131I) in patients with papillary and follicular thyroid cancer and the issue of remnant ablation: a consensus report. *Eur J Endocrinol.* 2005;153:651-659.

184. Verkooijen RB, Verburg FA, van Isselt JW, Lips CJ, Smit JW, Stokkel MP. The success rate of I-131 ablation in differentiated thyroid cancer: comparison of uptake-related and fixed-dose strategies. *Eur J Endocrinol.* 2008;159:301-307.

185. Torlontano M, Attard M, Crocetti U, et al. Follow-up of low risk patients with papillary thyroid cancer: role of neck ultrasonography in detecting lymph node metastases. *J Clin Endocrinol Metab.* 2004;89:3402-3407.

186. David A, Blotta A, Rossi R, et al. Clinical value of different responses of serum thyroglobulin to recombinant human thyrotropin in the follow-up of patients with differentiated thyroid carcinoma. *Thyroid.* 2005;15:267-273.

187. Giovanella L. Highly sensitive thyroglobulin measurements in differentiated thyroid carcinoma managemen. *Clin Chem Lab Med.* 2008;46:1067-1073.

188. Frasoldati A, Pesenti M, Gallo M, Caroggio A, Salvo D, Valcavi R. Diagnosis of neck recurrences in patients with differentiated thyroid carcinoma. *Cancer.* 2003;97:90-96.

189. Davies L, Welch HG. Increasing incidence of thyroid cancer in the United States, 1973-2002. *JAMA.* 2006;295:2164-2167.

190. Hay ID, McConahey WM, Goellner JR. Managing patients with papillary thyroid carcinoma: insights gained from the Mayo Clinic's experience of treating 2,512 consecutive patients during 1940 through 2000. *Trans Am Clin Climatol Assoc.* 2002;113:241-260.

191. Mazzaferri EL. Managing small thyroid cancers. *JAMA.* 2006;295:2179-2182.

192. Pujol P, Daures JP, Nsakala N, Baldet L, Bringer J, Jaffiol C. Degree of thyrotropin suppression as a prognostic determinant in differentiated thyroid cancer. *J Clin Endocrinol Metab.* 1996;81:4318-4323.
193. Jonklaas J, Sarlis NJ, Litofsky D, et al. Outcomes of patients with differentiated thyroid carcinoma following initial therapy. *Thyroid.* 2006;16:1229-1242.
194. McGriff NJ, Csako G, Gourgiotis L, Lori CG, Pucino F, Sarlis NJ. Effects of thyroid hormone suppression therapy on adverse clinical outcomes in thyroid cancer. *Ann Med.* 2002;34:554-5564.
195. Hovens GC, Stokkel MP, Kievit J, et al. Associations of serum thyrotropin concentrations with recurrence and death in differentiated thyroid cancer. *J Clin Endocrinol Metab.* 2007;92:2610-2615.
196. Hay ID, McDougall IR, Sisson JC. Perspective: the case against radioiodine remnant ablation in patients with well-differentiated thyroid carcinoma. *J Nucl Med.* 2008;49:1395-1397.
197. Sawka AM, Brierley JD, Tsang RW, et al. An updated systematic review and commentary examining the effectiveness of radioactive iodine remnant ablation in well-differentiated thyroid cancer. *Endocrinol Metabl Clin North Am.* 2008;37:457-480.
198. Hay ID. Selective use of radioactive iodine in the postoperative management of patients with papillary and follicular thyroid carcinoma. *J Surg Oncol.* 2006;94:692-700.
199. Sawka AM, Goldstein DP, Thabane L, et al. Basis for physician recommendations for adjuvant radioiodine therapy in early-stage thyroid carcinoma: principal findings of the Canadian-American thyroid cancer survey. *Endocr Pract.* 2008;14:175-184.
200. Brown AP, Chen J, Hitchcock YJ, Szabo A, Shrieve DC, Tward JD. The risk of second primary malignancies up to three decades after the treatment of differentiated thyroid cancer. *J Clin Endocrinol Metab.* 2008;93:504-515.
201. Rubino C, de Vathaire F, Dottorini ME, et al. Second primary malignancies in thyroid cancer patients. *Br J Cancer.* 2003;89:1638-1644.
202. Sawka AM, Thephamongkhol K, Brouwers M, Thabane L, Browman G, Gerstein HC. Clinical review 170: a systematic review and metaanalysis of the effectiveness of radioactive iodine remnant ablation for well-differentiated thyroid cancer. *J Clin Endocrinol Metab.* 2004;89:3668-3676.
203. Robbins RJ, Srivastava S, Shaha A, et al. Factors influencing the basal and recombinant human thyrotropin-stimulated serum thyroglobulin in patients with metastatic thyroid carcinoma. *J Clin Endocrinol Metab.* 2004;89:6010-6016.
204. Serhal DI, Nasrallah MP, Arafah BM. Rapid rise in serum thyrotropin concentrations after thyroidectomy or withdrawal of suppressive thyroxine therapy in preparation for radioactive iodine administration to patients with differentiated thyroid cancer. *J Clin Endocrinol Metab.* 2004;89:3285-3289.
205. Mazzaferri EL, Kloos RT. Is diagnostic iodine-131 scanning with recombinant human TSH useful in the follow-up of differentiated thyroid cancer after thyroid ablation? *J Clin Endocrinol Metab.* 2002;87:1490-1498.
206. Eustatia-Rutten CF, Smit JW, Romijn JA, et al. Diagnostic value of serum thyroglobulin measurements in the follow-up of differentiated thyroid carcinoma, a structured meta-analysis. *Clin Endocrinol (Oxford).* 2004;61:61-74.
207. Schlumberger M, Pacini F, Wiersinga WM, et al. Follow-up and management of differentiated thyroid carcinoma: a European perspective in clinical practice. *Eur J Endocrinol.* 2004;151:539-548.
208. Unger J, Van Heuverswyn B, Decoster C, Cantraine F, Mockel J, Van Herle A. Thyroglobulin and thyroid hormone release after intravenous administration of bovine thyrotropin in man. *J Clin Endocrinol Metab.* 1980;51:590-594.
209. Schlumberger M, Ricard M, De Pouvourville G, Pacini F. How the availability of recombinant human TSH has changed the management of patients who have thyroid cancer. *Nat Clin Pract Endocrinol Metab.* 2007;3:641-650.

210. Phan HT, Jager PL, van der Wal JE, et al. The follow-up of patients with differentiated thyroid cancer and undetectable thyroglobulin (Tg) and Tg antibodies during ablation. *Eur J Endocrinol.* 2008;158:77-83.

211. Pacini F, Pinchera A. Serum and tissue thyroglobulin measurement: clinical applications in thyroid disease. *Biochimie.* 1999;81:463-467.

212. Rotman-Pikielny P, Reynolds JC, Barker WC, Yen PM, Skarulis MC, Sarlis NJ. Recombinant human thyrotropin for the diagnosis and treatment of a highly functional metastatic struma ovarii. *J Clin Endocrinol Metab.* 2000;85:237-244.

213. Machens A, Holzhausen HJ, Dralle H. The prognostic value of primary tumor size in papillary and follicular thyroid carcinoma. *Cancer.* 2005;103:2269-2273.

214. Passler C, Scheuba C, Prager G, et al. Prognostic factors of papillary and follicular thyroid cancer: differences in an iodine-replete endemic goiter region. *Endocr Relat Cancer.* 2004;11:131-139.

215. Rosário PW, de Faria S, Bicalho L, et al. Ultrasonographic differentiation between metastatic and benign lymph nodes in patients with papillary thyroid carcinoma. *J Ultrasound Med.* 2005;24:1385-1389.

216. Pacini F, Fugazzola L, Lippi F, et al. Detection of thyroglobulin in fine needle aspirates of nonthyroidal neck masses: a clue to the diagnosis of metastatic differentiated thyroid cancer. *J Clin Endocrinol Metab.* 1992;74:1401-1404.

217. Uruno T, Miyauchi A, Shimizu K, et al. Usefulness of thyroglobulin measurement in fine-needle aspiration biopsy specimens for diagnosing cervical lymph node metastasis in patients with papillary thyroid cancer. *World J Surg.* 2005;29:483-485.

218. Boi F, Baghino G, Atzeni F, Lai ML, Faa G, Mariotti S. The diagnostic value for differentiated thyroid carcinoma metastases of thyroglobulin (Tg) measurement in washout fluid from fine-needle aspiration biopsy of neck lymph nodes is maintained in the presence of circulating anti-Tg antibodies. *J Clin Endocrinol Metab.* 2006;91:1364-1369.

219. Snozek CL, Chambers EP, Reading CC, et al. Serum thyroglobulin, high-resolution ultrasound, and lymph node thyroglobulin in diagnosis of differentiated thyroid carcinoma nodal metastases. *J Clin Endocrinol Metab.* 2007;92:4278-4281.

Chapter 8
Thyroid Function Testing in Ambulatory Practice

Angela M. Leung and Alan P. Farwell

Thyroid function tests are commonly obtained by both primary care physicians and various specialists in ambulatory practice for both the evaluation of symptomatic and screening assessment of asymptomatic thyroid disease. Abnormalities of thyroid function testing, including those which may not be clinically apparent, are common in the general population. Epidemiological studies have identified hypothyroidism (subclinical and overt) in 4.6–9.5% and hyperthyroidism (subclinical and overt) in 1.3–2.2% of individuals [1], while the incidence of mild/subclinical dysfunction in certain populations is much more common [2–4].

Health care practitioners are presented with a wide spectrum of serological tests in the evaluation of thyroid dysfunction (discussed in depth in Chaps. 4, 5, 6, and 7). Current laboratory testing allows measurement of the three major components of the thyroid-pituitary axis: thyroxine (T4); 3,5,3'-triiodothyronine (T3); and thyrotropin/thyroid stimulating hormone (TSH). Some clinicians may additionally opt to obtain titers of thyroid autoantibodies (e.g., thyroid peroxidase [TPO] and/or thyroglobulin [Tg] antibodies) in certain patients suspected to be at risk for autoimmune thyroid disease. An understanding of the appropriate indication for obtaining a specific test is paramount in the interpretation and management of the abnormal results that are found.

Here we review the approach to using thyroid function testing in ambulatory practice as it pertains to the recommendations of choosing initial tests, diagnostic evaluation of symptomatic patients, use for monitoring in treated thyroid diseases, and considerations of screening in targeted subsets of and in the general population.

A. P. Farwell (✉)
Division of Endocrinology, Diabetes and Nutrition, Boston University School of Medicine,
Boston Medical Center, Boston, MA 01583, USA
e-mail: alan.farwell@bmc.org

G. A. Brent (ed.), *Thyroid Function Testing,*
DOI 10.1007/978-1-4419-1485-9_8, © Springer Science+Business Media, LLC 2010

8.1   Choice of Tests in Thyroid Function Testing

The serum TSH assay is the most reliable test to assess thyroid dysfunction in the healthy ambulatory patient and is the initial laboratory test of choice of both internists and specialists, often measured along with free T4 (discussed in Chaps. 4 and 5). The serum TSH assay is a widely available and relatively inexpensive tool in the detection of thyroid function abnormalities [5]. When obtained in the ambulatory setting, the sensitivity and specificity of the TSH assay can approach 98% and 92%, respectively [6]. Further, individuals found to have an initial normal TSH level are unlikely (with as low as 2% probability) to have an abnormal measurement when testing is repeated within 5 years [7].

While TSH measurements have been utilized for many years to diagnose hypothyroidism, TSH assays developed in the last three decades have increased the sensitivity in the low end of the range and permitted the use of serum TSH in the evaluation of thyrotoxicosis. The lower limit of the serum TSH assay used should be 0.02 mU/L or less [5], which is generally standard in most laboratories and uniformly available. Because the relationship between serum TSH and peripheral thyroid hormone (T4 and T3) levels is logarithmic, abnormal TSH results should prompt confirmatory testing with other thyroid function tests. Assessment of serum T4 concentrations should be the first step after an abnormal TSH result. Because the concentration of total T4 is susceptible to changes in the levels and binding affinities of serum thyroid hormone binding proteins [8], assessment of free T4 concentrations should be performed by either the analog method (FT4) or in association with the assessment of thyroid binding globulin (TBG) stores (i.e., FT4 index [FTI]; discussed in depth in Chap. 5). Measurement of serum T3 concentrations should be a secondary test and reserved, for the most part, for the evaluation of suspected hyperthyroidism. Because serum free T3 concentrations are generally lower than those of free T4, their measurement is more difficult [9] and not as widely used.

The two most common thyroid autoantibodies that are measured clinically are TPO and Tg antibodies, with TPO antibody titers the most closely correlated with autoimmune thyroid disease (discussed in depth in Chap. 6). The presence of significant titers of these antibodies may suggest an increased risk for present or future thyroid dysfunction. Thyroid autoimmune antibody positivity may also suggest the presence of other concurrent autoimmune disease processes, such as type 1 diabetes mellitus, vitiligo, and celiac disease, although titers should not be obtained solely for this purpose. TPO antibody titers can be detected in approximately 11% of the general population [1], and only 12% of these individuals will have TSH levels greater than 6 mU/L after 4 years [10]. Thus, isolated measurements of thyroid antibodies without evidence of thyroid dysfunction is not recommended, with the possible exception of the woman suffering from recurrent miscarriages (see below).

Clinicians in ambulatory practice may also be presented with the option of measuring Tg concentrations (discussed in depth in Chap. 7). Tg is a key protein in the thyroid hormone synthetic pathway within the thyroid [11]. Circulating levels of Tg are used primarily in the assessment of thyroid cancer recurrence after surgery and radioactive iodine ablation. Tg measurement has a limited role in the evaluation of thyroid dysfunction in the nonthyroid cancer patient and should be reserved for specialized circumstances, such as the diagnosis of thyrotoxicosis factitia.

Finally, clinical judgment of each individual patient should dictate whether thyroid function testing should be performed in certain situations. Alterations in thyroid function are possible in the setting of recent large iodine loads, and consideration should be given to defer testing in these situations if there is otherwise no urgency. Thyroid function test abnormalities can be seen for up to 2 months after the administration of intravenous contrast media [12]. Similarly, thyroid function testing results may be altered in the setting of even a mild, concurrent nonthyroidal illness. Unless there is a strong clinical indication, thyroid function testing should also be deferred until the patient has recovered from the illness, as the alterations of thyroid hormone economy in sick euthyroid syndrome may make thyroid function measurements difficult to interpret [13, 14].

8.2 Evaluation of the Symptomatic Patient

The symptoms of thyroid dysfunction, especially hypothyroidism, are general and nonspecific. Manifestations vary greatly between individuals, and clinically apparent disease may further be masked by use of concurrent medications, particularly in the elderly. Although severe clinical consequences are possible, most patients follow an insidious progression of disease.

The spectrum of common signs, symptoms, risk factors, and other clues for hyperthyroidism and hypothyroidism are summarized, respectively, in Tables 8.1 and 8.2. It may be reasonable to pursue thyroid function testing when one or more of these clues are present when interpreted in combination with clinical judgment.

Table 8.1 Clues to thyrotoxicosis

Signs and symptoms
Weight loss
Palpitations
Heat intolerance diarrhea
Muscle weakness
Dyspnea
Insomnia
Diaphoresis or sweating
Anxiety or nervousness
Tremor
Tachycardia or atrial tachyarrhythmias
Skin moistness
Abnormalities of common laboratory tests
Hypercalcemia
Elevation in hepatocellular enzymes
Elevation of alkaline phosphatase

Table 8.2 Clues to
hypothyroidism

Signs and symptoms
Weight gain
Bradycardia
Cold intolerance
Constipation
Muscle cramps
Myalgias
Menstrual irregularity
Fatigue
Coarse or dry skin
Coarse or dry hair
Depression
Dementia
Edema
Hypothermia
Abnormalities of common laboratory tests
Hyperlipidemia
Anemia
Elevation lactate dehydrogenase
Hyponatremia
Elevation of creatine phosphokinase
Hyperprolactinemia

Moreover, since there may be associations between thyroid dysfunction and several common comorbidities, including osteoporosis, atrial fibrillation, and obesity, the evaluating clinician should also consider thyroid function testing when there is an otherwise unidentifiable etiology to these and other diseases. An algorithm to the evaluation of a patient with suspected thyroid dysfunction is presented in Fig. 8.1.

8.2.1 Suspected Thyrotoxicosis

When thyrotoxicosis is suspected clinically, further biochemical testing of thyroid function is required to confirm the diagnosis. As discussed above, the initial thyroid function test in suspected thyrotoxicosis should be a serum TSH level, as almost all etiologies of thyrotoxicosis will result in TSH suppression. If the TSH is undetectable or below the lower limit of the reference range, it should be followed with a free T4 or FTI level and/or total T3, which, if elevated, confirms the diagnosis of hyperthyroidism (Fig. 8.1). If the peripheral (T3 or T4) hormone levels are normal in the setting of a subnormal TSH level, differential diagnoses include subclinical hyperthyroidism, early pregnancy (first-trimester gestational thyrotoxicosis), the early phase of sick euthyroid syndrome, recent exposure to an exogenous iodine load (e.g., intravenous iodinated contrast dye, amiodarone, kelp), recent glucocorticoid administration, and central hypothyroidism.

Although a normal serum TSH level usually does not warrant follow-up testing with T3 or T4 levels, this may be performed when there is a suspicion of a thyroid

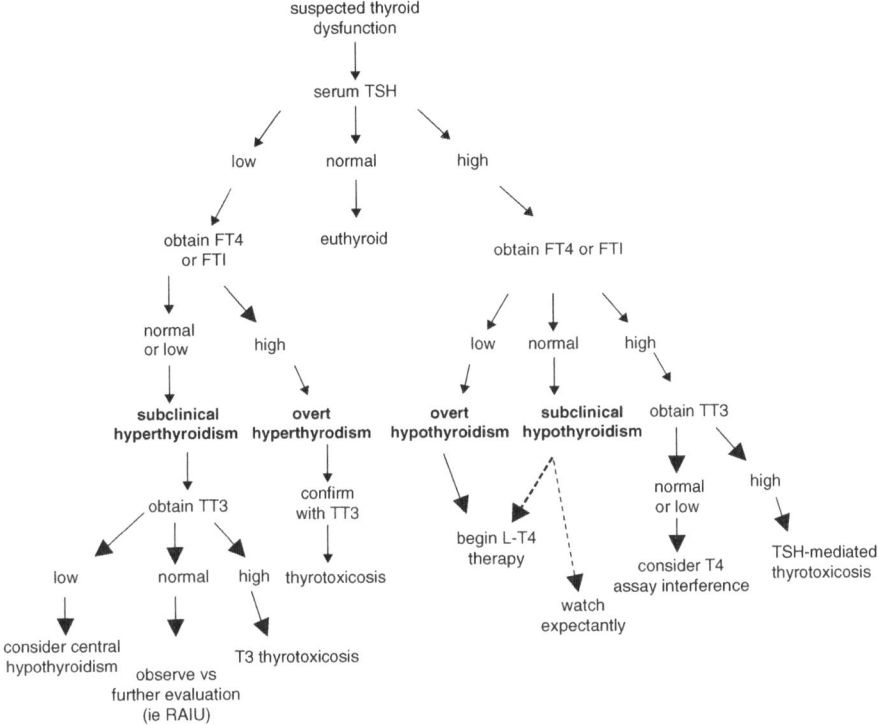

Fig. 8.1 Evaluation of suspected thyroid dysfunction

hormone protein binding abnormality. In such cases, one may encounter elevated total T3 and T4 concentrations in the setting of a normal serum TSH level. This pattern suggests the diagnosis of euthyroid hyperthyroxinemia and should be confirmed by ensuring the free T3 and free T4 levels are within their respective reference ranges. The most common etiology to this thyroid function testing pattern is TBG excess. Elevated TBG levels are seen in hereditary disorders, including familial dysalbuminemic hyperthyroxinemia [15]; increased estrogen states, including pregnancy and the use of oral contraceptive or hormone replacement pills [16]; hepatitis [17]; and the use of certain medications [18]. Patients with euthyroid hyperthyroxinemia are clinically euthyroid and should not be treated for hyperthyroidism. Rarely, serum T4 and T3 levels may be elevated in the presence of elevated TSH concentrations. This constellation of labs may be seen with TSH-secreting pituitary adenomas [19], TSH resistance [20], and peripheral thyroid hormone resistance [21].

8.2.2   Suspected Hypothyroidism

Signs and symptoms of an underactive thyroid (Table 8.2) often progress slowly and can be particularly nonspecific. Many features of hypothyroidism, such as fatigue, weight gain, and constipation, are common in the euthyroid general population. Similar to the scenario of suspected thyrotoxicosis, a serum TSH should be the initial test obtained in suspected hypothyroidism (Fig. 8.1). An elevated TSH level should then be followed with a free T4 or FTI level. Overt primary hypothyroidism is diagnosed with an elevated TSH level and low free T4 or FTI concentrations, while subclinical hypothyroidism refers to the pattern of an elevated TSH level and a normal free T4 or FTI concentration. Patients with overt hypothyroidism should be started on levothyroxine replacement, but the recommendation to begin thyroid replacement therapy in those with subclinical hypothyroidism is controversial [22]. In individuals with subclinical hypothyroidism, it may be reasonable to obtain TPO antibody titers which may predict the course of thyroid failure and eventual dysfunction [23].

Other reasons to consider for an isolated abnormally high TSH level are resolving sick euthyroid syndrome [14] and use of certain medications, including dopamine antagonists [24] and amiodarone [25]. While an elevated TSH is almost always indicative of hypothyroidism, TSH-mediated thyrotoxicosis may rarely be observed, as noted above.

Analogous to the entity of euthyroid hyperthyroxinemia, it is possible to encounter the pattern of euthyroid hypothyroxinemia, in which total T3 and T4 concentrations are decreased and TSH, free T3, and free T4 levels are normal. The isolated reductions in total T3 and T4 concentrations can be the result of TBG deficient states, such as hereditary causes [26], elevated androgen levels [27], glucocorticoid use [28], nephrotic syndrome in children [29], use of certain medications [18], and displacement of T4 from binding proteins by medications including salicylates [30]. Similar to the diagnosis of euthyroid hyperthyroxinemia, patients with euthyroid hypothyroxinemia are clinically euthyroid and should not be treated for hypothyroidism.

8.2.3 Nodular Goiter

Thyroid function testing is often utilized upon the detection of a thyroid nodule, although most patients with nodules are euthyroid. Palpable thyroid nodules are estimated to be present in 4–7% of the US population, with women affected more frequently than men [31]. The risk of developing a nodule has been estimated to be 0.1% per year, with a lifetime expectancy of 10% [31]. When ultrasound is used, up to 45% of women and 25% of men may be shown to harbor a thyroid nodule. The American Thyroid Association recommends the assessment of thyroid function for nodules greater than 1 cm [31].

The initial thyroid function test in a patient with a thyroid nodule should be a serum TSH, which is obtained to rule out biochemical evidence of hyperthyroidism. If the TSH level is low, the confirmatory tests should be performed as discussed above and nuclear thyroid imaging may be considered. Once biochemical euthyroidism is confirmed in the setting of a nodular goiter, there is no need for future serial measurements of TSH levels for the development of nodule autonomy.

8.3 Use of Thyroid Function Tests to Monitor Treated Thyroid Dysfunction

8.3.1 Monitoring Hypothyroidism

Patients with primary hypothyroidism who are treated with levothyroxine replacement require periodic assessments of thyroid function to ensure dose adequacy. For patients on a stable dose, a serum TSH level assessed annually is reasonable. This can be performed more or less frequently at the discretion of the clinician. An altered TSH (increase or decrease) in a patient who had previously been on a stable dose of levothyroxine should raise the possibility of one of a variety of interactions (Table 8.3). For example, high estrogen states that elevate TBG (i.e., birth control pill usage, estrogen replacement therapy, raloxifene, or pregnancy) or interference with levothyroxine absorption (i.e., concomitant administration of iron and/or calcium, history of gastric bypass surgery) may result in an elevation in TSH and require a dose increase. On the

Table 8.3 Factors that may alter levothyroxine dosing in hypothyroidism	**Reduced Absorption**
	Ferrous Sulfate
	Calcium
	Cholestyramine resin
	Colestipol
	Soybean formula
	Aluminum hydroxide
	Gastric bypass surgery
	Short bowel syndrome
	Celiac disease
	Altered metabolism
	Rifampin
	Carbamazepine
	Phenobarbitol
	Amiodarone
	Sertraline
	Sorafanib
	Sunitinib
	Altered hormone binding
	Estrogen (i.e., OCPs, ERT, Pregnancy)
	Raloxifene
	Phenytoin
	NSAIDs (i.e., Salicylate)
	Altered potency
	Change in Levothyroxine brand
	Change to generic Levothyroxine preparation
	Transient alterations
	Intercurrent illness
	Patient compliance

other hand, stopping birth control pills or the interference with levothyroxine binding to TBG (e.g., discontinuation of phenytoin) may lead to a decreased TSH and a dose reduction. Another complicating factor has become prevalent since the Food and Drug Administration (FDA) approved generic levothyroxine products in 2001. Physicians should be aware that generic levothyroxine preparations may be interchanged by pharmacists without provider notification despite the possibility of up to 15% difference in the potency of the differing brands [32, 33]. Current recommendations are to recheck thyroid function tests in patients switched to a generic levothyroxine preparation after 6–8 weeks of the change, although the FDA has recently removed this as a Black Box warning. Transient etiologies for altered TSH values in patients on levothyroxine include intercurrent illnesses and changes in patient compliance.

In general, dose adjustments should not exceed 25 µg with each titration, with the possible exception of during pregnancy (see below). Serum TSH values reflect steady state concentrations of levothyroxine, and dose adjustments will not reach new steady state levels until 4–6 weeks after a change in levothyroxine brand or dose.

There are no guidelines regarding the use of serial thyroid function testing for the monitoring of subclinical hypothyroidism if levothyroxine treatment is not initiated. New signs or symptoms suggestive of thyroid dysfunction should prompt repeat testing, but otherwise it is reasonable to repeat testing on an annual basis. It is interesting that one recent study has found that increasing the frequency of interval between follow-up visits was associated with a lower prevalence of subclinical hypothyroidism over 1 year [34].

There are special considerations to the management of hypothyroidism in women of childbearing age and in pregnant women (discussed in depth in Chap. 11). In studies by Haddow et al. [35] and Pop et al. [36], infants born to mothers with elevated TSH values or hypothyroxinemia, respectively, had worse neurocognitive outcomes as compared to controls. Thus, women with preexisting hypothyroidism should have a TSH and, in most cases, an FT4 or FTI measured as soon as pregnancy is confirmed. Alternatively, it has been suggested that the levothyroxine dose be empirically increased by approximately 30% as soon as pregnancy is confirmed [37]. The levothyroxine dose should be titrated to maintain a TSH in the first trimester of pregnancy of less than 2.5 mU/L and less than 3.0 mU/L during the second and third trimesters [38, 39]. Measuring TSH and FT4 or FTI values every 4–6 weeks during the first half of pregnancy and once in the third trimester is a reasonable approach. Following delivery, levothyroxine requirements typically decrease to prepregnancy levels. The levothyroxine dose should be returned to the prepregnancy dose and serum TSH levels should be monitored closely [40].

8.3.2 Monitoring Hyperthyroidism

Thyroid function testing is used to assess the response to antithyroid medication in the treatment of hyperthyroidism. Hyperthyroid patients who undergo definitive treatment with radioactive iodine ablation or surgery frequently become permanently hypothyroid and should be followed similarly to those with primary hypothyroidism as described above.

The monitoring of the effectiveness of antithyroid medication therapy should initially be done with serial serum total T3 and total T4 levels. Certain types of hyperthyroidism, such as Graves' disease, usually produce greater elevations in serum T3 concentrations relative to serum T4. TSH levels are often misleading in the initial stages of therapy, as they can continue to be suppressed for up to several months despite the initiation of treatment and subsequent normalization of serum T4 and T3 concentrations. Once within the normal range, TSH levels can also be used to titrate doses of antithyroid medication. The recommended frequency of obtaining T3 and T4 levels is dependent on the degree of their elevation prior to antithyroid medication initiation and in accordance with the clinical status of each individual patient.

8.4 Screening of the General Population for Thyroid Dysfunction

Several large population-based studies have demonstrated that serum thyroid function abnormalities are common in otherwise healthy asymptomatic individuals. Measurements of TSH levels from the Third National Health and Nutrition Examination Survey (NHANES III, 1988–1994) detected hypothyroidism in 4.6% (4.3% subclinical, 0.3% clinical) and hyperthyroidism in 1.3% (0.5% clinical, 0.7% subclinical) of the US population [1]. The Colorado Health Study, a cross-sectional analysis of 25,862 participants at a state health fair, reported elevated TSH levels in 9.5% and decreased TSH levels in 2.2% of the study population [2]. The Whickham Survey, a large cross-sectional assessment of thyroid dysfunction conducted in Great Britain during the late 1970s, found the prevalence of an elevated TSH value in 7.5% of women and 2.8% of men [3]. The recent 20-year follow-up report of the survivors of the original Whickham study demonstrated that the mean incidence of hypothyroidism over this time period was 4.1/1000 survivors per year (95% CI 3.3–5.0) in women and 0.6/1000 survivors per year (95% CI 0.3–1.2) in men, while the mean incidence of hyperthyroidism was 0.8/1000 survivors per year (95% CI 0.5–1.4) in women and negligible in men [41].

Despite the increased frequency of abnormal TSH values, recommendations for screening asymptomatic healthy adults for thyroid dysfunction have been controversial. Some have advocated the use of a targeted case-finding approach, in which clinicians perform thyroid function testing only in patients presenting with signs, symptoms, or other clues of thyroid disease. Others have argued for a more generalized screening method to detect potentially more individuals with nonclinically overt disease [42].

The American Thyroid Association recommends screening of adults beginning at age 35 with repeat measurements every 5 years thereafter using serum TSH [5]. The American College of Physicians recommends screening in women over the age of 50 when at least one symptom possibly attributable to thyroid disease is present

[43]. The American Academy of Family Physicians recommends against routine screening in asymptomatic individuals less than 60 years old [44]. The US Preventive Services Task Force has found insufficient evidence for routine thyroid disease screening (grade I recommendation) [6] based on multiple observational and controlled studies examining the benefits of treating subclinical thyroid disease [45]. Finally, the Institute of Medicine has recommended against Medicare coverage of routine thyroid screening [46].

8.5   Screening of Targeted Populations

Identification of risk factors for thyroid disease in the asymptomatic patient may be helpful in narrowing the focus in the decision to pursue thyroid function testing. These risk factors include previous thyroid dysfunction, goiter, history of surgery or radiotherapy affecting the thyroid gland, diabetes mellitus, vitiligo, pernicious anemia, leukotrichia (prematurely gray hair), and use of iodine-containing medications or agents (including amiodarone hydrochloride, radiocontrast agents, expectorants containing potassium iodide, and kelp) [47]. A family history of thyroid dysfunction is associated with a higher incidence of Graves' disease and Hashimoto's thyroiditis [48].

Thyroid nodules are also common and found more often in certain subsets of the population. As iodine is an essential component in thyroid hormone synthesis, iodine-deficient populations are more likely to have nodular goiters than those residing in iodine-sufficient areas. The presence of a nodular goiter prompts thyroid function testing for nodules greater than 1 cm [31], but there are currently no guidelines which recommend the screening of the general population for the detection of thyroid nodules.

Certain populations may be especially susceptible to thyroid dysfunction and warrant a targeted assessment to ensure normal thyroid function. In this section we discuss the indications to screen for thyroid dysfunction in the ambulatory setting for (1) women of childbearing age, pregnant women, lactating women; (2) the elderly; and (3) patients with specific comorbid conditions.

8.5.1   Women of Childbearing Age, Pregnant Women, and Lactating Women

The assurance of normal maternal thyroid function is imperative, as maternal hypothyroidism is adversely related to several important neurodevelopmental infant outcomes [36]. Women of childbearing age, pregnant women, and lactating women may thus require targeted screening to ensure normal biochemical thyroid function [49]. Indeed, one study has suggested that screening all women in the first trimester of pregnancy for thyroid autoimmunity has been found to be cost effective as compared to not screening [50].

In addition to serum TSH, measuring TPO autoantibodies in early pregnancy has been shown to be a good predictor of postpartum thyroiditis and can be used to identify those at higher risk for thyroid dysfunction after delivery [49, 51–54]. Not only can maternal thyroid autoantibody positivity status be suggestive of present or eventual maternal hypothyroidism, but the presence of TPO autoantibodies alone in euthyroid pregnant women has been suggested to have adverse obstetrical outcomes [55, 56]. Further, levothyroxine treatment in euthyroid women with positive TPO autoantibodies has been shown in one study to lower the chance of miscarriage and premature delivery [55].

Regarding the population subsets of women of childbearing age and pregnant women, the American Association of Clinical Endocrinologists recommends screening with a serum TSH in all women of childbearing age either before pregnancy or in the first trimester [57], and the American College of Obstetricians and Gynecologists recommends that physicians be aware of the symptoms and risk factors of postpartum thyroid disease and to obtain thyroid function tests when indicated [58]. The Endocrine Society recommends aggressive case finding, but not screening, among pregnant women (Table 8.4) [39]. However, case finding alone in pregnant women has limitations; it has been reported that screening pregnant women with a family or personal history of thyroid disease or other autoimmune disease would fail to identify 30% of women with overt or subclinical hypothyroidism [59]. In one study of primary care practices in Maine, screening of thyroid dysfunction during pregnancy was performed in 48% of primary care settings and employed the serum TSH assay, although the reference ranges between these were variable [60].

8.5.2   Elderly

The presentation of thyroid dysfunction can be especially subtle in older individuals, and clinicians should consider screening for thyroid disease, particularly in those at high risk (discussed in depth in Chap. 12). The prevalence of thyroid dysfunction is

Table 8.4 Endocrine Society recommendations on conditions that warrant screening for thyroid dysfunction in pregnant women [39]

History of hyperthyroid or hypothyroid disease, postpartum thyroiditis, or thyroid lobectomy
Family history of thyroid disease
Presence of goiter
Thyroid antibodies (when known)
Symptoms or clinical signs suggestive of thyroid underfunction or overfunction, including anemia, elevated cholesterol,and hyponatremia
Type I diabetes
Other autoimmune disorders
Infertility should have screening with TSH aspart of their infertility work-up
Prior therapeutic head or neck irradiation
Prior history of miscarriage or preterm delivery

higher in the elderly than in younger patients. In one study of 258 individuals more than 60 years old, followed serially for 4 years, TSH values > 4 mU/L were seen in 13.2% of individuals [4]. Of those with an elevated TSH but normal T4 concentrations, 33% progressed to overt hypothyroidism within the observation period. It has been postulated that the mechanisms for this phenomenon include the age-dependent processes of a decrease in thyrotropin-releasing hormone hypothalamic synthesis and release, a decrease in T4 degradation, and the impaired activity of the type I deiodinase (D1) [61, 62].

8.5.3 Patients with Specific Comorbidities

There are several well-established associations between thyroid dysfunction and certain comorbid conditions frequently encountered in the ambulatory setting. Clinical consideration of each patient on an individual basis should guide the decision to pursue thyroid function testing in the setting of specific concurrent diseases.

Both overt and subclinical hyperthyroidism have effects on bone and cardiovascular health. Recent data using the NHANES III database demonstrated that postmenopausal women with TSH values in the low–normal reference range were nearly five times as likely to have osteoporosis and three times as likely to have osteopenia, as compared to women with high–normal TSH values [63]. Thyrotoxicosis can also have serious cardiovascular consequences, including various arrhythmias. One study has reported the association of male sex, increasing age, ischemic heart disease, congestive heart failure, and heart valve disease with an increased risk of atrial fibrillation or flutter in hyperthyroid patients [64]. In older adults, those with subclinical hyperthyroidism have a greater incidence of atrial fibrillation than those with no thyroid dysfunction [65].

Patients with hypothyroidism, including those with subclinical disease, also have an increased chance of having specific comorbid conditions. Hypothyroidism has been positively associated with hyperlipidemia [66], obesity [67], and psychiatric disease [68]. Some [69], but not all [70], studies have found an increased risk of cardiovascular disease in those with subclinical hypothyroidism. Some have argued against population-based screening for detecting subclinical thyroid disease [71], while others have suggested the utility of aggressive screening and treatment of subclinical hypothyroidism if detected [72].

Although thyroid autoimmunity status has been correlated with other autoimmune processes, there is no utility of assessing thyroid antibody titers solely for this reason. However, in the presence of symptoms, evaluation for other conditions may be reasonable. The prevalence of thyroiditis is increased [73], with an estimated prevalence of 38.6%, in children with type 1 diabetes mellitus [74]. Interestingly, in diabetic patients (both types 1 and 2), TSH levels may be better predictors of thyroid dysfunction than thyroid autoantibodies [75].

Finally, the use of many medications can also alter thyroid function testing results, and confirmation of normal thyroid function prior to beginning these agents will enable interpretation of any future potential abnormal test results (discussed in depth in Chap. 13). Amiodarone, used as a Class III antiarrhythmic agent, is 37% iodine by weight, has an extremely long half-time of approximately 100 days, and releases 6 mg of inorganic iodine (in comparison to daily dietary intakes on average of 100–500 μg iodine) per 200 mg of amiodarone ingested [76]. It may produce an iodine-induced hyperthyroidism (amiodarone-induced thyrotoxicosis, type I) as well as an inflammatory destructive thyroiditis (amiodarone-induced thyrotoxicosis, type II). Large iodine loads, such as those administered with intravenous contrast dye and oral cholecystographic radiopaque agents (e.g., iopanoic acid, sodium ipodate), can also produce alterations in thyroid function within several days [77]. Drugs which induce changes in thyroid function tests through various mechanisms include interferon-alpha, lithium, phenytoin, carbamazepine, rifampin, glucocorticoids, and propanolol [18].

8.6   Conclusions

While thyroid function testing is commonly performed in ambulatory practice, the indications for thyroid function measurements in the nonhospitalized patients are varied. The interpretation of test results is dependent on the individual's clinical status, degree of suspicion for thyroid disease, reason for which the tests were performed, and recent use of medications or other agents which may alter thyroid function test findings.

In this chapter, we have reviewed the use of thyroid function testing in the recommended approach to initial testing, use in evaluation of symptomatic and asymptomatic patients, evidence for screening in targeted populations, and screening guidelines in the general population. A knowledgeable, systematic approach integrating these areas will best utilize the tool of thyroid function testing in ambulatory practice.

References

1. Hollowell JG, Staehling NW, Flanders WD, et al. Serum TSH, T(4), and thyroid antibodies in the United States population (1988 to 1994): National Health and Nutrition Examination Survey (NHANES III). *J Clin Endocrinol Metab.* 2002;87:489-499.
2. Canaris GJ, Manowitz NR, Mayor R, et al. The Colorado thyroid disease prevalence study. *Arch Intern Med.* 2000;160:526-534.
3. Tunbridge WM, Evered DC, Hall R, et al. The spectrum of thyroid disease in a community: the Whickham survey. *Clin Endocrinol (Oxford).* 1977;7:481-493.
4. Rosenthal MJ, Hunt WC, Garry PJ, Goodwin JS. Thyroid failure in the elderly. Microsomal antibodies as discriminant for therapy. *JAMA.* 1987;258:209-213.
5. Ladenson PW, Singer PA, Ain KB, et al. American Thyroid Association guidelines for detection of thyroid dysfunction. *Arch Intern Med.* 2000;160:1573-1575.
6. U.S. Preventive Services Task Force. Screening for thyroid disease: recommendation statement. *Ann Intern Med.* 2004;140:125-127.

7. Meyerovitch J, Rotman-Pikielny P, Sherf M, et al. Serum thyrotropin measurements in the community. Five year follow-up in a large network of primary care physicians. *Arch Intern Med.* 2007;167:1533-1538.
8. Grüning T, Zöphel K, Wunderlich G, et al. Influence of female sex hormones on thyroid parameters determined in a thyroid screening. *Clin Lab.* 2007;53:547-553.
9. Toft AD, Beckett GJ. Measuring serum thyrotropin and thyroid hormone and assessing thyroid hormone transport. In: Braverman LE, Utiger RD, eds. *Werner and Ingbar's The Thyroid.* 9th ed. Philadelphia, PA: Lippincott Williams & Wilkins; 2005:333.
10. Tunbridge WMG, Brewis M, French JM, et al. Natural history of autoimmune thyroiditis. *Br Med J (Clin Res Ed).* 1981(282):258-262.
11. Arvan P, Di Jeso B. Thyroglobulin structure, function, and biosynthesis. In: Braverman LE, Utiger RD, eds. *Werner and Ingbar's The Thyroid.* 9th ed. Philadelphia, PA: Lippincott Williams & Wilkins; 2005:77.
12. van der Molen AJ, Thomsen HS, Morcos SK, et al. Effect of iodinated contrast media on thyroid function in adults. *Eur Radiol.* 2004;14:902-907.
13. Camacho PM, Dwarkanathan AA. Sick euthyroid syndrome. What to do when thyroid function tests are abnormal in critically ill patients. *Postgrad Med.* 1999;105:215-219.
14. Farwell AP. Sick euthyroid syndrome. *J Intensive Care Med.* 1997;12:249-260.
15. Petitpas I, Petersen CE, Ha CE, et al. Structural basis of albumin-thyroxine interactions and familial dysalbuminemic hyperthyroxinemia. *Proc Natl Acad Sci U S A.* 2003;100: 6440-6445.
16. Ain KB, Mori Y, Refetoff S. Reduced clearance rate of thyroxine-binding globulin (TBG) with increased sialyation: a mechanism for estrogen-induced elevation of serum TBG concentration. *J Clin Endocrinol Metab.* 1987;65:689-696.
17. Pagliacci MC, Pelicci G, Francisci D, et al. Thyroid function tests in acute viral hepatitis: relative reduction in seru, thyroxine levels due to T4-TBG binding inhibitors in patients with severe liver cell necrosis. *J Endocrinol Invest.* 1989;12:149-153.
18. Surks MI, Sievert R. Drugs and thyroid function. *N Engl J Med.* 1995;333:1688-1694.
19. Foppiani L, Del Monte P, Ruelle A, et al. TSH-secreting adenomas: rare pituitary tumors with multifaceted clinical and biological features. *J Endocrinol Invest.* 2007;30:603-609.
20. Tonacchera M, Di Cosmo C, De Marco G, et al. Identification of TSH receptor mutations in three families with resistance to TSH. *Clin Endocrinol (Oxford).* 2007;67:712-718.
21. Refetoff S. Resistance to thyroid hormone: one of several defects causing reduced sensitivity to thyroid hormone. *Nat Clin Pract Endocrinol Metab.* 2008;4:1.
22. Lazarus JH. Aspects of treatment of subclinical hypothyroidism. *Thyroid.* 2007;17:313-316.
23. Karmisholt J, Laurberg P. Serum TSH and serum thyroid peroxidase antibody fluctuate in parallel and high urinary iodine excretion predicts subsequent thyroid failure in a 1-year study of patients with untreated subclinical hypothyroidism. *Eur J Endocrinol.* 2008;158:209-215.
24. Seki K, Nagata I. Effects of a dopamine antagonist (metoclopramide) on the release of LH, FSH, TSH and PRL in normal women throughout the menstrual cycle. *Acta Endocrinol (Copenhagen).* 1990;122:211-216.
25. Gheri RG, Pucci P, Falsetti C, et al. Clinical, biochemical and therapeutic aspects of amiodarone-induced hypothyroidism (AIH) in geriatric patients with cardiac arrhythmias. *Arch Gerontol Geriatr.* 2004;38:27-36.
26. Mannavola D, Vannucchi G, Fugazzola L, et al. TBG deficiency: description of two novel mutations associated with complete TBG deficiency and review of the literature. *J Mol Med.* 2006;84:864-871.
27. Arafah BM. Decreased levothyroxine requirement in women with hypothyroidism during androgen therapy for breast cancer. *Ann Intern Med.* 1994;121:247-251.
28. Bános C, Takó J, Salamon F, et al. Effect of ACTH-stimulated glucocorticoid hypersecretion on the serum concentrations of thyroxine-binding globulin, thyroxine, triiodothyronine, reverse triiodothyronine and on the TSH-response to TRH. *Acta Med Acad Sci Hung.* 1979;36:381-394.

29. Ito S, Kano K, Ando T, et al. Thyroid function in children with nephrotic syndrome. *Pediatr Nephrol.* 1994;8:412-425.
30. Wang R, Nelson JC, Wilcox RB. Salsalate and salicylate binding to and their displacement of thyroxine from thyroxine-binding globulin, transthyrin, and albumin. *Thyroid.* 1999;9: 359-364.
31. Cooper DS, Doherty GM, Haugen BR, et al. Management guidelines for patients with thyroid nodules and differentiated thyroid cancer: the American Thyroid Association guidelines task-force. *Thyroid.* 2006;16:109-142.
32. Hennessey JV. Levothyroxine dosage and the limitations of current bioequivalence standards. *Nat Clin Pract Endocrinol Metab.* 2006;2:474-475.
33. Burman K, Hennessey J, McDermott M, Wartofsky L, Emerson C. The FDA revises requirements for levothyroxine products. *Thyroid.* 2008;18:487-490.
34. Karmisholt J, Andersen S, Laurberg P. Interval between tests and thyroxine estimation method influence outcome of monitoring of subclinical hypothyroidism. *J Clin Endocrinol Metab.* 2008;93:1634-1640.
35. Haddow JE, Palomaki GE, Allan WC, et al. Maternal thyroid deficiency during pregnancy and subsequent neuropsychological development of the child. *N Engl J Med.* 1999;341: 549-555.
36. Pop VJ, Brouwers EP, Vader HL, et al. Maternal hypothyroxinaemia during early pregnancy and subsequent child development: a 3-year follow-up study. *Clin Endocrinol (Oxford).* 2003;59:282-288.
37. Alexander EK, Marqusee E, Lawrence J, et al. Timing and magnitude of increases in levothyroxine requirements during pregnancy in women with hypothyroidism. *N Engl J Med.* 2004;15:292-294.
38. Mandel SJ, Spencer CA, Hollowell JG. Are detection and treatment of thyroid insufficiency in pregnancy feasible? *Thyroid.* 2005;15:44-53.
39. Abalovich M, Amino N, Barbour LA, et al. Management of thyroid dysfunction during pregnancy and postpartum: an Endocrine Society Clinical Practice Guideline. *J Clin Endocrinol Metab.* 2007;92:S1-S47.
40. Mandel SJ, Larsen PR, Seely EW, et al. Increased need for thyroxine during pregnancy in women with primary hypothyroidism. *N Engl J Med.* 1990;323:91-96.
41. Vanderpump MP, Tunbridge WM, French JM, et al. The incidence of thyroid disorders in the community: a twenty-year follow-up of the Whickham Survey. *Clin Endocinol (Oxf).* 1995;43:55-68.
42. Stockigt JR. Case finding and screening strategies for thyroid dysfunction. *Clin Chim Acta.* 2002;315:111-124.
43. Clinical guideline, part 1. Screening for thyroid disease. American College of Physicians. *Ann Intern Med.* 1998;129:141-143.
44. American Academy of Family Physicians. *Summary of Policy Recommendations for Periodic Health Examinations. Reprint no. 510.* Leawood, KS: American Academy of Family Physicians; 2002.
45. Helfand M; U.S. Preventive Services Task Force. Screening for subclinical thyroid dysfunction in nonpregnant adults: a summary of the evidence for the U.S. Preventive Services Task Force. *Ann Intern Med.* 2004;140:128-141.
46. Committee on medicare coverage of routine thyroid screening. *Medicare Coverage of Routine Screening for Thyroid Dysfunction.* Washington, DC: The National Academies Press; 2003.
47. Ladenson PW, Singer PA, Ain KB, et al. American Thyroid Association Guidelines for Detection of Thyroid Dysfunction. *Arch Intern Med.* 2000;160:1573-1575.
48. Manji N, Carr-Smith JD, Boelaert K, et al. Influences of age, gender, smoking, and family history on autoimmune thyroid disease phenotype. *J Clin Endocrinol Metab.* 2006;91: 4873-4880.
49. Stagnaro-Green A. Can a high-risk care-finding aproach identify all women with thyroid dysfunction during pregnancy? *Nat Clin Pract Endocrinol Metab.* 2007;2:216-217.

50. Dosiou C, Sanders GD, Araki SS, et al. Screening pregnancy women for autoimmune thyroid disease: a cost-effectiveness analysis. *Eur J Endocrinol.* 2008;158:841-851.
51. Premawardhana LD, Parkes AB, John R, et al. Thyroid peroxidase antibodies in early pregnancy: utility for predictor of postpartum thyroid dysfunction and implications for screening. *Thyroid.* 2004;14:610-615.
52. Stagnaro-Green A. Postpartum thyroiditis. *Best Pract Res Clin Endocrinol Metab.* 2004;18: 303-316.
53. Stagnaro-Green A, Chen X, Bogden JD, Davies TF, Scholl TO. The thyroid and pregnancy: a novel risk factor for very preterm delivery. *Thyroid.* 2005;15:351-357.
54. Stagnaro-Green A, Glinoer D. Thyroid autoimmunity and the risk of miscarriage. *Best Pract Res Clin Endocrinol Metab.* 2004;18:167-181.
55. Negro R, Formoso G, Mangieri T, et al. Levothyroxine treatment in euthyroid pregnant women with autoimmune thyroid disease: effects on obstetrical complications. *J Clin Endocrinol Metab.* 2006;91:2587-2591.
56. Negro R, Formoso G, Coppola L, et al. Euthyroid women with autoimmune disease undergoing assisted reproduction technologies: the role of autoimmunity and thyroid function. *J Endocrinol Invest.* 2007;30:3-8.
57. AACE Thyroid Task Force. American Association of Clinical Endocrinologists medical guidelines for clinical practice for the evaluation and treatment of hyperthyroidism and hypothyroidism. *Endocr Pract.* 2002;8:457-469.
58. American College of Obstetricians and Gynecologists. ACOG Practice Bulletin, Clinical management guidelines for obstetrician-gynecologists, Thyroid disease in pregnancy. *Obstet Gynecol.* 2002;100:387-396.
59. Vaidya B, Anthony S, Bilous M, et al. Detection of thyroid dysfunction in early pregnancy: universal screening or targeted high-risk case finding? *J Clin Endocrinol Metab.* 2007;92: 203-207.
60. Haddow JE, McClain MR, Palomaki GE, et al. Screening for thyroid disorders during pregnancy: results of a survey in Maine. *Am J Obstet Gynecol.* 2006;194:471-474.
61. Weissel M. Disturbances of thyroid function in the elderly. *Wien Klin Wochenschr.* 2006;118: 16-20.
62. Sawin CT. Thyroid dysfunction in older persons. *Adv Intern Med.* 1992;37:223-248.
63. Morris MS. The association between serum thyroid-stimulating hormone in its reference range and bone status in postmenopausal American women. *Bone.* 2007;40:1128-1134.
64. Frost L, Vestergaard P, Mosekilde L. Hyperthyroidism and risk of atrial fibrillation or flutter: a population-based study. *Arch Intern Med.* 2004;164:1675-1678.
65. Cappola AR, Fried LP, Arnold AM, et al. Thyroid status, cardiovascular risk, and mortality in older adults. *JAMA.* 2006;295:1033-1041.
66. Pearce EN. Hypothyroidism and dyslipidemia: modern concepts and approaches. *Curr Cardiol Rep.* 2004;6:451-456.
67. Moulin de Moraes CM, Mancini MC, de Melo ME, et al. Prevalence of subclinical hypothyroidism in a morbidly obese population and improvement after weight loss induced by Roux-en-Y gastric bypass. *Obes Surg.* 2005;15:1287-1291.
68. McGaffee J, Barnes MA, Lippmann S. Psychiatric presentations of hypothyroidism. *Am Fam Physician.* 1981;23:129-133.
69. Walsh JP, Bremner AP, Bulsara MK, et al. Subclinical thyroid dysfunction as a risk factor for cardiovascular disease. *Arch Intern Med.* 2005;165:2467-2472.
70. Pirich C, Müllner M, Sinzinger H. Prevalence and relevance of thyroid dysfunction in 1922 cholesterol screening participants. *J Clin Epidemiol.* 2000;53:623-629.
71. Surks MI, Ortiz E, Daniels GH, et al. Subclinical thyroid disease. Scientific review and guidelines for diagnosis and management. *JAMA.* 2004;291:228-238.
72. Ayala AR, Wartofsky L. The case for more aggressive screening and treatment of mild thyroid failure. *Cleve Clin J Med.* 2002;69:313-320.

73. Mantovani RM, Mantovani LM, Dias VM. Thyroid autoimmunity in children and adolescents with type 1 diabetes mellitus: prevalence and risk factors. *J Pediatr Endocrinol Metab.* 2007;20:669-675.
74. Karagüzel G, Simşek S, Değer O, et al. Screening of diabetes, thyroid and celiac disease-related autoantibodies in a sample of Turkish children with type 1 diabetes and their siblings. *Diabetes Res Clin Pract.* 2008;80:238-243.
75. Warren RE, Perros P, Nyirenda MJ, et al. Serum thyrotropin is a better predictor of future dysfunction than thyroid antibody status in biochemically euthyroid patients with diabetes: implications for screening. *Thyroid.* 2004;14:853-857.
76. Basaria S, Cooper DS. Amiodarone and the thyroid. *Am J Med.* 2005;118:706-714.
77. Gartner W, Weissel M. Do iodine-containing contrast media induce clinically relevant changes in thyroid function parameters of euthyroid patients within the first week? *Thyroid.* 2004;14:521-524.

Chapter 9
Assessing Thyroid Function in Infants and Children

Alicia G. Marks and Stephen H. LaFranchi

9.1 Introduction

This chapter will review assessment of thyroid function through measurement of serum thyroid hormone and thyroid stimulating hormone (TSH) levels in infants and children. There are aspects of thyroid function that are unique to infants and children, as compared to thyroid function in adults. While serum TSH is the single most accurate test to diagnose hypo- or hyperthyroidism [1], age-related normal ranges are higher and vary with age more in infants and children as compared to adults [2]. Further, a TSH level alone is not adequate to diagnose central hypothyroidism or thyroid hormone resistance. In addition, in the early stages of thyroid dysfunction, a serum TSH abnormality will precede an abnormality in thyroid hormone levels, e.g., mild or subclinical hypo- or hyperthyroidism. For all of these reasons, pediatric endocrinologists prefer to measure both serum TSH and serum free thyroxine (T4; or total T4) in the evaluation of patients with suspected thyroid dysfunction.

There also are some unique differences in thyroid function between infants and children. In the newborn infant, there is a TSH surge shortly after birth that results in elevation of serum T4 and triiodothyronine (T3) levels in the first week of life to the range generally associated with hyperthyroidism. The levels fall over the first 2–4 weeks of life to the values characteristic of early childhood, but still somewhat higher than of older children. In addition, infants born preterm have their own unique set of thyroid function tests. Serum T4 levels (and to a lesser extent free T4 levels) are reduced in preterm infants, with levels directly correlated with gestational age and birth weight [3]. We will organize the chapter as the clinician might approach assessment of thyroid function, i.e., with a clinical suspicion of either hypothyroidism or hyperthyroidism, first in infants and then in children.

S. H. LaFranchi (✉)
Department of Pediatrics, Division of Endocrinology,
Oregon Health & Science University, Portland, OR 97239, USA
e-mail: lafrancs@ohsu.edu

G. A. Brent (ed.), *Thyroid Function Testing,*
DOI 10.1007/978-1-4419-1485-9_9, © Springer Science+Business Media, LLC 2010

9.2 Infants

9.2.1 Hypothyroidism

9.2.1.1 Primary Hypothyroidism

Primary or congenital hypothyroidism in infants almost universally is detected by routine newborn screening programs, as obvious clinical manifestations typically do not develop until after 3–6 months of life. Screening newborns for congenital hypothyroidism is routine in all 50 states in the United States, as well as most developed countries, with a birth prevalence of approximately 1:3,000 [4]. In the United States, 4 million newborns are screened annually, while worldwide it is estimated that 25% of the birth population of 130 million babies undergo screening tests. Whole blood is collected onto special filter paper cards by heel prick, typically between 2 and 5 days of life. Some programs collect a routine second specimen between 2 and 6 weeks of life. The filter paper cards are then sent to a centralized laboratory for testing. Blood spots are "punched" and whole blood is eluted for testing.

There are two main approaches to newborn thyroid testing: initial T4 measurement with a follow-up TSH determination on those infants whose T4 is below a set cutoff, or a primary TSH determination. Serum thyroid function undergoes dramatic changes after birth. Serum TSH rises from cord levels of approximately 6 uIU/mL (6 mU/L) at birth to a peak of 60–80 uIU/L (60–80 mU/L) 30 minutes after delivery. This TSH surge leads to a rise in serum T4 from cord levels of approximately 10 ug/dL (129 nmol/L) at birth to a peak of 16 ug/dL (206 nmol/L) at 24 hours of age (see Fig. 9.1). Serum TSH levels fall abruptly over the first 24 hours of life to

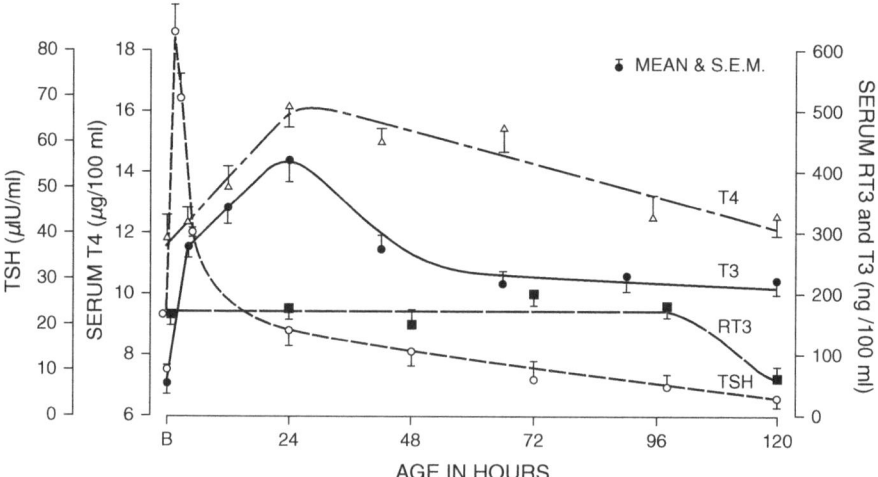

Fig. 9.1 Changes in serum TSH, T4, T3 and reverse T3 at birth and the first 120 hours of life. (From [26])

about 20 uIU/mL (20 mU/L) and then more slowly over the first week of life to about 6–10 uIU/mL (6–10 mU/L). Serum T4 levels also fall over the first week of life to approximately 10–16 ug/dL (129–206 nmol/L). Screening programs that use a primary T4 test set a statistical cutoff, typically <10th percentile for each assay. The absolute T4 level will vary depending on the age of the newborns when the specimen was obtained; at 2 days of age, the 10th percentile correlates with a serum T4 of approximately 10 ug/dL (129 nmol/L). The serum TSH cutoff, both in programs that do a follow-up TSH test and those that do a primary TSH screening test, varies with the age when the specimen was obtained. A typical TSH cutoff is >25 uIU/mL (>25 mU/L) in babies >48 hours of age [5].

Once an infant is detected to have a low filter paper T4 and elevated TSH, or an elevated TSH, a call is made to their primary care physician to examine the infant and obtain blood tests to confirm the diagnosis of congenital hypothyroidism. The recommended confirmatory serum tests are a TSH and free T4 determination, or T4 (total) determination and some measure of serum binding proteins, e.g., T3 resin uptake [6]. Measurement of serum T3 (total or free) is not useful in assessing thyroid function in infancy as it is often normal in primary hypothyroidism. Given the higher normal TSH and T4 levels present in the first few weeks of life, it is important to compare the patient's test results to the normal range for age (see Table 9.1). Between 1 and 4 weeks of life, the normal TSH range is approximately 1.7–9.1 uIU/mL (1.7–9.1 mU/L); the free T4 range is 0.9–2.3 ng/dL (12–30 pmol/L), while the T4 (total) range is approximately 7.2–15.7 ug/dL (93–202 nmol/L).

The finding of an abnormally elevated serum TSH and low serum free T4 or total T4 for age confirms the diagnosis of primary hypothyroidism. As in adults, an elevated serum TSH with a normal free T4 or total T4 is diagnostic of subclinical hypothyroidism. Because of the critical dependence of the developing central nervous system on adequate amounts of T4, most clinicians choose to treat infants with subclinical hypothyroidism. In these unique cases, it may be helpful to undertake imaging tests of the thyroid, such as a radionuclide uptake and scan or an ultrasound examination. The most common etiology of congenital hypothyroidism is thyroid

Table 9.1 Normal range for thyroid function tests in infants and children. (From [2, 27] and Esoterix Laboratory Services (Endocrine Sciences), CA, USA)

Age	Free T4 (ng/dL)	T4 (ug/dL)	Free T3 (pg/dL)	T3 (ng/dL)	TSH (mU/L)	TBG (mg/dL)
Cord blood	0.9–2.2	7.4–13.0		15–75	1.0–17.4	2.5–5.1
1–4 days	2.2–5.3	14.0–28.4	180–760	100–740	1.0–39.0	
2–20 weeks	0.9–2.3	7.2–15.7	185–770	105–245	1.7–9.1	2.1–6.0
5–24 months	0.8–1.8	7.2–15.7	215–770	105–269	0.8–8.2	
2–7 years	1.0–2.1	6.0–14.2	215–700	94–241	0.7–5.7	2.0–5.3
8–20 years	0.8–1.9	4.7–12.4	230–650	80–210	0.7–5.7	1.8–4.2
21–45 years	0.9–2.5	5.3–10.5	210–440	70–204	0.4–4.2	1.8–4.2

To convert free T4 from ng/dL to pmol/L and to convert T4 from ug/dL to nmol/L, multiply by 12.87. To convert free T3 from pg/dL to pmol/L, multiply by 0.1536; to convert T3 from ng/dL to pmol/L, multiply by 15.361. TSH uIU/mL = mU/L. To convert TBG from mg/dL to mg/L, multiply by 10.000

dysgenesis, and some infants with subclinical hypothyroidism may have a hypo-plastic and/or ectopic gland. Finding such an abnormality would support true mild hypothyroidism and the importance of thyroid hormone treatment. Most cases of subclinical hypothyroidism have a normal "gland-in-situ"; such cases may be asso-ciated with an inborn error in thyroid hormone biosynthesis (dyshormonogenesis). In other cases where imaging has not been done or does not disclose an abnormality, after 3 years of age thyroid hormone treatment can be discontinued for a month and thyroid function reevaluated.

Some primary T4 test programs choose to follow-up infants with persistently low filter paper T4 test results, even though the screening TSH is not elevated. When serum thyroid function tests are obtained, some of these infants have mild primary hypothy-roidism, with serum TSH in the 10–20 uIU/mL (10–20 mU/L) range (keep in mind that the filter paper TSH cutoff is typically >25 uIU/mL [>25 mU/L]). This screening follow-up approach will also detect infants with secondary or central hypothyroidism [7]. Serum thyroid tests will show a low serum free T4 or total T4 for age and either a normal or low TSH level (see "Secondary or Central Hypothyroidism" for details). A low serum total T4 and normal TSH level are also seen in infants with low serum binding proteins, most commonly due to hereditary thyroxine binding globulin (TBG) deficiency. For this reason, it is important to obtain some measure of serum thyroid hormone binding proteins when measuring a total T4, such as a T3 resin uptake. In cases of decreased binding protein, the T3 resin uptake will be elevated. Congenital TBG deficiency is a benign, X-linked recessive disorder, occurring in approximately 1:4,000 newborns, mostly males. Such infants are euthyroid, with normal free T4 and TSH levels and no treatment is indicated. Finally, preterm infants and infants with nonthyroidal illness syndrome will also have a "low T4—nonelevated TSH" finding (see discussion of "Hypothyroxinemia in the Preterm Infant" for details).

Monitoring Treatment of Primary Hypothyroidism

The American Academy of Pediatrics (AAP) recommends serum TSH and free T4 (or total T4) testing 2 and 4 weeks after initiation of treatment, every 1–2 months in the first 6 months of life, every 3–4 months between 6 months and 3 years of age, and 4 weeks after any change in l-thyroxine (l-T4) dose [6]. Infants with congenital hypothyroidism require more frequent monitoring than, for example, children with acquired hypothyroidism. Infants undergo rapid growth and development, and it is important to try and prevent any prolonged periods of under- or overtreatment dur-ing the first 3 years of life, the critical period of brain dependence on normal thyroid hormone levels. Thyroid function target ranges are [6]:

- Free T4 1.4–2.3 ng/dL (18–30 pmol/L)
- T4 (total) 10–16 ug/dL (130–206 nmol/L)
- TSH 0.5–2.0 uIU/mL (0–2.0 mU/L)

Treatment of most infants with congenital hypothyroidism will result in serum thyroid function tests in the target ranges. However, some infants will manifest a persistently elevated serum TSH level, typically in the 8–20 uIU/mL (8–20 mU/L) range, despite free T4 or T4 in the upper half of the normal range. If the l-T4 dose is raised to normalize the TSH level, the free T4 or T4 level will be elevated above the normal range and some patients will manifest thyrotoxic symptoms. This mild pituitary-thyroid resistance is speculated to be a result of *in utero* hypothyroidism resulting in resetting of the hypothalamic-pituitary-thyroid axis [8]. If there is evidence for this mild pituitary-thyroid resistance, we recommend using the free T4 or T4 level and clinical assessment to adjust the thyroid hormone dose, allowing the serum TSH to remain slightly elevated. Most cases of altered feedback resolve by age 10 years [8].

It should also be kept in mind that some infants with congenital hypothyroidism will manifest an elevated serum TSH with free T4 or T4 in the upper half of the normal range as a result of irregular compliance. The explanation for these findings appears to be irregular administration of l-T4 until just before an appointment and blood testing, when missed doses are quickly made up. Under these circumstances, serum free T4 or T4 will increase quickly, over 24 hours, while serum TSH may take several weeks to fall into the normal range [1]. These infants usually will have had normalization of serum TSH in the past, and so they can be separated from infants with resistance to thyroid hormone and abnormal feedback relationships described above.

9.2.1.2 Secondary or Central Hypothyroidism

A suspicion of secondary or central hypothyroidism resulting from TSH deficiency may occur because of clinical features or because of "low T4–nonelevated TSH" results from newborn screening tests (see above). TSH deficiency in infancy may be isolated, but more commonly it occurs in infants with congenital hypopituitarism (incidence approximately 1:25,000 to 1:100,000 [7]). In this situation, clinical features of hypothyroidism may be present, but more commonly the clinical manifestations are the result of other pituitary hormone deficiencies, such as hypoglycemia resulting from growth hormone deficiency or micropenis and undescended testes in males resulting from gonadotropin deficiency. In addition, TSH deficiency may be seen in congenital syndromes with mid-line defects, such as septo-optic dysplasia (presenting with vision defects), cleft lip and/or palate, or it may follow birth trauma or asphyxia.

Serum thyroid tests will show either a normal or low TSH level combined with a low serum free T4 or total T4 for age. While one might expect the serum TSH to be below the lower range of normal, studies show that the TSH is subnormal only in approximately 25% of cases of proven central hypothyroidism [1]. One explanation is that increased sialylation of the TSH molecule results in decreased bioactivity, but immunoactivity is preserved [9]. In the face of a low free or total T4, the TSH is "inappropriately" normal. If a thyrotropin releasing hormone (TRH) stimulation test is performed, it may show a delayed, lower TSH peak. With the current, sensitive third generation TSH assays, results from TRH stimulation tests generally do not add to the diagnosis (in addition, TRH is not currently commercially available in the United States).

As noted above, if one chooses to measure the total T4 level, it is important to combine this with some measure of serum thyroid hormone binding proteins, such as a T3 resin uptake, to be sure low serum binding proteins are not the cause of the low total T4. Lastly, some automated, one-step analog free T4 assays may give false low levels in infants (discussed in depth in Chap. 5). This is particularly likely if serum protein levels are low, or in the presence of the nonthyroidal illness syndrome. For these reasons, in the setting of possible central hypothyroidism we recommend repeating the free T4 measurement by the more accurate equilibrium dialysis method before a decision is made to start thyroid hormone treatment.

Monitoring Treatment in Central Hypothyroidism

The goal of treatment is to maintain the serum free T4 or total T4 in the upper half of the normal range for age. For the reasons described above, serum TSH determinations are not useful in monitoring treatment in patients with central hypothyroidism.

9.2.2   Hypothyroxinemia in the Preterm Infant

Preterm infants have a disproportionate number of "low T4–nonelevated TSH" test results in newborn screening programs. Fetal thyroid development begins in the first trimester, with increasing serum T4 production occurring from mid-gestation until delivery at term. As such, cord blood T4 levels are proportional to gestational age and birth weight [3]. After birth, preterm infants undergo the same changes in thyroid function as term infants, but the postnatal TSH surge is reduced and consequently the postnatal T4 increase is smaller. Preterm infants born at 23–27 weeks gestation actually experience a fall in serum T4 levels after birth rather than the rise seen in more mature infants [10]. This "hypothyroxinemia of prematurity" is the result of several factors: loss of the maternal T4 contribution to the fetus (amounting to approximately 5 ug/dL [64 nmol/L] at term), immaturity of the hypothalamic-pituitary stimulation of the thyroid gland, immaturity of each of the steps involved in thyroid hormone production, and lastly some infants receiving only IV nutrition may not receive adequate iodine intake (RDA = 90 μg/day). Further, some of the common drug treatments in preterm babies affect the hypothalamic-pituitary-thyroid axis. Both dopamine and steroids inhibit TSH release, and steroids inhibit thyroid hormone secretion. Acutely ill infants may be exposed to iodine-containing skin antiseptics. Absorption of excess iodine may result in transient primary hypothyroidism. Finally, infants who are acutely ill (either preterm or term) may manifest features of nonthyroidal illness.

For the above reasons, newborn screening programs often make requests for either repeat filter paper specimen or serum thyroid function tests in preterm infants.

In the typical case, serum T4 levels gradually rise to the normal range seen in term infants. If serum protein levels are low, which is not unusual in preterm infants, a serum free T4 determination will give a more accurate indication of thyroid function than a total T4 measurement [11]. As noted above, some automated, one-step analog free T4 assays may give false low levels in infants with low serum protein levels, whereas a method employing dialysis or filtration to physically separate thyroid hormone from its binding proteins will give a more accurate result. Conversely, falsely high free T4 results may occur with exposure of the specimen to heparin, either in the collection tube or in blood drawn from an incompletely flushed line. Heparin increases lipoprotein lipase, resulting in production of free (nonesterified) fatty acids, which result in dissociation of T4 form binding proteins and elevation of the apparent free T4 level [12].

Serum TSH levels are normal in the vast majority of infants born preterm. Some screening programs report an "atypical hypothyroidism" characterized by a low T4 and normal TSH level on initial screening, followed by an elevated TSH on repeat screening tests. This finding is more common in very low birth weight infants (<1500 g, incidence 1:294) as compared to low birth weight (1500–2500 g, incidence 1:4,224), or normal birth weight infants (>2500 g, incidence 1:77,820) [13]. When these abnormal filter paper tests are followed up with serum testing, the elevated TSH level normalizes in most of these low birth weight infants. However, this pattern of "delayed TSH rise" appears to be associated with permanent primary hypothyroidism in approximately 1:18,000 infants [14]. While there is good evidence to treat the preterm infants with an elevated serum TSH level, there is not convincing evidence that infants with transient hypothyroxinemia (without TSH elevation) benefit from thyroid hormone treatment.

9.2.3 Hyperthyroidism

9.2.3.1 Neonatal Graves' Disease

A clinical suspicion of hyperthyroidism in infancy occurs most commonly in the setting of maternal Graves' disease with possible neonatal Graves' disease. Neonatal Graves' disease (incidence approximately 1:25,000) is more likely when the maternal thyrotropin receptor stimulating antibody (TRSAb) test activity is >500% of the values seen in the normal population [15]. TRSAbs are typically determined by either a thyroid stimulating immunoglobulin (TSI) or thyrotropin binding inhibitor immunoglobulin (TBII) measurement.

In cases of suspected neonatal Graves' disease, serum TSH, free T4, and T3 should be measured in cord blood or shortly after birth. If the infant's mother has been treated with antithyroid drugs, testing in the first day or two of life may show results consistent with euthyroidism or hypothyroidism. However, most cases of neonatal Graves' disease will show hyperthyroidism at birth, with elevation of serum free T4 or T4 levels, elevation of T3 or free T3 levels, and suppression of TSH. Again, it is important to compare test results to the normal range for age, as serum T4, free T4, T3 and free T3 levels are higher in the first few weeks after birth (see Table 9.1).

Monitoring Treatment in Neonatal Graves' Disease

Serum free T4, T3, and TSH levels should be followed serially to monitor the effect of antithyroid drug treatment in the neonate. As the serum TRSAb activity falls, serum free T4 and T3 levels will also decrease, leading to a reduction in antithyroid drug dose. Most cases of neonatal Graves' hyperthyroidism resolve somewhere between 4 and 12 weeks of life. Serum TSH may stay suppressed for several weeks or months after euthyroidism occurs, and so generally it is not useful in monitoring treatment. In some cases, TSH will stay low indefinitely, serum free T4 or T4 will fall below normal, and so it appears the infants now have central hypothyroidism [16]. This outcome appears to be the result of *in utero* hyperthyroidism resulting in suppression of TSH during a critical period of hypothalamic-pituitary-thyroid axis development.

Rare cases of hyperthyroidism in infants are not associated with maternal Graves' disease, are permanent rather than transient, and may be caused by activating mutations of the TSH receptor or of the alpha subunit of the G protein, as seen in McCune–Albright syndrome.

9.3   Children

9.3.1   *Hypothyroidism*

9.3.1.1   Primary Hypothyroidism

A clinical suspicion of hypothyroidism in a child is usually the result of clinical manifestations, such as decreased growth velocity or a goiter, though sometimes screening may be done because the child has risk factors such as autoimmunity. The most common cause of primary hypothyroidism in children is autoimmune thyroiditis, otherwise known as Hashimoto thyroiditis. Other causes include exposure to excessive iodine, iodine deficiency, thyroid irradiation, and cystinosis.

Regardless of the cause of the hypothyroidism, serum TSH and free T4 or total T4 should be measured. As mentioned previously in the section on infants, if total T4 is used, it should be accompanied by a measure of serum thyroid hormone binding proteins. This is important because most cases of TBG deficiency are not identified at birth and because TBG concentrations can be altered by acute illnesses and by taking estrogens and androgens. As is true for both infants and adults, findings of free T4 or total T4 below the lower end of normal for age and TSH above the upper end of normal for age are consistent with a diagnosis of hypothyroidism. Measurement of T3 is not useful in evaluating for hypothyroidism because it is normal in a large portion of patients with hypothyroidism [17].

It is possible to measure antithyroid peroxidase antibodies and antithyroglobulin antibodies to confirm a diagnosis of autoimmune thyroiditis. Because of the frequency of autoimmune thyroiditis and the fact that obtaining antibody levels does not change clinical management in most cases of confirmed hypothyroidism, measuring antibodies is not necessary, although some families are interested in knowing the underlying etiology. Antibody levels may be useful in very mild cases of hypothyroidism because some of these cases can revert back to normal thyroid function. Those with high antibody levels are unlikely to revert to normal.

9.3.1.2 Subclinical Hypothyroidism

Subclinical hypothyroidism is relatively common in children. The 1988–1994 National Health and Nutrition Examination Survey (NHANES III) found that 2% of children 12–19 years old had an elevated TSH (defined in the study as a TSH >4 uIU/mL [>4 mU/L]), but the majority had a normal T4 level [18]. Findings in subclinical hypothyroidism are a normal free T4, normal total T4, normal free T3, normal total T3, and elevated TSH level. As changes in TSH precede changes in free T4 and total T4 in early hypothyroidism, this may represent very early hypothyroidism. Because of the risk of developing overt hypothyroidism, thyroid function in these patients should be monitored. Also, because those who have high antithyroid antibodies are more likely to progress to overt hypothyroidism [19, 20], measuring antibodies is useful in helping to assess risk of progression. Whether or not to treat subclinical hypothyroidism in children who are older than 3 years old is still an area of debate.

The other scenario that could result in an elevated TSH with a normal free T4 or total T4 is irregular administration of thyroid medication. The tendency is to try to make up for missed doses right before the appointment, resulting in normalization or even elevation of the free T4 and total T4. However, the TSH usually does not have enough time to normalize before blood is drawn.

Monitoring Treatment of Primary Hypothyroidism

When treatment with thyroid hormone is started, free T4 and total T4 normalize more quickly than TSH. Free T4 and total T4 can normalize in as little as 1–2 weeks. TSH takes 4–6 weeks to normalize. As a result, it is recommended that the first check of thyroid function on treatment be 4–6 weeks after the initiation of treatment. Also thyroid function should be checked 4–6 weeks after a dose change. After a stable dose is established, T4 and TSH should be checked every

6–12 months until growth is completed [6]. The goal of treatment is to keep the TSH in the lower end of the normal range for age and T4 in the upper end of the normal range for age [1].

9.3.1.3   Secondary or Central Hypothyroidism

As is the case for infants, isolated TSH deficiency in children is rare. Usually it occurs in association with hypopituitarism. Any child who has a history of septo-optic-dysplasia, head trauma, brain tumors, radiation to the brain, or central nervous system infections should be monitored for deficiency of the pituitary hormones including TSH. The laboratory findings are the same for children with central hypothyroidism as they are for infants: TSH that is low or normal for age and free T4 or total T4 that is low for age.

Monitoring Treatment of Secondary Hypothyroidism

As was mentioned previously in the section on infants, monitoring is based on free T4 or total T4. TSH is not useful in monitoring. The goal of treatment in children with secondary hypothyroidism is the same as in infants: maintain the free T4 or total T4 in the upper half of the normal range for age. The frequency of monitoring is the same as in primary hypothyroidism: routine monitoring every 6–12 months until growth is complete and 4–6 weeks after any dose changes.

9.3.2   Hyperthyroidism

9.3.2.1   Primary Hyperthyroidism

A clinical suspicion of hyperthyroidism is most often prompted by symptoms and findings on physical examination, including diffuse enlargement of the thyroid gland and possible eye signs of Graves' disease. In children, the most common cause of hyperthyroidism is Graves' disease (incidence approximately 1:5,000 [21]). Graves' hyperthyroidism is an autoimmune disease that involves elevated TRSAb. In most cases of hyperthyroidism, TSH is suppressed below normal for age, free T4 and total T4 are high for age, and free T3 and total T3 are high for age. However, there are some cases in which free T4 and total T4 are normal for age and only T3 is elevated [22, 23]. In these cases, a free T3 or total T3 level can help make the diagnosis.

Another scenario in which patients can have symptoms of hyperthyroidism, elevated T4, elevated T3, and suppressed TSH is ingestion of thyroid hormone. In cases in which the form of thyroid hormone ingested is T4, both T4 and T3 will be elevated, but the rise in T4 will be greater than the rise in T3 [17]. If the form of thyroid hormone taken is T3, T4 will be low while T3 will be elevated [17]. In either case, serum thyroglobulin levels will be low because endogenous production of thyroid hormone is suppressed [24].

Other rare causes of elevated T3 and T4 are infectious thyroiditis (subacute or chronic granulomatous), TSH secreting adenomas, and thyroid hormone resistance. In infectious thyroiditis causing hyperthyroidism, the TSH is suppressed and T3 and T4 are elevated. However, in contrast to hyperthyroidism from ingestion of thyroid hormone, the serum thyroglobulin level is elevated. In TSH secreting adenomas and thyroid hormone resistance, TSH is elevated along with T3 and T4.

9.3.2.2 Subclinical Hyperthyroidism

Children with subclinical hyperthyroidism have few to no symptoms of hyperthyroidism. Thus, this diagnosis is generally made based on screening that is done for other reasons. In subclinical hyperthyroidism, free T4, total T4, free T3, and total T3 are in the normal range for age, whereas, TSH is below the normal range for age. This may occur because TSH is very sensitive to small changes in T3 and T4. Thus a small increase in T3 and T4 can be enough to cause TSH to drop below the normal range for age. There is no evidence-based medicine to guide management of subclinical hyperthyroidism in children. The recommendation for young adults, observation and follow-up testing, is likely appropriate for children [25].

9.3.2.3 Monitoring Treatment of Hyperthyroidism

Monitoring treatment in Graves' disease is dependent on the choice of treatment. In cases where thyroidectomy or I-131 ablation is the treatment, the patient most frequently becomes hypothyroid and is started on thyroid hormone replacement. Thus the monitoring and goals of therapy become the same as in primary hypothyroidism.

Antithyroid drugs inhibit hormone formation, not release. As a result, T3 and T4 can be elevated and continue to suppress TSH for several weeks after starting therapy while the hormone stored in the thyroid gland is released. Once all of the stored hormone is released, T3 and T4 levels drop and TSH rises. The duration of this process is approximately 4–6 weeks. Rechecking thyroid function studies, including free T4 or total T4 and T3, for adequacy of treatment should occur after the initial 4–6 weeks have elapsed. The goal of therapy is to maintain TSH, T4, and T3 in the normal ranges for age. It is recommended that thyroid function tests be checked every 3–4 months after thyroid function has been normalized. Also, thyroid function should be checked 4–6 weeks after a dose change. In children who have gone into remission, there is a risk of relapse as well as a risk of hypothyroidism. As a result, lifelong monitoring is important. It is recommended that thyroid function be checked every 6 months until growth and puberty are completed and then every year thereafter.

References

1. Baloch Z, Carayon P, Conte-Devolx B, et al. Guidelines Committee, National Academy of Clinical Biochemistry, Laboratory medicine practice guidelines. Laboratory support for the diagnosis and monitoring of thyroid diseases. *Thyroid.* 2003;13:3-126.
2. Nelson JC, Clark SJ, Borut DL, et al. Age-related changes in serum thyroxine during childhood and adolescence. *J Pediatr.* 1993;123:889-905.
3. Murphy N, Hume R, van Toor H, et al. The hypothalamic-pituitary-thyroid axis in preterm infants; changes in the first 24 hours of postnatal life. *J Clin Endocrinol Metab.* 2004;89: 2824-2831.
4. National Newborn Screening and Genetics Resource Center. *National Newborn Screening Report—2000.* Austin, TX: NNSGRC; February, 2003.
5. Verkerk PH, Buitendijk SE, Verloove-Vanhorick SP. Congenital hypothyroidism screening and the cutoff for thyrotropin measurement: recommendations from the Netherlands. *Am J Pub Health.* 1993;83(6):868-871.
6. American Academy of Pediatrics; Rose SR, Section on Endocrinology and Committee on Genetics, American Thyroid Association; Brown RS, Public Health Committee, Lawson Wilkins Pediatric Endocrine Society, et al. Update of newborn screening and therapy for congenital hypothyroidism. *Pediatrics.* 2006;117:2290.
7. Hanna CE, Krainz PL, Skeels MR, et al. Detection of congenital hypopituitary hypothyroidism: ten-year experience in the Northwest Regional Screening Program. *J Pediatr.* 1986;109:959-964.
8. Fisher DA, Schoen EJ, La Franchi S, et al. The hypothalamic-pituitary-thyroid negative feedback control axis in children with treated congenital hypothyroidism. *J Clin Endocrinol Metab.* 2000;85:2722-2727.
9. Oliveira JH, Persani L, Beck-Peccoz P, Abucham J. Investigating the paradox of hypothyroidism and increased serum thyrotropin (TSH) levels in Sheehan's syndrome: characterization of TSH carbohydrate content and bioactivity. *J Clin Endocrinol Metab.* 2001;86: 1694-1699.
10. Williams FL, Mires GJ, Barnett C, et al. Transient hypothyroxinemia in preterm infants: the role of cord sera thyroid hormone levels adjusted for prenatal and intrapartum factors. *J Clin Endocrinol Metab.* 2005;90:4599-4606.
11. Deming DD, Rabin CW, Hopper AO, et al. Direct equilibrium dialysis compared with two non-dialysis free T4 methods in premature infants. *J Pediatr.* 2007;151:404-408.
12. Stockigt JR. Free thyroid hormone measurement. A critical appraisal. *Endocrinol Metab Clin North Am.* 2001;2:265-289.
13. Mandel SJ, Hermos RJ, Larson CA, et al. Atypical hypothyroidism and the very low birthweight infant. *Thyroid.* 2000;10:693-695.
14. Hunter MK, Mandel SH, Sesser DE, et al. Follow-up of newborns with low thyroxine and nonelevated thyroid-stimulating hormone-screening concentrations: results of the 20-year experience in the Northwest Regional Newborn Screening Program. *J Pediatr.* 1998;132:70.
15. Zakarija M, McKenzie JM. Pregnancy-associated changes in the thyroid-stimulating antibody of Graves' disease and the relationship to neonatal hyperthyroidism. *J Clin Endocrinol Metab.* 1983;57:1036-1040.
16. Kempers MJE, van Tijn DA, van Trotsenburg P, et al. Central congenital hypothyroidism due to gestational hyperthyroidism: detection where prevention failed. *J Clin Endocrinol Metab.* 2003;88:5851-5857.
17. Toft A, Beckett G. Measuring serum thyrotropin and thyroid hormone and assessing thyroid hormone transport. In: Braverman L, Utiger R, eds. *Werner and Ingbar's The Thyroid.* Philadelphia, PA: Lippincott Williams & Wilkins; 2005:329-344.
18. Hollowell J, Staehling N, Flanders W, et al. Serum TSH, T4, and thyroid antibodies in the United States population (1988–1994): National Health and Nutrition Examination Survey (NHANES III). *J Clin Endorinol Metab.* 2002;87:489-499.

19. Cooper D. Subclinical hypothyroidism. *N Engl J Med.* 2001;345:260-265.
20. Vanderpump M, Tunbridge W, French J, et al. The incidence of thyroid disorders in the community: a twenty-year follow-up of the Whickham Survey. *Clin Endocrinol (Oxford).* 1995;43:55-68.
21. Barnes H, Blizzard R. Antithyroid drug therapy for toxic diffuse goiter (Graves disease): thirty years experience in children and adolescents. *J Pediatr.* 1977;91:313-320.
22. Seth J, Beckett G. Diagnosis of hyperthyroidism: the newer biochemical tests. *Clin Endocrinol Metab.* 1985;14:373-396.
23. Harland P, McArthur R, Fawcett D. T3 toxicosis in children. *Acta Paediatr Scand.* 1977;66: 405-438.
24. Cohen J, Ingbar S, Braverman L. Thyrotoxicosis due to ingestion of excess thyroid hormone. *Endocr Rev.* 1989;10:113-124.
25. McDermott M, Woodmansee W, Haugen B, et al. The management of subclinical hyperthyroidism by thyroid specialists. *Thyroid.* 2003;13:1133-1139.
26. Fisher DA. Thyroid physiology in the perinatal period. Mead Johnson Symposium on Perinatal and Developmental Medicine. No.8. Marco Island, Florida; 1975.
27. Elmlinger MW, Kuhnel W, Lambrecht HG, et al. Reference intervals from birth to adulthood for serum thyroxine (T4), triiodothyronine (T3), free T3, free T4, thyroxine binding globulin (TBG), and thyrotropin (TSH). *Clin Chem Lab Med.* 2001;39:973-979.

Chapter 10
Assessing Thyroid Function in Hospitalized Patients

Jonathan S. LoPresti and Komal S. Patil

10.1 Introduction

Severe nonthyroidal illness requiring hospitalization in an individual without a history of preexisting thyroid disease produces a series of well-orchestrated and predictable alterations in serum thyroid hormone indices. The changes in circulating thyroid hormone values have come to be known as the nonthyroidal illness syndrome. Most commonly, these assume the form of a low triiodothyronine (T3) state in which serum total and free T3 concentrations are decreased in the face of normal circulating total and free thyroxine (T4) levels which, then, can progress to the low T3/T4 state in which both T3 and T4 values are reduced. This spectrum of change becomes more pronounced as the underlying disease transitions to more severe life-threatening illness. Concurrent with these alterations in T4 and T3 levels, a rise in the circulating reverse triiodothyronine (rT3) concentration is also observed. Despite the fall in T4 and T3 values, little clinical evidence of hypothyroidism can be found. In addition, serum thyrotropin (TSH) levels generally remain in the normal range [1–3]. It is interesting to note that all of these changes are reversible with resolution of the inciting event (Fig. 10.1). This constellation of biochemical changes and clinical findings has also led to the use of descriptor euthyroid sick syndrome, which is used interchangeably with the nonthyroidal illness syndrome [4]. However, with recent evidence demonstrating a more local tissue regulation rather than a global response in the thyroid hormone axis being responsible for the alterations in circulating thyroid hormone levels, it may be better to use the more general descriptive expressions of low T3 and low T3/T4 states. In addition, this begs the question as to whether serum thyroid hormone values accurately reflect the true thyroid status of the hospitalized patient.

The types of illnesses responsible for these alterations in serum thyroid hormone levels vary widely and include acute disease such as infection, sepsis, trauma, and

J. S. LoPresti (✉)
Keck School of Medicine, University of Southern California,
Los Angeles, CA 90089, USA
e-mail: jlopresti@socal.rr.com

G. A. Brent (ed.), *Thyroid Function Testing,*
DOI 10.1007/978-1-4419-1485-9_10, © Springer Science+Business Media, LLC 2010

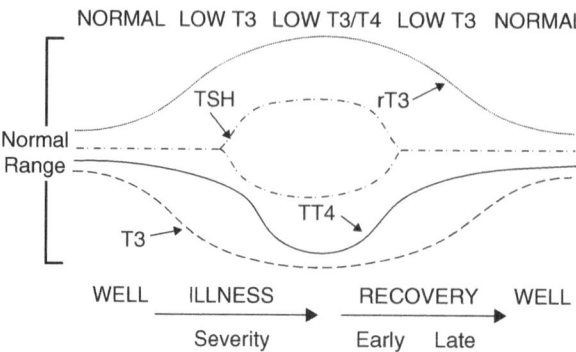

Fig. 10.1 The temporal changes in serum thyroid hormone indices with increasing severity of illness is shown. Note the predictable transition from the low T3 state (low serum T3, elevated rT3, and normal T4) to the low T3/T4 state (very low serum T3, markedly elevated rT3, and low T4) as illness becomes more severe. Serum TSH remains in the normal range until severe illness is superimposed leading to variable TSH levels. All thyroid tests normalize with resolution of the underlying illness

surgery; chronic disease, such as cardiac failure; and degenerative conditions as well as metabolic disorders, such as diabetes mellitus, undernutrition, and fasting [3]. Although the low T3 state represents a distinct alteration from normal, it is still uncertain as to the metabolic impact that these changes have on the affected individual. The most widely held view is that the reduction in circulating T3 levels acts to minimize protein losses and conserve energy sources in catabolic conditions, especially with caloric deprivation. This has a great deal of appeal as the characteristic alterations observed in the low T3 and low T3/T4 states do not occur as isolated events but rather take place in conjunction with a wide array of other endocrine alterations in response to illness or fasting. These include a reduction in insulin-like growth factor 1 and its binding protein, an acquired state of central hypogonadism as evidenced by a reduction in both gonadotropin and sex steroid concentrations, and a rise in serum adrenocorticotropic hormone (ACTH) and cortisol values. This integrated endocrine response aids in the adaptation to catabolic stress by decreasing the anabolic processes of growth and reproduction, facilitating catabolism and immune modulation as well as providing a mechanism to reduce metabolic demands and conserve overall energy sources.

In the clinical realm, it is important for the physician to distinguish between the changes in serum thyroid hormone concentrations due to nonthyroidal illness and those resulting from true thyroid dysfunction. This may be particularly difficult in the severely ill individual when serum T4, T3, and TSH values may all be abnormal. One approach would be to defer all thyroid testing until the patient is discharged from the hospital, but this would mean misdiagnosing and not treating individuals with true thyroid disease with its possible dire consequences. This chapter, thus, will focus on the typical changes seen in thyroid hormone levels in the hospitalized individual, speculate on their pathogenesis, and develop a paradigm for differentiating abnormal thyroid tests due to illness from those caused by intrinsic thyroid disease.

10.2   Low T3 State

The most common abnormality seen in patients hospitalized with a nonthyroidal illness is the low T3 state which is defined as low serum T3 levels, normal range circulating T4 and TSH values, and increased rT3 concentrations. This low T3 state of illness can be observed in up to 90% of hospitalized patients [1]. The magnitude of the fall in the serum T3 concentration is indicative of the severity of the underlying illness. These biochemical changes associated with illness are also seen in other catabolic conditions, including uncontrolled diabetes mellitus, administration of glucocorticoids, calorically restricted diets, and fasting. Alterations in peripheral thyroid hormone metabolism rather than changes in the secretory function of the thyroid gland appear to be pivotal in the genesis of low T3 state.

Three distinct deiodinase enzyme systems play a major role in the peripheral metabolism of thyroid hormone (discussed in depth in Chap. 1). These include the type 1 5'-deiodinase (D1) which can remove an outer-ring iodide from either T4 or rT3 to form T3 or T2, respectively, with rT3 serving as the preferred substrate for this enzyme, the type 2 5'-deiodinase (D2) which preferentially removes an outer-ring iodide from T4 to produce T3, and the type 3 5-deiodinase (D3) which appears to act as an inactivating enzyme by catalyzing deiodination of an inner-ring iodide from T4 to rT3 or T3 to T2. The interplay amongst these various deiodinase enzymes likely determines circulating thyroid hormone concentrations. Normally, about 80% of circulating T3 arises in peripheral tissues from the 5'-deiodination of T4 with the remaining 20% being from direct thyroidal secretion. The enzymatic source of circulating T3 has not been firmly identified in humans, but recent data suggest that the type 2 5'-deiodinase (D2) may be responsible for this conversion process [5, 6]. In contrast, almost all circulating rT3 is generated from T4 mediated by the type 3 5-deiodinase (D3) [7]. The type 1 5'-deiodinase (D1), at least in humans, plays a minor role in T3 generation and appears to be pivotal in overall thyronine disposal. With the onset of either illness or fasting, predictable changes in the peripheral metabolism of thyroid hormones occur. Kinetic analysis of tracer T3 in these conditions suggests that a decrease in the conversion of T4 to T3 takes place, presumably form an inhibition of the type 2 5'-deiodinase (D2) activity, while that for rT3 shows, not a diversion of T4 to rT3, but rather a reduction in the disposal of rT3 mediated by a decrease in the activity of the type 1 5'-deiodinase (D1). Tracer T4 studies in illness and fasting have shown no change in the production rate of T4 when compared to healthy, euthyroid control subjects [8]. The net result is the aforementioned serum thyroid hormone indices characteristic of the low T3 state, that is, low T3, high rT3, and normal T4 levels. Recent studies in both animal models of fasting and illness and postmortem humans who died in an intensive care unit (ICU) setting have lent considerable insight into the possible mechanisms responsible for the genesis of the alterations of the serum thyronines observed in the low T3 state [9].

It is well documented that the activity of type 1 5'-deiodinase (D1) is reduced in the low T3 state and likely plays a role in the thyroid hormone adaptation to illness [10]. Consistent with this finding is a similar slowing of the clearance and deiodination efficiency of tracer rT3 in humans undergoing a voluntary fast or critically ill in the ICU setting when compared to the effects of propylthiouracil (PTU), a specific type 1 5'-deiodinase (D1) inhibitor, administered to euthyroid volunteers [6, 11]. More recent investigations have demonstrated a similar inhibition in activity in this deiodinase when hepatocytes in cell culture are exposed to cytokines (TNF alpha, IL-1, and IL-6) [10]. Parenthetically, administration of these cytokines to humans produces a drop in serum T3 and rise in rT3 concentrations, while T4 and TSH levels remain relatively normal [12, 13]. Recent studies carried out in postmortem liver samples have also shown a marked reduction in hepatic type 1 5'-deiodinase (D1) activity in patients who died in an ICU setting [14]. Thus, it appears that both fasting and illness decrease the type 1 5'-deiodinase (D1) activity in the liver and this decline likely plays a pivotal role in the genesis of the low T3 state of illness.

In contrast to the type 1 5'-deiodinase (D1), T4 is the preferred substrate of the type 2 5'-deiodinase (D2) which removes an outer-ring iodide to produce T3. For years this enzyme was felt to be responsible for local tissue production of T3 from T4; however, recent studies strongly implicate the type 2 5'-deiodinase (D2) as the source of circulating T3 in healthy, well-fed humans [5, 6]. Little data, however, exist as to the role that the type 2 5'-deiodinase (D2) plays in the thyroid adaptation to illness/fasting. Initial studies completed suggested that little to no activity of the type 2 5'-deiodinase (D2) could be detected in postmortem muscle samples which was consistent with the notion that this decrease in enzyme activity contributes to the genesis of the low T3 state. A more recent study, on the other hand, demonstrated no reduction in either the activity or expression of the type 2 5'-deiodinase (D2) with acute illness and, in fact, a frank increase in both when the illness is more protracted [15]. This provocative study strongly implies that the type 2 5'-deiodinase (D2) may have little direct role, but rather facilitates the genesis of the low T3 state.

The third deiodinase enzyme responsible for thyronine deiodination and peripheral thyroid hormone metabolism is the type 3 5-deiodinase (D3). This enzyme appears to play more of an inactivating role in peripheral thyroid hormone metabolism, as it is responsible for the generation of rT3, an inactive metabolite, from T4 and for the production of T2 from T3 [7]. Much like the type 2 5'-deiodinase (D2), little is known about its function in illness and fasting. Rodent models have demonstrated an increase in the activity of this deiodinase in states of acute and chronic inflammation [16]. In addition, a recent study has shown that with illness, expression of the type 3 5-deiodinase (D3) can be found both in liver and skeletal muscle samples from postmortem tissue obtained from patients who died in an ICU setting [14]. What is so intriguing about these observations is that no type 3 5-deiodinase (D3) activity could be detected in tissue samples in healthy humans. These results suggest that the type 3 5-deiodinase (D3) may play a role in the genesis of the low T3 state of illness in humans, possibly serving to inactivate T3 to T2 thereby reducing T3's entrance into the circulation.

The elegant work describing the changes in the various deiodinase activities in illness and fasting (summarized above) cannot fully explain the genesis of the low T3 state associated with illness in humans. Studies describing the kinetic handling of the various thyronines in fasting and illness have added an unexpected layer of complexity to the process. Normally, most T4 is metabolized to either T3 or rT3 in the healthy human. As the low T3 state develops, a presumed reduction in conversion of T4 to T3 occurs leading to a fall in serum T3 levels. Concurrent with the fall in T3, a rise in circulating rT3 is noted, but this increase results from an impaired clearance of rT3 rather than from an increase in production of rT3 from T4 [6]. As overall T4 production remains unaltered in the low T3 state, an increase in the production of alternate metabolites of thyroid hormone must occur to explain this accounting gap in T4 metabolism. The source of these alternate T4 metabolites has not been fully characterized, but one likely pathway is the formation of sulfated thyronines. One attractive product is triiodothyronine sulfate (T3S), a hormonally inactive metabolite produced when a sulfate moiety is added to T3 via the action of thyronine sulfotransferases. In fact, up to 50% of T3 disposal occurs via this route in healthy humans [17]. Elevations in serum T3S and diiodothyronine sulfate (T2S) have been measured in the low T3 state consistent with its enhanced formation from T3 [18–21]. This enhanced T3S generation would act to shift T3 away from the circulation and contribute to the low T3 state similar to that seen for T3 undergoing deiodination to T2. Another T3 metabolite, triiodothyroacetic acid (TA3), a naturally occurring metabolite of T3 may also play a role in the genesis of the low T3 state. Normally, TA3 formation is a very minor component of overall T3 metabolism in healthy humans, but its enhanced formation in the low T3 state, if it occurs, would also help lower serum T3 concentrations leading to a low T3 state. The unaltered or even enhanced type 2 5′-deiodinase (D2) activity recently described suggests that local tissue production of T3 may be unaltered in the low T3 state, and that the actual fall in T3 is due to shunting of T3 through these alternate pathways of metabolism as well as to T2. Evidence for augmentation in these alternate pathways

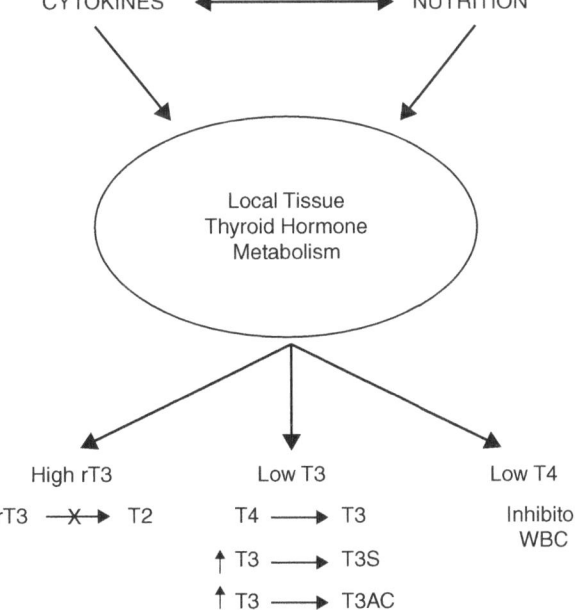

Fig. 10.2 Proposed mechanisms for the genesis of the low T3 and low T3/T4 states of illness are described. Cytokines and nutritional status are the likely mediators of the alterations in thyroid hormone metabolism observed in illness (see text for details)

in the genesis of the low T3 state in illness and fasting was recently seen when it was noted that serum T3 levels fell within a few hours into a surgical procedure despite no reduction in type 2 5′-deiodinase (D2) activity. Consistent with augmentation of these alternate pathways was the demonstration of a marked increase in the urinary excretion of both TA3 and T3S in fasting humans. A proposed model for the genesis of the low T3 state of illness is depicted in Fig. 10.2.

10.3   Low T3/T4 State

A transition from the low T3 to the low T3/T4 state is observed in patients as any given illness progresses to more severe conditions, including overwhelming infection, sepsis and septic shock, and major trauma. In contrast to the low T3, high rT3, and normal range T4 and TSH values characteristic of the low T3 state, the low T3/T4 state is defined by even lower T3 and higher rT3 levels, the onset of a fall in the T4 concentration, and more variable TSH values. This decline in the serum T4 value is strongly correlated with an overall increase in mortality.

What is responsible for the decline in serum T4 noted in critically ill patients? In contrast to the unaltered T4 clearance and production noted in the low T3 state, the metabolic clearance rate of T4 is enhanced while its production rate falls [22]. Three possibilities have been hypothesized for the genesis of the low T3/T4 state. The first is a change in the molecular structure of thyroxine binding globulin (TBG) such that the affinity of TBG for T4 is reduced thereby decreasing its binding which facilitates disposal from the circulation. Second is the "inhibitor theory" of nonthyroidal illness [23]. This states that substance(s) produced from tissues during severe illness, possibly oleic acid, is released into the circulation, whereby it interferes with the binding of T4 to TBG with the resultant defect leading to the decline in serum T4 levels. This has inherent appeal, as this inhibitor can also interfere with leukocyte function which could explain the loose association between the absolute drop in T4 in the low T3/T4 state and overall mortality. However, this has fallen somewhat out of favor as, depending on how serum samples are handled after being collected from ill patients, the presence of the inhibitor may or may not be detected. The final, and certainly most intriguing, hypothesis is the White Blood Cell (WBC)-mediated theory of the low T3/T4 state. It has been shown that TBG, a protein in the serpin class, is susceptible to degradation by enzymes known as elastases. Activated WBCs seen in sepsis, which are rich in elastases, take up the T4–TBG complex from the circulation. Once in the cell, this complex undergoes hydrolysis freeing up the bound T4 [24]. In addition to elastases, WBCs also have the capability to catalyze ether link cleavage of the unbound T4 producing diiodotyrosines which would serve as a source of iodine for free radical generation in phagocytosing leukocytes. This free iodine within the WBCs likely will iodinate bacteria facilitating their killing by the activated WBCs. Several studies in humans have given evidence corroborating this theory. The low T4 state in meningococcal sepsis has been associated with lower serum TBG levels when compared to those without the low T4 state.

Further analysis demonstrated a strong inverse correlation between the low TBG levels and elastase activity [25, 26]. This reduction in T4 also portended a higher mortality. Thus, thyroid hormone, besides its purported role in energy conservation in illness and fasting, may, in addition, be a crucial player in the body's defense mechanism of infection. Figure 10.2 also depicts the theoretical pathogenesis of the low T3/T4 state of illness.

10.4   Measurement of Thyroid Hormones in Illness

Controversy exists as to the accuracy of free thyroid hormone measurements in hospitalized patients [27] (discussed in depth in Chap. 5). Ultrafiltration and dialysis methodologies offer the most precise and reliable assessment of free thyronine concentrations. In fact, free T4 values are reported to be normal in fasting and illness consistent with the notion that T4 production rates are unchanged when they have been determined. It is interesting to note that free T3 determinations also have been reported to be normal when employing these methods [28]. In spite of this, the routine use of either ultrafiltration or dialysis is impractical as they are complex and costly to perform. To combat these limitations, analog tests to estimate free T4 and T3 values have been developed and have gained widespread acceptance as they are both cost effective and give reproducible results in healthy outpatients. However, the ability to accurately measure free thyroid hormone levels in the face of a nonthyroidal illness has recently come into question. This has been highlighted in studies comparing various analog methods in their ability to accurately determine free T4 and T3 concentrations. When serum samples from sick patients are run concurrently in the different assays, little to no agreement amongst the methods could be shown, with the lack of reproducibility being worse for T3 than for T4. This lack of accuracy may reflect a problem with either the quantity or structure of the protein in the sample, as varying the protein content in the assays can produce variable and inconsistent results [29]. One, then, has to ask if any free thyronine measurement is accurate in the sick patient? Finally, there is no role for the routine determination of free T3 in the hospitalized patient as the serum T3 appears to be a poor indicator of intracellular T3 concentration. In addition, the assays currently available to measure free T3 are even less reliable than those for free T4 due to these protein matrix problems making the interpretation of any given value challenging.

What, then, is to be done if thyroid hormone indices need to be determined in the sick patient? Because of the limitations in newly developed methodologies (cost and complexity of ultrafiltration/dialysis and lack of reliability of analog assays), perhaps a return to the more traditional and robust free T4 estimate by a free T4 index determination (the product of the total serum T4 and T3 uptake [T3U]) should be considered. This would minimize matrix problems (total T4) as well as give an assessment of the severity of the illness as evidenced by lack of TBG binding (the higher the T3U value, the greater the binding defect).

10.5   TSH Regulation in the Low T3 and Low T3/T4 States

In the healthy subject, the serum TSH concentration is the net effect of the stimulatory effect of the hypothalamic hormone thyrotropin releasing hormone (TRH) on the synthesis and release of TSH and the inhibitory effect of thyroid hormone on TSH production in the thyrotroph (discussed in depth in Chap. 4). In contrast, the hallmark of the euthyroid sick syndrome is, for the most part, a normal range serum TSH concentration in the face of either low circulating T3 or T4 levels [1–3]. This observation has remained an enigma until recently when a series of elegant studies have begun to unravel the mechanisms responsible for this seeming paradox in serum thyroid hormone indices in illness and fasting. The first piece of the puzzle came when it was observed that patients who demonstrated low T3/T4 state and died from their illness showed a decrease in the hypothalamic gene expression of TRH [30]. Subsequent investigations have begun to understand the genesis of the reduction in TRH in both illness and fasting. Induction of limited tissue inflammation by local turpentine administration or an acute systemic illness by lipopolysaccharide injection produces distinct and predictable changes in deiodinase activities within the hypothalamus [31]. The first is an up regulation in the activity and expression of the type 2 5′-deiodinase (D2) in the tanycytes, cells that line the third ventricle. In addition to this increase in type 2 5′-deiodinase (D2) activity, the same maneuvers lead to a reduction in type 3 5-deiodinase (D3) in the hypothalamus rather than the previously described induction in the type 3 5-deiodinase (D3) seen in liver and skeletal muscle associated with acute illness [32]. The net effect of the increase in type 2 5′-deiodinase (D2) and inhibition of the type 3 5-deiodinase (D3) is an increase in local hypothalamic T3 production which, in turn, down regulates TRH gene expression leading to the paradoxically normal TSH levels observed in illness.

Fasting of healthy, euthyroid individuals also produces a predictable decline in serum TSH levels in the face of the low T3 state, though the values remain in the normal range [33]. Despite the fact that the changes in TSH are not as well delineated as that for illness, some insights have been gained in describing this paradox. Leptin levels fall dramatically with the onset of fasting and it has been well documented that these lower leptin levels in fasting stimulate the activity and expression of the same type 2 5′-deiodinase (D2) level in the hypothalamus that immune activation appears to do in illness [34, 35]. The net result of this enhanced hypothalamic enzymatic activity is a local increase in T3, which, in turn, contributes to the decrease in TSH values. Thus, in the low T3 and T3/T4 states, the regulation of TSH is not as dependent on circulating thyroid hormone levels as seen in the healthy individual, but rather via the hypothalamus sensing systemic signals that induce local type 2 5′-deiodinase (D2) and reduce type 3 5-deiodinase (D3) enzyme activities leading to a decrease in TRH and a subsequent fall in serum TSH levels characteristic of these conditions [36, 37]. This begs the question, then, as to the role of serum TSH determinations in assessing the thyroid status of hospitalized patients.

10.6 Interpretation of Thyroid Tests in the Hospitalized Patient

Alterations in serum thyroid hormone indices in the form of either the low T3 or low T3/T4 state can be seen in up to 90% of hospitalized patients making interpretation of thyroid status difficult in this setting. When and how to evaluate a patient with nonthyroidal illness for the presence of thyroid disease now becomes a diagnostic challenge. Because of the frequency of these changes one cannot advocate routine screening of hospitalized patients for thyroid disease. On the other hand, it would not seem prudent to delay thyroid testing until resolution of the underlying illness occurs. In order to minimize diagnostic difficulty, thyroid testing should be limited to those situations where clinical thyroid disease is suspected, such as the presence of a goiter, tachycardia and bradycardia, atrial fibrillation, or poor response to appropriate medical therapy.

The strong inverse relationship between free T4 and log TSH described in the healthy human is no longer seen between free T4 and log TSH in sick patients (Fig. 10.3). This likely reflects the aforementioned hypothalamus sensing systemic illness leading to a local change in deiodinase activities producing changes in TRH leading to alterations of serum TSH independent of circulating thyroid hormone levels. Further complicating the ability to assess thyroid status is the inherent variability in serum TSH levels seen in the low T3/T4 state of illness (Fig. 10.4). Fifteen percent of hospitalized patients will display either frankly elevated (3.5–20 mU/L) or low (0.1–0.5 mU/L) TSH concentrations. In addition, about 3% of these patients have markedly elevated (>20 mU/L) or suppressed (<0.01 mU/L) TSH values that may or may not reflect thyroid disease (Figs. 10.5 and 10.6) [38]. These variations likely reflect the inherent lability of TSH secretion in response to or recovery from illness as well as the local hypothalamic effects on TRH secretion [39]. In addition, the administration or cessation of drugs known to influence TSH

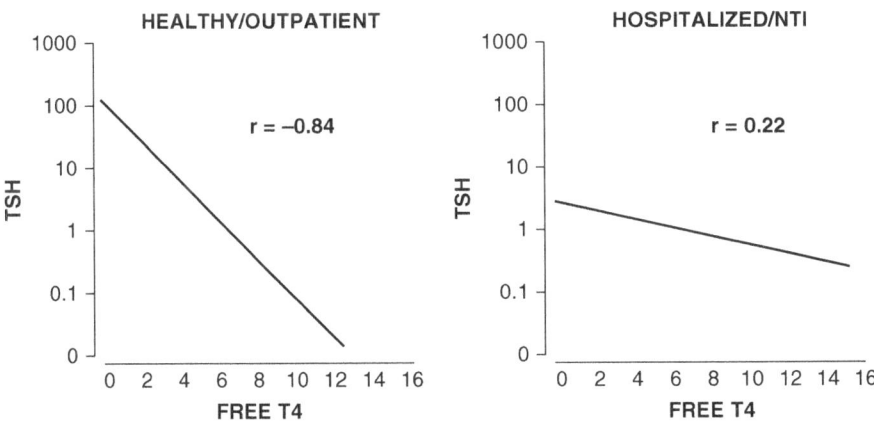

Fig. 10.3 Free T4/TSH relationship in healthy outpatients and hospitalized individuals is depicted. Note the loss of the inverse relationship between free T4 and TSH in the hospitalized setting

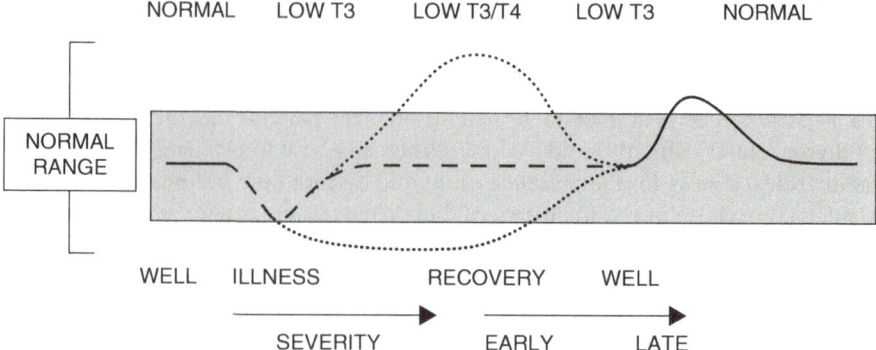

Fig. 10.4 This figure describes the various serum TSH patterns seen in illness. Note that with mild illness (low T3 state) TSH remains in the normal range while with severe illness (low T3/T4) serum TSH becomes variable with values above and below the normal range. TSH normalizes with resolution of illness

levels, such as dopamine and glucocorticoids, may also play a role in these TSH changes in illness [40, 41].

How, then, does one approach the diagnosis of thyroid disease in the hospitalized patient? Combined measurements of T4 and TSH would seem to offer the most cost effective and useful approach to thyroid testing in the hospitalized setting, which contrasts with the utility of a sole TSH determination to asses thyroid status in the healthy patient in the outpatient venue. If both free T4 and TSH levels are in the normal range, it can reasonably be concluded that the hospitalized patient

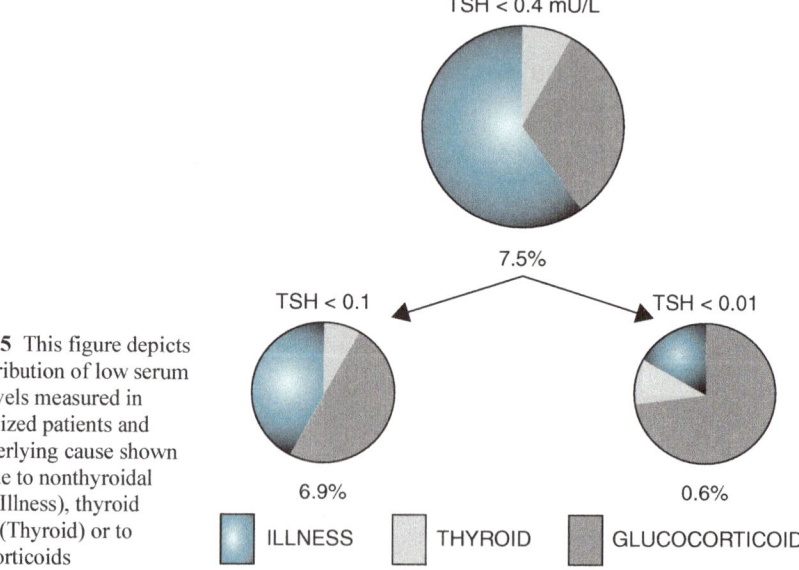

Fig. 10.5 This figure depicts the distribution of low serum TSH levels measured in hospitalized patients and the underlying cause shown to be due to nonthyroidal illness (Illness), thyroid disease (Thyroid) or to Glucocorticoids

Fig. 10.6 This figure depicts the distribution of elevated serum TSH levels in hospitalized patients and the underlying cause shown to be due to nonthyroidal illness (Illness) or to thyroid disease (Thyroid)

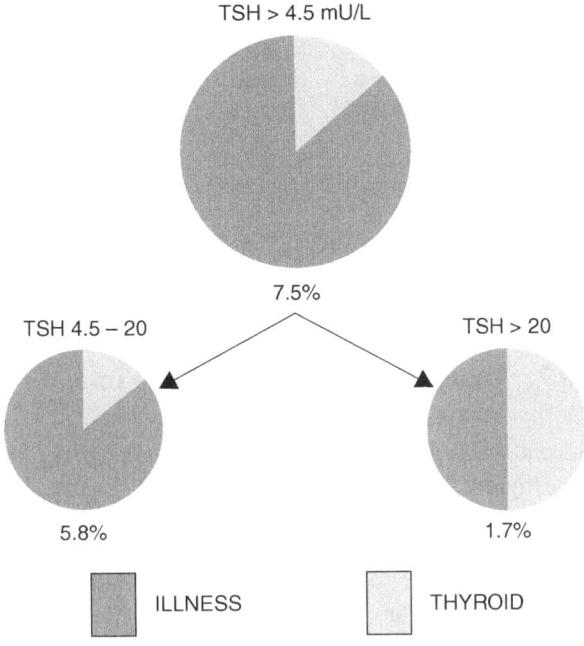

is euthyroid. Conversely, if the serum TSH is either slightly low (0.1–0.5 mU/L) or high (3.5–20 mU/L) and the serum free T4 is normal, the most likely diagnosis is abnormal tests due to nonthyroidal illness. As previously mentioned, these isolated alterations in serum TSH concentrations are seen in about 15% of hospitalized patients. On the other hand, if the serum TSH value is markedly high or low, then it makes sense that if the free T4 shows a reciprocal change with the TSH level the presence of underlying thyroid disease is likely. Severe but isolated changes in TSH levels are more consistent with illness alone (Tables 10.1 and 10.2). One clinical situation of a low free T4 and normal range TSH in the sick patient needs attention. Does this represent the low T3/T4 state of illness or does it reflect pituitary disease? The most reliable means to distinguish between the two is to determine a serum cortisol level where the value would be elevated in illness and be inappropriately low in pituitary disease. As mentioned earlier, much of this confusion can be avoided if thyroid testing is limited to those clinical situations where the presence of inherent thyroid disease is strongly suspected.

Table 10.1 describes the spectrum of thyroid status associated with low serum TSH during illness.

Table 10.1 Interpretation of low serum TSH levels during illness

TSH (mIU/mL)	Normal	0.1–0.4	0.01–0.1	<0.01	<0.01
Free T4	Normal	Normal	Normal	Low/Normal	High
Thyroid Status	Euthyroid	Euthyroid	Likely euthyroid	Likely hyperthyroid	
Treatment	None	None	None	Antithyroid drugs	

Table 10.2 Interpretation of high serum TSH levels during illness

TSH (mIU/mL)	Normal	5–20	5–20	>20	>20
Free T4	Normal	Normal	Low	Normal	Low
Thyroid Status	Euthyroid	Likely euthyroid	Likely hypothyroid	Likely euthyroid	Hypothyroid
Treatment	None	None	Levothyroxine	None	Levothyroxine

Table 10.2 describes the spectrum of thyroid status associated with high serum TSH during illness.

10.7 Drugs that Affect Thyroid Function Tests

Several drugs that are commonly administered to the hospitalized patient can influence thyroid function tests making it more difficult to assess the thyroid status of that patient (discussed in depth in Chap. 13). Obtaining a good drug history is extremely important in order to most accurately assess the true thyroid status of any given patient. In addition, serum thyroid hormone indices, if indicated, should be obtained prior to initiating any drug therapy. A brief discussion on the effects of some of the most commonly used drugs in hospitalized patients on thyroid function tests are summarized below. A more detailed accounting of the effects of these drugs, as well as others, on serum thyroid function tests can be found in Chap. 13.

Table 10.3 outlines and summarizes the patterns of thyroid function tests that occur with the administration of certain drugs.

10.7.1 Glucocorticoids

Pharmacologic doses of glucocorticoids are administered in a variety of clinical scenarios in hospitalized patients, including asthma and rheumatic disease, and are also increasingly given in stress doses for the treatment of presumed adrenal insufficiency in the ICU setting. Prolonged glucocorticoid administration in critically ill patients will exacerbate the low T3 and high rT3 state presumably via its stimulatory effects on the type 3 5-deiodinase (D3) enzyme [42]. Glucocorticoids are also known to reduce TSH secretion at the level of both the hypothalamus (via inhibition of TRH release) and the pituitary leading to low serum TSH levels [43, 44]. In fact, up to 50% of hospitalized patients with a serum TSH level <0.1 mU/L and 10% with a TSH value <0.01 mU/L have received glucocorticoids (Fig. 10.5).

10.7.2 Dopamine

Dopamine is a naturally occurring hormone and neurotransmitter that is commonly used in the ICU for its pressor effects. Administering dopamine acutely suppresses

Table 10.3 Predictable patterns of thyroid function tests with drugs

Drug	Mechanism of action	TSH	T4	T3	rT3
Amiodarone	Acute: ↓ T4 clearance from circulation Chronic: inhibits 5′-DI	↑ TSH initially, then normalizes after 3 months	↑ T4	↓ T3	↑ rT3
Glucocorticoids	Inhibits TRH release at HT ↓ TSH secretion from pituitary Stimulates type 3 5′-DI	↓ TSH	Normal T4	↓ T3	↑ rT3
Dopamine (DA)	Suppresses serum TSH Inhibits T4 secretion in response to ↓ TSH	↓ TSH	↓ T4	↓ T3	
UFH	↑ FFA levels due to LPL & hepatic lipase release from vascular endothelium Displacement of T4 from TBG	Normal TSH	↑ T4	Normal T3	Normal rT3
LMWH (Enoxaparin)	↑ FFA levels due to LPL & hepatic lipase release from vascular endothelium Displacement of T4 from TBG	Unknown	Single dose: ↑ T4 by 60% Multiple doses: ↑ T4 by 170%	Unknown	Unknown
DPH	Displacement of T4 from TBG (acute) Chronic use ↑ hepatic metabolism	Normal TSH	Acute: ↑ T4 Chronic: ↓ T4	Normal T3	Normal rT3

5′-DI 5′-deiodinase, *HT* hypothalamus, *LPL* lipoprotein lipase, *UFH* unfractionated heparin, *LMWH* low molecular weight heparin, *DPH* diphenylhydantoin serum TSH levels to the 0.1 mU/L range within hours after starting its infusion [41]. In addition, protracted dopamine use may exacerbate the low T4 state by decreasing the production of T4, possibly via an inhibition of T4 secretion by the thyroid gland in response to the low serum TSH concentrations. On the other hand, cessation of dopamine infusion resulted in a rapid normalization of TSH, T3, and T4 levels, and even a rebound in TSH giving a high serum TSH value [41].

10.7.3 Amiodarone

Amiodarone is a class III antiarrhythmic agent used in the management of refractory supraventricular and ventricular arrhythmias as well as severe congestive heart failure. The acute administration of amiodarone reduces the egress of T4 from the circulation leading to an increase in serum free T4 levels by 15% and total T4 values by 12% above baseline [45]. In addition, amiodarone inhibits the various 5'-deiodinase enzymes resulting in a rise in serum rT3 and a fall in serum free T3 values by 12% and total T3 levels by 18% [45]. Because of these effects on thyroid hormone metabolism an increase in the serum TSH concentration by 39% at 24 hours and 65% at 48 hours is also observed [45], giving a picture of T4/TSH discordance. After 3 months of treatment with amiodarone, the serum TSH returns to normal/high to normal range [45, 46], whereas serum total T4 and rT3 remain elevated (113% and 219% of baseline, respectively) and total T3 continues to be low (87% of baseline) [45].

10.7.4 Heparin and Low Molecular Weight Heparins

Unfractionated heparin is a naturally occurring polysaccharide whereas low molecular weight (LMW) heparin is synthetically derived and consists of shorter chains of polysaccharides. Both agents are commonly used in the inpatient setting for anticoagulation. The administration of intravenous unfractionated heparin increases free fatty acid concentrations secondary to release of lipoprotein lipase and hepatic lipase from the vascular endothelium [47, 48]. These fatty acids then displace T4 from TBG causing a transient increase in the serum free T4 concentration [49].

The literature that exists for the effects of LMW heparins on free T4 values is more varied. Studies to date show conflicting results on serum thyroid hormone indices. Depending on the type of LMW heparin that is utilized and the time at which the serum free T4 assay is performed in relation to when the specimens are collected influences the effect on the final measurements. The two LMW heparins studied to date include enoxaparin (Lovenox) and dalteparin (Fragmin). A marked increase in free T4 values (~60%) was observed in individuals administered a single dose of enoxaparin, while patients receiving chronic enoxaparin demonstrated an even greater rise in free T4 values (~170%) [49]. These alterations appeared to be related to the effect of the drug on lipoprotein lipase activity and subsequent fatty acid release. To minimize this influence, specimens should be drawn more than 10 hours after the last injection, and the assays should be performed within 24 hours of receiving the sample. In contrast, dalteparin was found to have a substantially lower lipolytic effect in comparison to unfractionated heparin, and may not increase free T4 values [50].

10.7.5 Diphenylhydantoin

Diphenylhydantoin (Dilantin) is an antiepileptic agent that is commonly used in both the outpatient and hospital settings for the treatment of seizures. There are specific changes in thyroid hormone indices that occur with both the acute and chronic administration of Dilantin. Loading doses of Dilantin given for new onset seizure activity have been shown to displace T4 from its TBG binding sites leading to a transient rise in free T4 measurements, usually resolving within 24 hours of administration [51, 52]. However, chronic Dilantin therapy and its resultant effect on the hepatic metabolism of thyroid hormone produces frankly low and low normal serum T4 and free T4 values [2, 53], while serum T3, free T3 and TSH remain in the normal range [54].

10.8 Variants of Nonthyroidal Illness

10.8.1 HIV and Thyroid Function

Patients infected with HIV do not have an increase in the overall prevalence of thyroid disease. However, there are identifiable patterns of thyroid function abnormalities that are common in the different stages of HIV infection. The prevalence of overt thyroid disease is seen in up to 2% of patients affected with HIV, but as many as 35% of these patients may have aberrant thyroid function tests [55, 56]. In addition, the pattern of thyroid hormone indices varies according to whether or not highly active antiretroviral therapy (HAART) is employed in these patients. This remains an issue as most HIV positive patients that are hospitalized with an AIDS or non-AIDS related illness are either HAART naïve or not taking the medical regimen.

The characteristic alterations in thyroid function tests in patients seropositive for HIV but not receiving HAART therapy include significant increases in serum T4 concentrations with normal range serum T3 and TSH levels. In contrast, with the superimposition of severe illness, HIV positive patients do not display the typical fall in serum T3 values previously described in patients without HIV and only demonstrate the expected low T3 state as a preterminal event [57]. Much like the unexpected stability of T3 levels in the face of a superimposed illness, rT3 concentrations did not show the expected rise in hospitalized HIV positive patients until death was imminent [57]. No change in T4 values was noted, suggesting that this unique group of patients does not generate the signals responsible for both the low T3 and low T3/T4 states of illness [57].

10.8.2   Liver Disease and Thyroid Function

Predictable patterns in thyroid function tests have been demonstrated in patients with acute and chronic liver disease. The alterations in the plasma concentrations of TSH, T3, and T4 depend on the type of liver disease and the level of dysfunction (mild vs. end-stage). Much as described for untreated HIV positive patients, in individuals with compensated liver disease (acute and chronic) serum total T4 levels are elevated secondary to elevation of plasma TBG levels. TSH has also been shown to be higher at baseline in patients with liver cirrhosis, though still within the normal range (3 ± 1.2 μU/mL vs. 1.6 ± 0.73 μU/mL) [58]. Plasma T3 concentrations, however, usually remain within the normal range, and rT3 levels are found to be slightly depressed in compensated liver disease [59]. The exception to normal serum T3 is seen in patients who have acute viral hepatitis—T3 levels are elevated in these patients [59]. However, when patients with liver disease decompensate, the expected low T3 state of illness is seen where serum T3 levels are decreased and plasma rT3 concentrations are increased [60]. Depending on the severity of liver disease, there may also be a decrease in serum T4 levels.

10.8.3   Hyperemesis Gravidarum

Hyperemesis gravidarum (HG) occurs in up to 1.5% of all pregnancies, and is characterized by prolonged and severe vomiting and weight loss that causes a 5% loss of body weight, dehydration, and ketosis [61, 62]. It usually presents early in pregnancy (6–9 weeks gestation) and resolves without treatment by 18–20 weeks gestation [63]. Thyroid function tests consistent with biochemical hyperthyroidism are common in the setting of HG—66% of women will have either a low or suppressed serum TSH or an elevated serum free T4 value [62], while free T3 levels are elevated in only 12–20% of patients [64]. These changes likely occur secondary to beta-human chorionic gonadotropin (hCG) stimulation of the thyroid gland. In fact, a correlation between beta-hCG levels and the degree of thyroid stimulation in patients with HG when compared to normal patients has been reported in the literature [64]. Initially hyperthyroidism was implicated as the cause of HG, but nausea and vomiting have been shown to persist despite treatment with antithyroid medications. At this time, the recommendation is to clinically observe patients with thyroid function test abnormalities and HG, as the TSH, T4, and T3 will normalize on resolution of HG.

10.8.4   Psychiatric Illness and Thyroid Function

Extremes of overt thyroid dysfunction, either severe hypothyroidism or thyrotoxicosis, have been shown to exacerbate psychiatric illness. It has also been demonstrated that treatment of these entities leads to clinical improvement in psychiatric disorders. However, there are some recognizable alterations in serum thyroid hormone indices in response to depression and other psychiatric illnesses that do not reflect systemic thyroid disease.

One of the most commonly appreciated alterations in the hypothalamic-pituitary-thyroid axis is the low circulating serum TSH value. This is likely the result of a down regulation of the TRH receptor on the thyrotroph, making it more resistant to TRH stimulation. In fact, a blunted TSH response to TRH stimulation has been reported [65, 66]. This abnormality in the TSH values has been demonstrated in 25–30% of depressed patients [67].

Another common perturbation of the thyroid axis is an increase in total T4 and/or free T4 levels from baseline [68], as seen with both depression and acute psychotic decompensation. The serum T4 concentrations return to normal after treatment and resolution of depression [68]. It has also been shown that patients hospitalized for acute manifestations of psychiatric illnesses have a transient rise in T4 outside of the normal range that resolves without treatment [69].

Psychiatrists currently advocate the assessment of thyroid hormone indices in all patients with psychiatric infirmities [67], but given the cost of these laboratory analyses and the frequency of "psych-induced" changes in thyroid hormone values, this approach is not currently recommended. Thus, analysis of thyroid function tests should be limited to hospitalized patients in whom thyroid disease is suspected or in those who manifest the extremes of psychiatric illness. Prompt treatment of overt thyroid dysfunction can help alleviate severe manifestations in patients with underlying psychiatric disorders.

10.9   Concluding Remarks

The low T3 and T3/T4 states of nonthyroidal illness represent an altered state of thyroid hormone metabolism compared to that seen in a well-fed, healthy population. Recent studies suggest that these changes in serum thyroid hormone indices likely reflect alterations in local tissue rather than systemic thyroid hormone metabolism and can be triggered by both cytokines and undernutrition, thus suggesting that they may be adaptive in nature. Because of the frequency and scope of the changes in thyroid function tests in hospitalized patients, it seems imperative to test for thyroid abnormalities only if thyroid disease is strongly suspected and not on a routine basis. Compared to the outpatient setting where a single TSH determination is usually adequate to assess thyroid status, if one is testing in the hospital setting, an estimate of both T4 and TSH levels should be obtained. Physicians also need to be aware that commonly administered drugs can influence serum thyroid hormone indices making the task of interpreting thyroid function tests in the hospitalized patient even more difficult. In addition, certain diseases give "variant" patterns of serum thyroid function tests. The challenge remains to properly assess the thyroid status in a hospitalized patient, but if one restricts thyroid function testing to those strongly suspected of having concurrent thyroid dysfunction and ordering tests for both T4 and TSH levels, then this daunting task will be made easier.

References

1. Adler SM, Wartofsky L. The nonthyroidal illness syndrome. *Endocrinol Metab Clin N Am.* 2007;36:657-672.
2. Burman KD, Wartoksky L. Thyroid function in the intensive care setting. *Crit Care Clin.* 2001;17:43-57.
3. Wartofsky L, Burman KD. Alterations in thyroid function in patients with systemic illness: the "euthyroid sick syndrome". *Endocr Rev.* 1982;3:164-217.
4. Chopra IJ. Clinical review 86: euthyroid sick syndrome: is it a misnomer? *J Clin Endocrinol Metab.* 1997;82:329-334.
5. Bianco AC, Kim BW. Deiodinases: implications of the local control of thyroid hormone action. *J Clin Invest.* 2005;116:2571-2579.
6. LoPresti JS, Eigen A, Kaptein E, et al. Alterations in 3,3',5'-triiodothyronine metabolism in response to propylthiouracil, dexamethasone, and thyroxine administration in man. *J Clin Invest.* 1989;84:1650-1656.
7. Huang SA. Physiology and pathophysiology of type 3-deiodinase in humans. *Thyroid.* 2005;15:875-881.
8. Faber J, Francis-Thomsen H, Lumholtz IB, et al. Kinetic studies of thyroxine, 3,5,3'-triiodothyronine, 3,3',5'-triiodothyronine, 3'5'-diiodothyronine, 3,3'-diiodothyronine, and 3'-monoiodothyronine in patients with liver cirrhosis. *J Clin Endocrinol Metab.* 1981;53:978-984.
9. Peeters RP, Wouters PJ, Kaptein E, et al. Serum 3,3',5'-triiodothyronine (rT3) and 3,5,3'-triiodothyronine/rT3 are prognostic markers in critically ill patients and are associated with postmortem tissue deiodinase activities. *J Clin Endocrinol Metab.* 2005;90:4559-4565.
10. Koenig RJ. Regulation of type 1 deiodinase in health and disease. *Thyroid.* 2005;15:835-840.
11. LoPresti JS, Gray D, Nicoloff JT. Influence of fasting and refeeding on reverse T3 metabolism (rT3) in man. *J Clin Endocrinol Metab.* 1991;72:130-136.
12. Chopra IJ, Sakane S, Teco GN. A study of the serum concentration of tumor necrosis factor-alpha in thyroidal and nonthyroidal illnesses. *J Clin Endocrinol Metab.* 1991;72:1113-1116.
13. Stouthard JM, van der Poll T, Endert E, et al. Effects of acute and chronic interleukin-6 administration on thyroid hormone metabolism in humans. *J Clin Endocrinol Metab.* 1994;79:1342-1346.
14. Peeters RP, Wouters PJ, Kaptein E, et al. Reduced activation and increased inactivation of thyroid hormone in tissues of critically ill patients. *J Clin Endocrinol Metab.* 2003;88:3202-3211.
15. Mebis L, Langouche L, Visser TJ, et al. The type II deiodinase is up-regulated in skeletal muscle during prolonged critical illness. *J Clin Endocrinol Metab.* 2007;92:3330-3333.

16. Boelen A, Kwakkel J, Alkemade A, et al. Induction of type 3 deiodinase activity in inflammatory cells of mice with chronic local inflammation. *Endocrinology.* 2005;146:5128-5134.
17. LoPresti JS, Nicoloff JT. 3,5,3'-triiodothyronine sulfate (T3S): a major metabolite of T3 metabolism in man. *J Clin Endocrinol Metab.* 1994;78:688-694.
18. Chopra IJ, Wu S-Y, Chua Teco GN, Santini F. A radioimmunoassay for measurement of 3,5,3'-triiodothyronine sulfate: studies in thyroidal and nonthyroidal diseases, pregnancy, and neonatal life. *J Clin Endocrinol Metab.* 1992;75:189-194.
19. Chopra IJ. A radioimmunoassay for measurement of 3,3'-diiodothyronine sulfate: studies in thyroidal and nonthyroidal diseases, pregnancy, and fetal/neonatal life. *Metabolism.* 2004;53:538-543.
20. Peeters RP, Kester MH, Wouters PJ, et al. Increased thyroxine sulfate levels in critically ill patients as a result of decreased hepatic type 1 deiodinase activity. *J Clin Endocrinol Metab.* 2005;90:6460-6465.
21. Wu S-Y, Green WL, Huang W-S, et al. Alternate pathways of thyroid hormone metabolism. *Thyroid.* 2005;15:943-958.
22. Kaptein EM, Grieg D, Spencer CA, et al. Thyroxine metabolism in the low thyroxine state of critical nonthyroidal illness. *J Clin Endocrinol Metab.* 1981;53:764-771.
23. Chopra IJ, Huang TS, Hurd RE, et al. A competitive ligand binding inhibitor assay for measurement of thyroid hormone-binding inhibitor in serum and tissues. *J Clin Endocrinol Metab.* 1984;58:619-628.
24. Jirasakuldeck B, Schussler GC, Yap MG, et al. A characteristic serpin cleavage product of thyroxine-binding globulin appears in sepsis sera. *J Clin Endocrinol Metab.* 2000;85:3994-3999.
25. Meinhold H, Gramm HJ, Meissner W, et al. Elevated serum diiodotyrosine (DIT) in severe infections and sepsis: DIT, a possible new marker of leukocyte activity. *J Clin Endocrinol Metab.* 1991;72:945-953.
26. den Brinker M, Joosten KF, Visser TJ, et al. Euthyroid sick syndrome in meningococcal sepsis: the impact of peripheral thyroid hormone metabolism and binding proteins. *J Clin Endocrinol Metab.* 2005;90:5613-5620.
27. Kaptein EM, Macintyre SS, Weiner JM, et al. Free thyroxine estimates in nonthyroidal illness: comparison of eight methods. *J Clin Endocrinol Metab.* 1981;52:1073-1077.
28. Chopra IJ. Simultaneous measurement of free thyroxine and free 3,5,3'-triiodothyronine in undiluted serum by direct equilibrium dialysis/radioimmunoassay: evidence that free triiodothyronine and free thyroxine are normal in many patients with the low triiodothyronine syndrome. *Thyroid.* 1998;8:249-257.
29. Joldy E, Locsei Z, Szabolcs I, Bezzegl A, Kovacs GL. Protein interference in thyroid assays: an in vitro study with in vivo consequences. *Clini Chim Acta.* 2005;352:93-104.
30. Fliers E, Guldenaar SE, Wiersinga WM, Swaab DF. Decreased hypothalamic thyrotropin-releasing hormone gene expression in patients with nonthyroidal illness. *J Clin Endocrinol Metab.* 1997;82:4032-4036.
31. Fekete C, Gereben B, Doleschall M, et al. Lipopolysaccharide induces type 2 iodothyronine deiodinase in the mediobasal hypothalamus: implications for the nonthyroidal illness syndrome. *Endocrinology.* 2004;145:1649-1655.
32. Boelen A, Kwakkel J, Wiersinga WW, Fliers E. Chronic local inflammation in mice results in decreased TRH and type 3 deiodinase mRNA expression in the hypothalamic paraventricular nucleus independently of diminished food intake. *J Endocrinol.* 2006;191:707-714.
33. Spencer CA, Lum SFC, Wilbur JF, et al. Dynamics of serum thyrotropin and thyroid hormone changes in fasting. *J Clin Endocrinol Metab.* 1983;56:883-888.
34. Schurgin S, Canavan B, Koutkia P, et al. Endocrine and metabolic effects of physiologic r-metHuLeptin administration during acute caloric deprivation in normal weight women. *J Clin Endocrinol Metab.* 2004;89:5402-5409.
35. Seoane LM, Carro E, Tovar S, Casanueva FF, Dieguez C. Regulation of in vivo TSH secretion by leptin. *Regul Pept.* 2000;92:25-29.
36. Fliers E, Alkemade A, Wiersinga WM, Swaab DF. Hypothalamic thyroid hormone feedback in health and disease. *Prog Brain Res.* 2006;153:189-207.

37. Lechan RM, Fekete C. Role of thyroid hormone deiodination in the hypothalamus. *Thyroid.* 2005;15:883-897.
38. Spencer CA, Eigen A, Shen, et al. Sensitive TSH tests: specificity limitations for screening thyroid disease in hospitalized patients. *Clin Chem.* 1987;33:1392-1399.
39. Bacci V, Schussler GC, Kaplan TB. The relationship between serum triiodothyronine and thyrotropin during systemic illness. *J Clin Endocrinol Metab.* 1882;54:1229-1235.
40. Brabant G, Brabant A, Ranft U, et al. Circadian and pulsatile thyrotropin secretion in euthyroid man under the influence of thyroid hormone and glucocorticoid administration. *J Clin Endocrinol Metab.* 1987;65:83-88.
41. Kaptein EM, Spencer CA, Kamiel MB, et al. Prolonged dopamine administration and thyroid hormone economy in normal and critically ill subjects. *J Clin Endocrinol Metab.* 1980;51:387-393.
42. LoPresti JS, Eigen A, Kaptein E, et al. Alterations in 3,3',5'-triiodothyronine metabolism in response to propylthiouracil, dexamethasone, and thyroxine administration in man. *J Clin Invest.* November 1989;84(5):1650-1656.
43. Wilber JF, Utiger RD. The effect of glucocorticoids on thyrotropin secretion. *J Clin Invest.* November 1969;48(11):2096-2103.
44. Nicoloff JT, Fisher DA, Appleman MD Jr. The role of glucocorticoids in the regulation of thyroid function in man. *J Clin Invest.* October 1970;49(10):1922-1929.
45. Iervasi G, Clerico A, Bonini R, et al. Acute effects of amiodarone administration on thyroid function in patients with cardiac arrhythmia. *J Clin Endocrinol Metab.* January 1997;82(1):275-280.
46. Melmed S, Nademanee K, Reed AW, et al. Hyperthyroxinemia with bradycardia and normal thyrotropin secretion after chronic amiodarone administration. *J Clin Endocrinol Metab.* 1981;53:997-1001.
47. Persson E, Ezban M, Shymko RM. Plasma lipolytic activity after subcutaneous administration of heparin and a low molecular weight heparin fragment. *Thromb Res.* 1987;46:697-704.
48. Bayer MF. Effect of heparin on serum free thyroxine linked to post-heparin lipolytic activity. *Clin Endocrinol.* 1983;19:591-596.
49. Stevenson HP, Archbold GPR, Johnston P, et al. Misleading serum free thyroxine results during low molecular weight heparin treatment. *Clin Chem.* 1998;44(5):1002-1007.
50. Myrmel T, Larsen TS, Reikerås O. Lipolytic effect of low-molecular-weight-heparin (Fragmin) and heparin/dihydroergotamine in thromboprophylactic doses during total hip replacement. *Scand J Clin Lab Invest.* November 1992;52(7):741-745.
51. Chin W, Schussler GC. Decreased serum free thyroxine concentration in patients treated with diphenylhydantoin. *J Clin Endocrinol Metab.* February 1968;28(2):181-186.
52. Larsen PR, Atkinson AJ Jr, Wellman HN, et al. The effect of diphenylhydantoin on thyroxine metabolism in man. *J Clin Invest.* June 1970;49(6):1266-1279.
53. Hansen JM, Skovsted L, Lauridsen UB, et al. The effect of diphenylhydantoin on thyroid function. *J Clin Endocrinol Metab.* 1974;39(4):785-789.
54. Smith PJ, Surks MI. Multiple effects of 5,5'-diphenylhydantoin in the thyroid hormone system. *Endocr Rev.* 1984;5(4):514-524.
55. Beltran S, Lescure FX, Desailloud R, et al. The thyroid and VIH (THYVI) group increased prevalence of hypothyroidism among human immunodeficiency virus-infected patients: a need for screening. *Clin Infect Dis.* August 2003;37(4):579-583.
56. Madeddu G, Spanu A, Chessa F, et al. Thyroid function in human immunodeficiency virus patients treated with highly active antiretroviral therapy (HAART): a longitudinal study. *Clin Endocrinol (Oxford).* April 2006;64(4):375-383.
57. LoPresti JS, Fried JC, Spencer CA, et al. Unique alterations of thyroid hormone indices in the acquired immunodeficiency syndrome (AIDS). *Ann Intern Med.* June 15, 1989;110(12):970-975.
58. Huang TS, Wu HP, Huang LS, et al. A study of thyroidal response to thyrotropin (TSH) in decompensated liver cirrhosis. *Thyroidology.* December 1989;1(3):119-125.

59. Yamanaka T, Ido K, Kimura K, et al. Serum levels of thyroid hormones in liver diseases. *Clin Chim Acta.* February 14, 1980;101(1):45-55.
60. Hepner GW, Chopra IJ. Serum thyroid hormone levels in patients with liver disease. *Arch Intern Med.* 1979;139:1117-1120.
61. Hershman JM. Physiological and pathological aspects of the effect of human chorionic gonadotropin on the thyroid. *Best Pract Res Clin Endocrinol Metab.* June 2004;18(2):249-265.
62. Goodwin TM, Montoro M, Mestman JH. Transient hyperthyroidism and hyperemesis gravidarum: clinical aspects. *Am J Obstet Gynecol.* September 1992;167(3):648-652.
63. Mestman JH, Goodwin TM, Montoro MM. Thyroid disorders of pregnancy. *Endocrinol Metab Clin North Am.* March 1995;24(1):41-71.
64. Goodwin TM, Montoro M, Mestman JH, et al. The role of chorionic gonadotropin in transient hyperthyroidism of hyperemesis gravidarum. *J Clin Endocrinol Metab.* November 1992;75(5):1333-1337.
65. Hein MD, Jackson IM. Review: thyroid function in psychiatric illness. *Gen Hosp Psychiatry.* July 1990;12(4):232-244.
66. Prange AJ Jr. Commentary. *Integr Psychiatry.* 1988;6:91-92.
67. Jackson IM. The thyroid axis and depression. *Thyroid.* October 1998;8(10):951-956.
68. Bauer M, Whybrow PC. Thyroid hormones and the central nervous system in affective illness: interactions that may have clinical significance. *Integr Psychiatry.* 1988;6:75-100.
69. Chopra IJ, Solomon DH, Huang TS. Serum thyrotropin in hospitalized psychiatric patients: evidence for hyperthyrotropinemia as measured by an ultrasensitive thyrotropin assay. *Metabolism.* 1990;39:538-543.

Chapter 11
Assessing Thyroid Function in Pregnancy

John H. Lazarus, Offie P. Soldin and Carol Evans

11.1 Importance of Thyroid Status in Pregnancy

The role of iodine in ensuring normal fetal development has been appreciated for more than 100 years [1]. Cretinism, defined as an infant or child with an IQ of 40 or less, was described in many severely iodine-deficient areas of the world and prevention of this state was achieved by iodine supplementation before or early in gestation [2]. It was not thought that thyroid hormone crossed the placental barrier to enter the developing fetus until the opposite was shown in 1989 [3]. Not only has this physiological fact now been verified, but there is now a wealth of data on the importance of maternal-derived thyroxine (T4) in fetal brain development (Table 11.1).

During the last two decades, advances in our understanding of thyroid physiology in pregnancy [5] has informed interpretation of thyroid function in gestation [6], and has led to a more rational approach to therapy of thyroid disease in pregnancy [7]. Central to treatment is an appreciation of the assessment of thyroid function in pregnancy which is the subject of the following discussion.

11.1.1 Thyroid Physiology in Pregnancy

Pregnancy has an appreciable effect on thyroid economy [5]. There are significant changes in iodine metabolism characterized by increased excretion of iodine in the urine accounting for the increase in thyroid volume even in areas of moderate dietary iodine intake [8]. Although thyroid size increases in areas of iodine deficiency,

J. H. Lazarus (✉)
Centre for Endocrine and Diabetes Sciences, University Hospital of Wales,
Cardiff CF14 4XN, Wales, UK
e-mail: lazarus@cardiff.ac.uk

G. A. Brent (ed.), *Thyroid Function Testing,*
DOI 10.1007/978-1-4419-1485-9_11, © Springer Science+Business Media, LLC 2010

Table 11.1 Physiology of thyroid hormone availability to fetal brain (from [4])

Before onset of fetal thyroid function	Between onset of fetal thyroid function and birth
T4 and T3 present in embryonic and fetal fluids and tissues	Maternal transfer continues
T4 and T3 are of maternal origin	Brain T3 dependent on local production of T3 from T4 by the action of D2
Nuclear receptors present and occupied by T3	Normal maternal T4 protects fetal brain from T3 deficiency
D2 and D3 expressed in brain	Normal T3 in low T4 mother does not prevent cerebral T3 deficiency

D2 5′ deiodinase Type 2, *D3* 5 deiodinase Type 3

it does not do so in those regions that are iodine sufficient [9]. There is ample evidence that iodine deficiency during pregnancy is associated with maternal goitre and reduced maternal T4 level, which is seen in areas of endemic cretinism [10]. Even in moderately iodine-deficient regions urinary iodine excretion is higher in all trimesters than in nonpregnant women, and may be causative in maternal goitre formation as assessed by ultrasound.

A daily iodine intake of 250 μg is recommended in pregnancy, but is not always achieved even in developed parts of the world [11]. Thus, to prevent fetal brain damage, additional iodine supplementation in pregnancy may be required in areas of suboptimal iodine nutrition.

Thyroid hormone transport proteins, particularly thyroxine binding globulin (TBG), increase due to enhanced hepatic synthesis and a reduced degradation rate due to oligosaccharide modification. Serum concentration of thyroid hormones has been reported to be decreased, increased, or unchanged during gestation by different groups depending on the assays used. However, there is general consensus that there is a transient rise in free T4 (FT4) in the first trimester due to the relatively high circulating human chorionic gonadotrophin (hCG) concentration and a decrease of FT4 in the second and third trimester, albeit within the normal reference range [6]. Changes in free triiodothyronine (FT3) concentration are also seen in which they broadly parallel the FT4, again within the normal range [6]. The precise reason for the decline in free thyroid hormones is not clear, but the interaction of TSH, estrogen, and thyroid binding proteins is of importance. In iodine-deficient areas (including marginal iodine deficiency seen in many continental European countries) the pregnant woman may become significantly hypothyroxinaemic with preferential T3 secretion. The thyroidal "stress" is also evidenced by a rise in the median TSH and serum thyroglobulin [5]. The increase in thyroid volume already referred to is substantially greater in iodine-deficient areas.

Thus, pregnancy is associated with significant but reversible changes in thyroid function (Table 11.2). The findings associated with the hypermetabolic state of normal pregnancy can overlap with the clinical signs and symptoms of thyroid disease.

Table 11.2 Physiologic changes in pregnancy that influence thyroid function tests (from [6])

Physiologic change	Thyroid function test change
↑ Thyroid binding globulin (TBG)	↑ Serum total T4 and T3 concentration
First trimester hCG elevation	↑ Free T4 and ↓ TSH
↑ Plasma volume	↑ T4 and T3 pool size
↑ D3 (inner-ring deiodination) due to increased placental mass	↑ T4 and T3 degradation resulting in requirement for increased hormone production
Thyroid enlargement (in some women)	↑ Serum thyroglobulin
↑ Iodine clearance	↓ Hormone production in iodine-deficient areas

11.2   Human Chorionic Gonadotrophin

The placenta secretes hCG, a glycoprotein hormone sharing a common alpha sub-unit with TSH but having a unique beta subunit, which confers specificity. Evidence derived from *in vitro* studies on thyroid tissue and on eukaryotic cells stably express-ing the human TSH receptor (TSHR) suggests that hCG, or a molecular variant, is able to act as a thyroid stimulating hormone (TSH) agonist [12], although this is contro-versial [13]. A screening study of more than 23,000 pregnant women has shown inci-dence of gestational transient hyperthyroxinemia of 0.285% which has been ascribed to elevated hCG levels [14]. No therapy is necessary for this condition. There is good evidence that hyperemesis gravidarum (HG), which sometimes requires hospitaliza-tion because of the development of dehydration and ketosis, may be associated with hyperthyroidism due to excess hCG stimulation [15]. The situation is complicated by the fact that the modification of carbohydrate structure attached to hCG may alter the biological activities of the molecule; for example, asialo-hCG plays a critical role in hyperthyroidism during pregnancy and has increased thyrotropic effects [16]. The precise relationship between hCG structure and bioactivity is not known, not only because of the number and complexity of hCG isoforms, but also because bioactiv-ity is difficult to measure in a way meaningful to human physiology. An important problem is the poor correlation between bioactivity as measured by *in vitro* and *in vivo* systems. Despite these reservations, it is noteworthy that the hCG produced by hydatiform mole tissue as well as that produced in the first trimester of normal ges-tation, is reported to have high thyroid stimulating specific activity [17]. Therefore the development of thyrotoxicosis in gestational trophoblastic neoplasia (GTN) and gestational thyrotoxicosis (GT) may be related not only to the high serum hCG con-centrations, but also to the nature of the hCG isoforms that are produced in these settings. The sensitivity of the TSH receptor to hCG has also been demonstrated by a unique case report of familial gestational hyperthyroidism caused by a mutant TSHR [18]. In this report, a woman and her mother were described who both had recur-rent gestational hyperthyroidism and normal serum hCG. Both were heterozygous

Fig. 11.1 Gestational variation in thyroid function in normal women

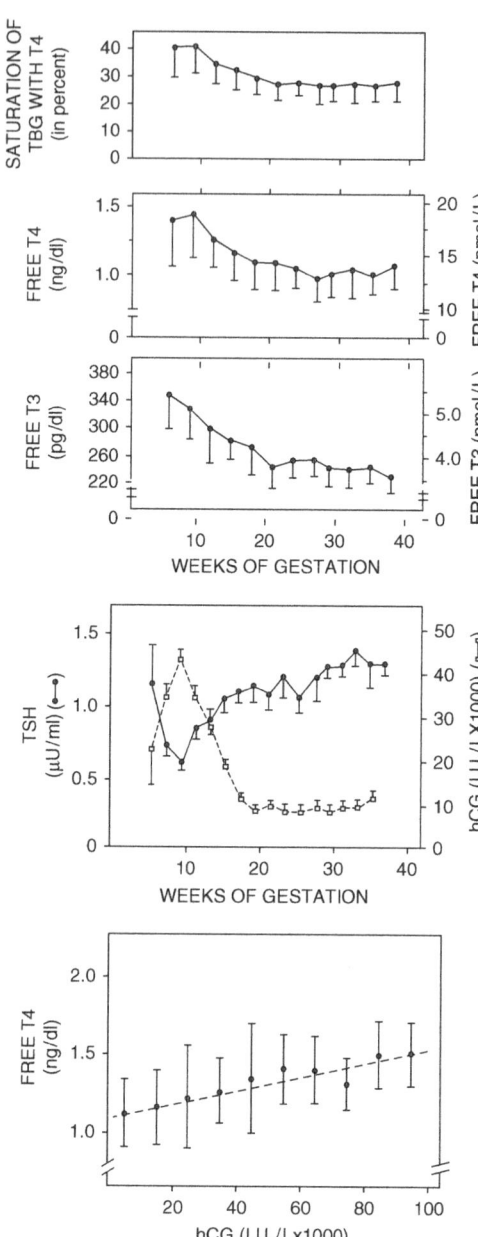

for a missense mutation in the extracellular domain of the TSHR, which was more sensitive to hCG than the wild-type receptor. The changes in TBG, thyroid hormones, and the relationship between hCG and TSH and FT4 are shown in Fig 11.1.

Data from 606 normal pregnancies show the rise in TBG (top panel) accompanied by the changes in FT4 and FT3 concentrations throughout gestation in a mildly iodine-deficient area (Brussels). The lower two panels show the relationship between serum TSH and hCG as a function of gestational age and the relation between FT4 and hCG in the first half of gestation [5].

11.3   Clinical Relevance of Assessing Thyroid Function in Pregnancy

There is good evidence that maternal thyroid dysfunction during pregnancy may affect maternal health, fetal health, and obstetric outcome. There is significant overlap between the symptoms experienced by normal euthyroid pregnant women and those with thyroid dysfunction (hyperthyroidism and hypothyroidism). Clinical diagnosis is therefore not straightforward making it essential to have reliable accurate tests of thyroid function in pregnancy. It is becoming clear that normative gestational related reference ranges for thyroid hormones are required for diagnosis.

11.3.1   Hyperthyroidism

Maternal complications of hyperthyroidism include miscarriage, placenta abruptio, and preterm delivery. Congestive heart failure and thyroid storm may also occur and the risk of preeclampsia is significantly higher in women with poorly controlled hyperthyroidism, and low birth weight may be up to nine times as common [19]. Neonatal hyperthyroidism, prematurity, and intrauterine growth retardation may be observed [20]. Women with thyroid hormone resistance who, despite being euthyroid, had high levels of circulating T4 had a significantly increased miscarriage rate compared to euthyroid unaffected couples [21]. Subclinical hyperthyroidism, comprising 1.7% of women, showed no significant adverse pregnancy outcomes suggesting that treatment of this condition in pregnancy is not warranted [22]. Nevertheless, it is clearly essential to diagnose and treat overt clinical and biochemical hyperthyroidism to lessen the rate of complications described above. Gestational amelioration of Graves' disease is often associated with a reduction in titer of TSHR antibody (TSHR Ab) and a change from stimulatory to blocking antibody activity [23]. A small number of newborns from mothers with Graves' disease develop central hypothyroidism characterized by low FT4 concentrations in combination with suppressed TSH levels and a blunted TSH response after thyropin releasing hormone (TRH) administration. This situation may arise because of passively transferred T4 from the mother who is hyperthyroid in the short term or as a result of longer term (1 month) neonatal hyperthyroidism due to passively transferred thyroid stimulating antibodies (TSAbs). There is a suggestion from the clinical description that maternal thyrotoxicosis before 32 weeks gestation may be an important time point for the development of central hypothyroidism in the baby. The syndrome provides some indication of the effect of excess maternal thyroid hormones on the development of the hypothalamic-pituitary-thyroid axis as well as the effect of excess neonatal thyroid hormones on the same system [24].

11.3.2   Hypothyroidism

The incidence of hypothyroidism during pregnancy is around 2.5% [25]. The etiology is usually autoimmune thyroiditis characterized by the presence of anti-thyroid peroxidase (TPO) antibodies. Significant titers of these antibodies are found in about 10% of women at about 14 weeks gestation. Other causes of hypothyroidism in pregnancy include postoperative thyroid failure and noncompliance with existing T4 therapy. In areas of iodine deficiency the circulating maternal T4 concentrations are low, although TSH is usually in the normal range. In this situation the incidence of thyroid abnormalities is higher and in particular thyroid autoimmunity may be associated with diminished thyroid reserve and an increase in spontaneous abortion.

The diagnosis of hypothyroidism is made by noting an elevated TSH accompanied by a low serum FT4. Subclinical hypothyroidism (mild hypothyroidism) is recognized to be as important in its adverse effects affecting mother and neonate as the full expression of the disease [26]. Maternal hypothyroxinemia (without increased TSH) is also being increasingly accepted as deleterious to the neuropsychological development of the child [27]. Care should be taken in the interpretation of TSH concentrations in early gestation due to the thyrotrophic effects of hCG already discussed.

Previous studies have documented the effects of hypothyroidism on maternal and fetal well-being, drawing attention to increased incidence of abortion, obstetric complications, and fetal abnormalities in untreated women [28]. Women already receiving T4 for hypothyroidism require an increased dose during gestation. This is critical to ensure adequate maternal T4 levels for delivery to the fetus, especially during the first trimester. The dose should normally be increased by 50–100 μg/day as soon as pregnancy is diagnosed; subsequent monitoring of TSH and FT4 is then necessary to ensure correct and timely replacement dosage [29].

11.4   Maternal Thyroid Disease in Pregnancy: Effect on Child Development

Thyroid hormones are major factors for the normal development of the brain. The mechanisms of actions of thyroid hormones in the developing brain are mainly mediated through two ligand-activated thyroid hormone receptor isoforms [30]. It is known that thyroid hormone deficiency may cause severe neurological disorders resulting from the deficit of neuronal cell differentiation and migration, axonal and dendritic outgrowth, myelin formation, and synaptogenesis [31]. This is the situation well documented in iodine-deficient areas where the maternal circulating T4 concentrations are too low to provide adequate fetal levels, particularly in the first trimester. However, concern has been raised that in an iodine-sufficient area maternal thyroid dysfunction (hypothyroidism, subclinical hypothyroidism or hypothyroxinemia) during pregnancy results in neuro-intellectual impairment of the child. For example, low thyroid hormone concentrations in early gestation have been associated with significant decrements of IQ of the children when tested at 7 years and 10 months respectively [32, 33], and maternal hypothyroxinemia during early gestation may be an independent determinant of neurodevelopmental delay [34]. Furthermore, when FT4 concentrations increase during gestation in women who have had low FT4 in early pregnancy, infant development is not adversely affected [34]. The neurodevelopmental impairment is similar to that seen in iodine-deficient areas and implies that iodine status should be normalized in regions of deficiency in addition to routine monitoring of thyroid function.

11.5 Clinical Implications of Thyroid Antibodies in Gestation

Although the measurement of thyroid antibodies (TPO antibodies [TPOAbs] and TSHR antibodies) does not give any indication as to thyroid function, their presence in pregnancy may have significant effects on mother and child. Their measurement is discussed in Chap. 6.

TPOAbs are a marker for an increased risk of infertility, miscarriage, and preterm delivery [7]. TPOAbs are found in around 10% of women in early pregnancy, and are also associated with decreased thyroid functional reserve during gestation with possible development of hypothyroidism. Their presence at 32 weeks gestation has also resulted in a significant IQ decrement in children even when the mothers were euthyroid [35]. It should also be remembered that the finding of TPOAbs in early pregnancy imparts a 50% risk for the development of postpartum thyroid dysfunction and the whole spectrum of postpartum thyroiditis [36].

TSHR antibodies are present only rarely in gestation (<1%), but do signify the presence of Graves' disease (see above).

11.6 Methods for Measuring Thyroid Function in Pregnancy

The profound changes that occur during the first few weeks following conception have consequences for thyroid hormone concentrations and thyroid function assessment. The increase in TBG concentrations is due to both an increase in hepatic synthesis of TBG and an estrogen-induced increase in sialylation, which increases the half-life of TBG [37, 38], leading to increases in total T4 concentrations early in gestation. At the same time, dramatic increases in serum hCG lead to thyroid-stimulating activity and decreases in TSH concentrations [39] and seem to be somewhat dependent on ethnicity [40]. In addition, pregnancy-related increases in plasma volume and glomerular filtration rate (by approximately 50%), as well as changes in deiodinase activity, can lead to decreases in serum iodine concentrations. Moreover, due to the general immunosuppressive state during pregnancy [41], thyroid autoimmune-related activity is decreased, leading to additional physiological changes that result in changes in serum thyroid hormone concentrations.

The limitations of thyroid hormone assessment in pregnancy are worth noting. Free hormone assays, based on analog methods that rely on the concentrations of binding proteins, are notoriously method-dependent and may give misleading FT4 and FT3 values in pregnancy. Direct assays with equilibrium dialysis are expensive, laborious to perform, and not widely available [42]. Also, gestation-specific reference intervals for thyroid function tests are not in use in most laboratories.

11.6.1 Total and Free Thyroid Hormone Measurements in Pregnancy

Circulating T4 and T3 are at equilibrium of free- and protein-bound hormones. The majority of thyroid hormones (>99%) are bound to transport proteins, mainly to TBG and to a lesser extent to transthyretin and albumin. Protein binding may prevent thyroid hormones from entering cells to exert their biological effects and also provide a storage reservoir. In contrast, the free hormones are present at much lower concentrations (picomolar compared to the nanomolar concentrations of total hormones) and are biologically active.

Due to their increased serum concentrations, it has been technically easier to develop assays for total thyroid hormones compared to free (free T4 measurements discussed in depth in Chap. 5). These assays tend to be regarded as more accurate and valid than free hormone assays. However, changes in the concentration of hormone binding proteins have a big effect on the total hormone concentration. In pregnancy, estrogen causes an increase in TBG and by the second trimester, total T4 concentration correspondingly increases to 1.5 times the concentration typical in the nonpregnant individual. Total T4 assays generally agree quite well resulting in better defined reference intervals in adults. Due to the changes in serum concentrations in pregnancy, gestation-specific reference intervals for total thyroid hormones need to be defined and used [43]. However, in most clinical laboratories total T4 testing has been replaced with free hormone assays.

The measurement of free hormones has the theoretical advantage that they measure the biologically active form of the hormone. However, there are difficulties, not least due to the lower concentration of analyte, in the requirement that the assay does not disturb the equilibrium between protein-bound and free hormone and that the assay is unaffected by the much higher concentrations of protein-bound hormone. Measurement of free hormones can be accomplished by immunoassay, or more recently using isotope dilution mass spectrometry [44] following physical separation of the free from protein-bound hormones by techniques such as equilibrium dialysis or ultrafiltration[45, 46]. These assays are technically demanding, are limited to specialized laboratories, and are not in routine clinical use. More often clinical laboratories employ commercially available immunoassays for FT4 and FT3 that estimate the free thyroid hormone concentrations without physical separation from protein-bound hormone [47]. However, recent evaluation of one such commercially available FT4 assay has shown that it correlates more closely to total T4 assays than to FT4 measured following physical separation from binding proteins [48]. In general, commercial FT4 immunoassays are affected to variable degrees by the physiological increase in TBG that occurs in pregnancy [49]. For this reason, there is significant method-dependant variation in FT4 measurement in pregnancy and it is difficult to establish pregnancy-related FT4 reference intervals [50, 51].

In view of the method-related differences and gestation-specific changes in thyroid hormone, it is recommend that method- and gestation-specific reference intervals are used for the interpretation of various laboratory results during pregnancy [47]. Furthermore, it is becoming increasingly recognized that iodine sufficiency of the reference population, as well as the background thyroid autoimmunity, should be taken into account and that the reference population be iodine-sufficient [52, 53]. To that end, most clinical laboratory reports only provide nonpregnant reference intervals for the interpretation of laboratory results. Unfortunately, few, if any, FT4 immunoassay manufacturers provide appropriate normal pregnancy-related reference intervals that are method-specific (specific to the method used for hormone analysis). It is therefore imperative that method- and gestation-specific reference intervals for FT4 are derived in the appropriate reference populations to prevent misinterpretation of thyroid status in pregnant women.

11.6.2 TSH Tests in Pregnancy

In general, serum TSH concentrations provide the first clinical indicator of thyroid dysfunction. Due to the log–linear relationship between TSH and FT4, very small changes in T4 concentrations will provoke very large changes in serum TSH. However, in pregnancy, thyroid and pituitary functions are less stable. During early gestation TSH is suppressed by 20–50% by week 10 due to the steep increase in hCG concentrations [54]. Therefore, maternal serum TSH does not provide a good indicator for the control of treatment of thyroid dysfunction, and can lead to maternal underreplacement with levothyroxine (L-T4) or overtreatment with antithyroid drugs, which can result in both maternal hypothyroidism and an increased risk of adverse fetal brain development. In women with depressed TSH yet normal FT4, the parents' hypermetabolic symptoms may be explained by the additional evaluation of FT3 and FT3 index (FT3I).

Reliable trimester-specific (or gestation-specific) reference intervals for TSH are now available. These reference intervals are based on a large enough sample size composed of iodine-sufficient, antibody-free populations, and use a reliable and sensitive detection method (Table 11.3). It is important to base these TSH intervals on women who have a singleton pregnancy and do not have high levels of hCG or hyperemesis.

Table 11.3 Selected trimester-specific, method-specific FT4, FT3, and TSH medians (± SD) or means* (± SE) and reference intervals

Country (ref)	Gestation (n =)	FT4 median (reference interval) or mean (± SEM)* pmol/L	TSH median (reference interval) or mean (± SEM) mIU/L	FT3 median (reference interval) or mean (± SEM) pmol/L	FT4/FT3 instrument
Australia 2008 [55] Means*	T1[a](1,817)	13.5 (10.4–17.8)	0.74 (0.02–2.15)	4.35 (3.3–5.7)	Abbott Architect i
	Nonpregnant (100)	(9.0–19.0)	(0.40–4.00)	(3.0–5.5)	
Canada[b] 2008 [56]	T1 (224)	15.0 (11.0–19.0)			Roche Cobas e601/E-170
	T2 (240)	13.5 (9.7–17.5)			
	T3 (211)	11.7 (8.1–15.3)			
China 2001[b] [57]	T1 (343)	16.2 (11.1–22.9)	0.8 (0.03–2.3)	4.0 (3.0–5.7)	Siemens/Bayer ACS 180
	T2 (343)	11.5 (8.1–16.7)	1.33 (0.03–3.7)	3.5 (2.8–4.2)	
	T3 (343)	11.6 (8.5–14.4)	1.28 (0.13–3.4)	3.4 (2.4–4.1)	
	Postpartum (63)	14.2 (10.7–18.0)	1.17 (0.39–3.51)	3.9 (3.3–6.2)	
Hong Kong 2000 [58] Mild ID	T1 (230)	13.4 (12.2–15.0)	0.49 (IQR[d] 0.12–1.00)		Siemens/Bayer ACS 180
	T2 (230)	11.9 (10.7–13.1)	0.96 (IQR[d] 0.62–1.28)		
	T3 (230)	11.7 (10.1–13.0)	0.95 (IQR[d] 0.60–1.36)		
	Postpartum (230)	14.4 (12.0–23.0)	1.14 (0.23–3.4)		
Hungary 2004 [59] Means Moderate ID	T2 (85)	10.4 (9.3–11.5) ELISA 14.3 (13.0–15.6) MEIA 12.7 (10.9–14.5) RIA	1.6 (0.8–2.4)		ELISA MEIA RIA
	T3 (72)	6.5 (5.4–7.6) ELISA 11.4 (9.9–12.9) MEIA 8.5 (6.5–10.5) RIA	1.7 (1.0–2.4)		
India 2008 [60] ID[b]	T1 (107)	14.46 (12.00–19.45)[d]	2.1 (0.60–5.00)[d]	4.4 (1.92–5.86)[d]	Roche Cobas e411/Elecsys
	T2 (137)	13.4 (9.48–19.58)[d]	2.4 (0.40–5.78)[d]	4.3 (3.20–5.70)[d]	
	T3 (87)	13.28 (11.30–17.71)[d]	2.1 (0.74–5.70)[d]	4.1 (3.30–5.18)[d]	

Table 11.3 (continued)

Country (ref)	Gestation (n =)	FT4 median (reference interval) or mean (± SEM)* pmol/L	TSH median (reference interval) or mean (± SEM) mIU/L	FT3 median (reference interval) or mean (± SEM) pmol/L	FT4/FT3 instrument
Italy 2002 [61] Mean Mild ID	T1 (86)	10.4 (10.1–10.7)	1.1 (0.3–1.9)	3.1 (3.01–3.19)	Lyso-Phase Kit
Japan 2005 [62] Means	T1 (119)	1.43c (0.21) ng/dL (1.16–1.95)	1.05 (0.97) (0.04–3.39)	3.60c (0.5) pg/mL (2.68–4.59)	Roche Cobas e411/Elecsys
	T2 (132)	1.11c (0.13) ng/dL (0.89–1.39)	1.51 (0.94) (0.17–3.72)	3.39c (0.44) pg/mL (2.56–4.11)	
	T3 (135)	1.02c (0.15) ng/dL (0.77–1.27)	1.23 (0.75) (0.04–3.30)	3.17c (0.43) pg/mL (2.53–4.10)	
	Postpartum (136)	1.08c (0.14) ng/dL (0.81–1.34)	2.96 (0.51) (0.90–5.81)	3.57c (0.55) pg/mL (2.62–4.46)	
Malaysia 1993 [63]	T1 (127)		(0.73–1.08)		Abbott AxSYM
	T2 (234)		(1.69–1.95)		
	T3 (248)		(1.82–2.05)		
Nigeria 1994 [64] Means Moderate ID	T1 (27)	TT4c 129.1 (34.1) nmol/L (61–197)	2.7 (0.9) (0.5–5.0)	TT3c 2.6 (0.48) nmol/L (1.7–3.5)	Boehringer Manheim Immuno-diagnostica
	T2 (27)	TT4c 157.2 (38.2) nmol/L (85–233)	2.12 (1.6) (0.5–5.0)	TT3c 2.7 (0.62) nmol/L (1.86–3.54)	
	T3 (27)	TT4c 173.1 (42.3) nmol/L (89–257)	2.29 (2.1) (0.5–5.0)	TT3c 2.91(0.51) nmol/L (1.9–3.94)	
	Postpartum (27)	TT4c 139.6 (35) nmol/L (70–210)	3.1 (1.9) (0.5–5.0)	TT3c 2.7 (0.52) nmol/L (1.66–3.64)	
Singapore 2001 [65] Iodine sufficient	T1 (500)		(0.36–3.24)	FT3 (5.8–8.7) TT3 (1.57–2.59)	VitrosECi

Table 11.3 (continued)

Country (ref)	Gestation (n =)	FT4 median (reference interval) or mean (± SEM)* pmol/L	TSH median (reference interval) or mean (± SEM) mIU/L	FT3 median (reference interval) or mean (± SEM) pmol/L	FT4/FT3 instrument
Sudan 2000 [66]	T1 (21)	11.4 (9.6–13.4)	1.1 (0.5–1.5)	TT3[c] 2.6 (2.1–3.2) nmol/L	Delfia TR-FIA
	T2 (21)	9.6 (8.6–10.8)	1.2 (0.7–1.8)	TT3 2.7 (2.2–3.5)	
	T3 (21)	10.2 (9.4–12.6)	1.0 (0.6–1.6)	TT3 2.6 (2.2–2.9)	
Sweden 2004 [67] Means Iodine sufficient	T1 (47)	FT4 12.3 (0.4) TT4[c] 127.7 (3.6) nmol/L (74.6–185.3)	0.89 (0.24–2.99)	TT3[c] 2.7 (0.09) (1.45–4.15) nmol/L	TT4 and TT3 by LC/MS/MS Sciex API 3000
	T2 (47)	FT4 10.5 (0.3) TT4[c] 127.7 (3.6) nmol/L (79.7–189.1)	1.17 (0.46–2.95)	TT3[c] 2.8 (0.1) (1.63–4.22) nmol/L	FT4 Dade Behring RxL Dimension
	T3 (47)	FT4 10.5 (0.2) TT4[c] 129.3 (3.6) nmol/L (74.6–182.7)	1.16 (0.43–2.78)	TT3[c] 3.2 (0.1) (1.58–4.57) nmol/L	
	Postpartum (47)	FT4 13.7 (0.5) TT4[c] 89.2 (2.9) nmol/L (60.4–154.5)	1.06 (0.07) (0.28–2.94)	TT3 1.9 (0.06) (1.2–3.34) nmol/L	
Switzerland 2007 [68] ID[b]	T1 (783)	13.79 (10.53–18.28) TT4[c] 110.64 (72.27–171.18) nmol/L	1.04 (0.88–2.83)	4.67 (3.52–6.22) TT3 1.78 (1.25–2.72)	Abbott Architect i2000SR
	T2 (528)	12.17 (9.53–15.68) TT4[c] 134.84 (94.77–182.51) nmol/L	1.02 (0.20–2.79)	4.47 (3.41–5.78) TT3 2.15 (1.43–3.16)	
	T3 (598)	11.08 (8.63–13.61) TT4[c] 136.65 (94.88–193.35) nmol/L	1.13 (0.31–2.90)	4.27 (3.33–5.59) TT3 2.19 (1.40–3.16)	

Table 11.3 (continued)

Country (ref)	Gestation (n =)	FT4 median (reference interval) or mean (± SEM)* pmol/L	TSH median (reference interval) or mean (± SEM) mIU/L	FT3 median (reference interval) or mean (± SEM) pmol/L	FT4/FT3 instrument
United Arab Emirates (UAE Arabs) 2006 [69]	T1 (97)	14.6 (8.9–24.6)	0.71 (0.06–8.3)		Abbott Architect i2000
	T2 (252)	12.7 (8.4–19.3)	1.04 (0.17–5.9)		
	T3 (52)	12.0 (8.0–18.0)	1.20 (0.21–6.9)		
Means					
United Arab Emirates (Other Arabs) 2006 [69]	T1 (122)	14.9 (10.5–22.3)	0.63 (0.04–9.3)		Abbott Architect i2000
	T2 (283)	13.3 (9.5–18.7)	1.1 (0.23–5.7)		
	T3 (60)	12.4 (8.8–17.4)	1.3 (0.31–5.30)		
Means					
United Arab Emirates (Asians) 2006 [69]	T1 (79)	15.7 (11.3–21.9)	0.95 (0.12–7.4)		Abbott Architect i2000
	T2 (174)	13.4 (9.7–18.5)	1.3 (0.3–5.5)		
	T3 (21)	12.1 (8.9–16.6)	1.1 (0.3–4.85)		
Means					
UK Asians 2001 [70]	T1 (20)	12.6 (11.8–13.4)	0.9 (0.6–1.3)	4.3 (4.1–4.6)	Bayer diagnostics ACS:180
	T2 (20)	11.5 (10.9–12.1)	1.3 (1.0–1.8)	4.1 (4.0–4.3)	
Means					
UK Caucasians 2001 [70]	T1 (50)	12.4 (12.0–12.8)	0.9 (0.7–1.1)	4.2 (4.1–4.4)	Bayer Diagnostics ACS:180
	T2 (50)	11.5 (11.2–11.8)	1.3 (1.2–1.5)	4.1 (4.0–4.2)	
Means Mild ID					
USA 2008 [71]	T1 (585)	9.9 (6.8–13.0)	1.1 (0.04–3.60)		Siemens Immulite 2000
USA 2008 [72]	T1 (9,562)	1.1c (1.00–1.20) ng/dL	1.05 (0.63–1.66)		Siemens Immulite 2000
	T2 (9,562)	1.01c (0.92–1.11) ng/dL	1.23 (0.82–1.78)		
USA 2007 (NHANES III) [73]	T1 (71)	TT4c 141.35 (3.07 nmol/L (123.64–158.29)	0.91 (0.17)		Roche
Means			0.28–1.06		
	T2 (83)	TT4c 152.95 (2.17) nmol/L (146.36–165.13)	1.03 (0.20) 0.57–1.28		
	T3 (62)	TT4c 142.64 (3.73) nmol/L (126.46–160.69)	1.32 (0.27) 0.69–2.87		

Table 11.3 (continued)

Country (ref)	Gestation (n =)	FT4 median (reference interval) or mean (± SEM)* pmol/L	TSH median (reference interval) or mean (± SEM) mIU/L	FT3 median (reference interval) or mean (± SEM) pmol/L	FT4/FT3 instrument
USA [74]	T1 (59)	FT4 1.13 (0.23) ng/dL TT4c 114.29 (34.36) nmol/L	1.13 (0.69)		LC/MS/MS API 4000
	T2 (35)	FT4 0.92 (0.30) ng/dL TT4c 137.32 (24.97) nmol/L	1.13 (0.54)		
	T3 (26)	FT4 0.86 (0.21) ng/dL TT4c 138.48 (25.74) nmol/L	1.04 (0.61)		
	Nonpregnant (26)	FT4 0.93 (0.25) ng/dL TT4c 91.63 (10.17) nmol/L	1.73 (1.13)		
USA 2007 [75]	T2 (2,551)	FT4 12.0 (9.3–15.2) TT4 128 (89.0–176.0)	1.14 (0.15–3.11)	FT3 4.85 (3.82–5.96) TT3 2.62 (1.82–3.68)	Abbot Architect i2000SR

*Means as marked. All are geometric means (± Standard error of the mean, SEM)

[a] T1 first trimester, gestation weeks (GW) 1–14; T2 second trimester, GW 15–28; T3 third trimester, GW 29–40

[b] Iodine nutrition status was not assessed in this study; iodine deficiency has not been ruled out

[c] To convert to SI units use www.unc.edu/~rowlett/units/scales/clinical_data.html. To convert to SI units: T4 μg/dL × 12.87 to nmol/L; T3 ng/dL × 0.0154 to nmol/L; FT4 ng/dL × 12.87 to pmol/L

[d] Reference interval is 90%

[e] IQR interquartile range

Some trimester-specific reference intervals are available for a specific population. These can be useful for others if the instrument and calibration standards are similar. More importantly, different populations may differ depending on dietary iodine intake, on individual genetic setpoints resulting in a narrow variability in intraindividual variability of the thyroid hormone levels, and the interindividual variation reflected by the reference interval. In some cases, serum anti-TPO antibodies, anti-thyroglobulin (Tg) and/or TSHR antibody levels can provide other information; TPOAbs can predict the risk of hypothyroidism. In pregnant women with low TSH hyperthyroidism this is accompanied by TSHR antibodies in 60–70% of the cases.

11.6.3   Free Thyroid Hormone Testing in Pregnancy

Laboratory assessment of thyroid function based on free thyroid hormone estimates would bypass the problem of increased serum TBG concentrations and correct for the 50% increase in serum binding proteins, as well as ruling out binding protein abnormalities. If free hormone concentrations are not sufficient, the analysis of total T4 and T3 may resolve or confirm some of the issues. Reanalysis of the samples in a different clinical laboratory is an option. The normal, expected changes in the hormonal milieu and added demands of pregnancy call for normative gestational age-related reference intervals for all thyroid function tests.

11.7   Development of Reference Intervals for Thyroid Hormones in Pregnancy

It has been established that diagnosing maternal thyroid dysfunction during pregnancy is of clinical importance for maternal and fetal health [76, 77]. This requires appropriate technology that can measure thyroid hormones with high specificity and sensitivity, normal intervals for comparison, and appropriate treatment regimen. Several national organizations have published guidelines e.g., Endocrine Society Clinical Practice Guideline and Laboratory Medicine Practice Guidelines [53, 78].

Many of the difficulties associated with the laboratory measurements of thyroid function tests result from the profound underlying (normal) physiological changes that occur during pregnancy. These changes are being unraveled by intense scientific research accompanied by global efforts in educating obstetricians, gynaecologists, and primary care physicians who are caregivers to women during pregnancy.

Laboratory analysis of serum thyroid hormones denotes results based on sex, age, ethnicity, genetics, and iodine sufficiency of the population tested and is method-specific. Until recently, all thyroid hormone assays were conducted using immunoassay techniques that do not provide a direct hormone measurement and are prone to interference from heterophilic antibodies and thyroid hormone antibodies

[50, 51]. A more reliable free thyroid hormone estimate is provided by measurement of total hormone concentrations (T3 and T4) and correction for the increased binding proteins by either direct measurement of TBG (to provide T4 to TBG or T3 to TBG ratios) or by a T3 or T4 uptake test to provide free thyroid hormone indices. Availability of these tests depends on the specific clinical biochemical laboratory. Total hormone measurements and free thyroid hormone measurements are the most reliable tests with the highest precision and accuracy. Very recently, free thyroid hormones have been measured by tandem mass spectrometry, which provides accurate, precise, fast, and simple measurements [67, 74, 79]. Such methods are technically complex, however not generally available yet, and most laboratories use immunoassays.

11.7.1   Trimester-Specific Method-Specific Reference Intervals

The Peer-reviewed publications provide numerous trimester-specific population-based reference intervals reflecting increasing total hormone concentration, decreasing FT4, and TSH suppressed in the first trimester [55–75]. Even though this approach will reduce the global variability of thyroid hormone assessment, it is important to stress that laboratory- and population-specific ranges are crucial, since measurements by different methods in different populations provide very different ranges (see examples shown in Table 11.3). The table is not exhaustive and illustrates that even in the same population different ethnicities will have slightly different results. In addition, the table illustrates that the results vary with different populations even when using the same method.

It should be noted that population-based reference ranges do not take into account that each individual has its own genetic setpoint [80, 81]. It was noted that while the intraindividual coefficient of variation (CV) was between 6 and 17% [80, 82], the interindividual CV was 11–25%. A more relevant way of evaluating this is through an individuality assessment, which was below 0.5 in these studies, indicating that thyroid function cannot be meaningfully assessed by population-based reference ranges [80–83]. Similarly, during pregnancy intraindividual changes may be more important than the specific single measurement in relation to a specific reference interval. Therefore, despite the reduction of total variability provided by applying gestation- and method-specific reference intervals, intraindividual variability should also be taken into consideration.

11.7.2   Trimester-Specific Thyroid Function Tests

The data provided in Table 11.3 present gestation-specific medians and means for different populations worldwide. Some provided reference intervals for FT4, FT3, and TSH for all three trimesters. For others total T4 (TT4) and total T3 (TT3) were available, or only two or one of the trimesters were reported. Iodine status was available for only some of the studies, making comparisons difficult and often clinically irrelevant. For pregnant women and women of childbearing age, urinary iodine levels reflecting iodine intake lower than recommended are reflected in higher TSH intervals and lower FT4.

Table 11.3 summarizes some trimester-specific thyroid function test data found in the literature. The table provides trimester-specific FT4, FT3, and TSH medians and means ± SEM (when indicated by the country name). The tables combine either longitudinal or cross-sectional studies. Comparison of these data suffers from several drawbacks, since some of the studies rely on very few subjects while others rely on hundreds and even thousands of participants. There are published cross-sectional studies that established mean concentrations for gestation weeks. However, these were based on less than ten subjects per week, and sample size was not noted for each of the weeks. Most studies did not determine iodine sufficiency, thyroid autoimmunity, multiple pregnancies, or hCG levels, all of which influence TSH and thyroid hormone levels. Furthermore, inclusion and exclusion criteria are not consistent, nor are statistical methods of analysis and in many of the studies some intervals are based on 2.5 and 97.5 percentiles (95% intervals), while others on 90% intervals. At times it is difficult to compare intervals due to the variation of units employed, therefore conversion factors are provided.

An increase in TSH levels is noted in the second and third trimesters in areas of iodine sufficiency, while FT4 and FT3 levels decrease. This is not the case in countries with populations that are not iodine-sufficient, as iodine-deficient populations will show TSH stimulation.

In areas of iodine sufficiency, total T4 levels reach a stable level within the first few weeks of pregnancy (approximately 40–50% higher than postpartum). In general, the trend for lower TSH in the first trimester persists throughout. Also, the increase in T4 relative to nonpregnancy and from first to second trimesters is seen in most studies. FT4 values need to be viewed with caution since FT4 methods of analysis are notorious for their variability in results even within the same study population [50, 51]. In summary, it has been recommended that specific reference intervals provide a guide for normal ranges of thyroid hormones, age-, sex-, and pregnancy-specific. However, for serum thyroid hormone levels to provide a useful measure of clinical and subclinical disease, there need to be appropriate reference intervals, namely method- and instrument-specific for the particular laboratory where samples were tested. A better understanding of thyroid hormone physiology during pregnancy, new developments in the technology for thyroid hormone analysis, and progress in defining pregnancy-specific reference intervals for thyroid hormones have advanced the detection of thyroid dysfunction in pregnancy. There are strengths and weaknesses to the available thyroid function tests as outlined in two recent guidelines provided by the Endocrine Society [53] and by the National Academy of Clinical Biochemistry [78]. Pregnancy-related physiological processes should affect TSH concentrations in the first trimester, total T4, T3, and possibly free hormone concentrations throughout gestation, and, therefore, normal reference intervals for pregnancy should be gestation-specific and method-specific and conducted on iodine-sufficient populations that do not include women with anti-TPO antibodies who are autoimmune. This can prevent misinterpretation of thyroid function test results during pregnancy.

Mild-to-moderate iodine deficiency is still present in certain counties or geographical areas despite national efforts to implement the mandatory use of iodized salt affecting T4 and TSH levels. Furthermore, iodine intake may vary unexpectedly because of significant variations in the natural iodine content of the local food and water and because of the variability in response to supplementation. Therefore, in comparing gestation-specific data it is important to note the methods of analysis; take into account iodine status, group sample size, subject inclusion and exclusion criteria, statistical methods used for data analysis, study design (cross-sectional or longitudinal); as well as note ethnicity, age, and singleton pregnancy status.

11.8   Screening for Thyroid Function in Pregnancy

It is clear from the information already discussed relating to the effects of thyroid dysfunction in pregnancy on both mother and fetus that consideration be given to screening thyroid function in pregnancy with the aim of interventional therapy if necessary. The development of normative reference ranges for thyroid hormone during pregnancy would assist this process considerably. Screening is a strategy to detect a disease in asymptomatic individuals in order to improve health outcomes by early diagnosis and treatment. The National Screening Committee (NSC) of the UK [84] has indicated appropriate criteria for implementation for the condition, the test, the treatment, and the screening program (Table 11.4).

With regard to the criteria for screening for thyroid function in pregnancy, it is noted that points 1 and 2 are satisfied; 3 is not completed and 4 is unknown. For the test, points 5 and 6 are in place and the tests would be acceptable. There is reasonable consensus on further testing (point 8). Although there is an effective treatment, there is no evidence available from point 10.

A limited number of screening studies for thyroid dysfunction in nonpregnant adults have been found to be cost effective [85, 86], but there has been no universal agreement from expert endocrine and thyroid associations (Table 11.5). Dosiou et al. [93] have conducted a cost-effective analysis of screening pregnant women for autoimmune thyroid disease using a state transition Markov model [94]. They concluded that screening pregnant women in the first trimester for TSH was cost effective compared with no screening. Screening using anti-TPO antibodies was also cost effective. Nevertheless, the recommendation of the clinical practice guideline published under the auspices of the Endocrine society is that targeted screening should be performed in those women at high risk for thyroid disease. In a study to

Table 11.4 Criteria for appraising the viability, effectiveness, and appropriateness of a screening program

The Condition

1. The condition should be an important health problem
2. The epidemiology and natural history of the condition, including development from latent to declared disease, should be adequately understood and there should be a detectable risk factor, disease marker, latent period, or early symptomatic stage
3. All the cost-effective primary prevention interventions should have been implemented as far as practicable
4. If the carriers of a mutation are identified as a result of screening, the natural history of people with this status should be understood, including the psychological implications

The Test

5. There should be a simple, safe, precise, and validated screening test
6. The distribution of test values in the target population should be known and a suitable cutoff level defined and agreed
7. The test should be acceptable to the population
8. There should be an agreed policy on the further diagnostic investigation of individuals with a positive test result and on the choices available to those individuals
9. If the test is for mutations, the criteria used to select the subset of mutations to be covered by screening, if all possible mutations are not being tested, should be clearly set out

The Treatment

10. There should be an effective treatment or intervention for patients identified through early detection, with evidence of early treatment leading to better outcomes than late treatment NSC/criteria

Table 11.5 Recommendations for thyroid screening in pregnancy by expert groups (from [92])

Authority	Year	Recommendation
American Association of Clinical Endocrinologists [87]	2002	Universal screening
Expert panel of American Thyroid Association, American Association of Clinical Endocrinologists, and The Endocrine Society [88]	2004	Case finding in high-risk group
Second panel of American Thyroid Association, American Association of Clinical Endocrinologists and The Endocrine Society [89]	2005	Universal screening
British Thyroid Association, Association of Foundation [90]	2006	Case finding in high-risk Clinical Biochemists and British Thyroid group
American College of Obstetric and Gynecology [91]	2007	Case finding in high-risk group
The Endocrine Society [53]	2007	Case finding in high-risk group

validate this strategy, Vaidya [95] found that restricting screening to these groups of women would miss about one third of women with significant thyroid dysfunction. Until the results of carefully controlled randomized prospective outcome studies are available the screening controversy will continue.

11.9   Conclusions

Evidence has been presented that thyroid disorders occurring during pregnancy have adverse effects on mother and fetus, which require active management. In view of this it is essential to make a correct diagnosis on the basis of the thyroid function tests. As thyroid physiology is altered in pregnancy, it has become clear that normative gestational reference ranges for thyroid hormone analytes are necessary. While "gold standard methodology" (e.g., tandem mass spectrometry) is useful for accurate standardization of values, in practice the use of kit assays for free thyroid hormones as well as routine estimation of total bound hormones are used. Gestational reference ranges for these hormones as well as TSH should be available in every hospital dealing with pregnancy. The current views on screening for thyroid function in early gestation are summarized. It is suggested that the guidelines of the endocrine society whereby only targeted case finding is used for screening are appropriate at this time, although there are emerging data to suggest that all women should be screened.

References

1. McCarrison R. Observations on endemic cretinism in the Chitral and Gilgit valleys. *Lancet.* 1908;2:1275-1280.
2. Pharoah POD, Connolly KJ. Iodine deficiency in Papua New Guinea. In: Stanbury JB, ed. *The Damaged Brain of Iodine Deficiency.* Elmsford, NY: Cognizant Communication Corporation; 1994:299-305.
3. Vulsma T, Gons MH, De Vijlder JJM. Maternal-fetal transfer of thyroxine in congenital hypothyroidism due to a total organification defect or thyroid agenesis. *N Engl J Med.* 1989;321:13-16.
4. Lazarus JH. Iodine and brain function. In: Lieberman HR, Kanarek RB, Prasad C, eds. *Nutritional Neuroscience.* Boca Raton, FL: CRC Press; 2005:261-274.
5. Glinoer, D. The regulation of thyroid function in pregnancy: pathways of endocrine adaptation from physiology to pathology. *Endocr Rev.* 1997;18:404-433.
6. Brent GA. Maternal thyroid function: interpretation of thyroid function tests in preganancy. *Clin Obstet Gynecol.* 1997;40(1):3-15.
7. Lazarus JH. Thyroid disease during pregnancy. In: Krassas GE, Rivkees SA, Kiess W, eds. *Diseases of the Thyroid in Childhood and Adolescence.* Basel, Switzerland: Karger Ltd; 2007:25-43.
8. Smyth PPA, Hetherton AMT, Smith DF, Radcliffe M. Maternal iodine status and thyroid volume during pregnancy: correlation with neonatal iodine intake. *J Clin Endoc Metab.* 1997;82:2840-2843.
9. Berghout A, Wiersinga W. Thyroid size and thyroid function during pregnancy: an analysis. *Eur J Endocrinol.* 1998;138(5):536-542.
10. Vermiglio F, Lo Presti VP, Scaffidi AG, et al. Maternal hypothyroxinemia during the first half of gestation in an iodine deficient area with endemic cretinism and related disorders. *Clin Endocrinol (Oxford).* 1995;42:409-415.
11. de Benoist B, Delange F, eds. Report of a WHO Technical Consultation. Prevention and control of iodine deficiency in pregnancy, lactation, and in children less than 2 years of age (Geneva, 24–26 January 2005). *Public Health Nutr.* 2007;12(A):1527-1611.

12. Yoshimura M, Nishikawa M, Yoshikawa N, et al. Mechanism of thyroid stimulation by human chorionic gonadotropin in sera of normal pregnant women. *Acta Endoc (Copenhagen)*. 1991;124:173-178.
13. Hoermann R, Poertl S, Liss I, Amir SM, Mann K. Variation in the thyrotropic activity of human chorionic-gonadotropin in Chinese-hamster ovary cells arises from differential expression of the human thyrotropin receptor and microheterogeneity of the hormone. *J Clin Endocrinol Metab*. 1995;80:1605-1610.
14. Tanaka S, Yamada H, Kato EH, et al. Gestational transient hyperthyroxinemia (GTH) screening for thyroid function in 23, 163 pregnant women using dried blood spots. *Clin Endocrinol (Oxford)*. 1998;49:325-329.
15. Kimura M, Amino N, Tamaki H, et al. Gestational thyrotoxicosis and hyperemesis gravidarum: possible role of hCG with higher stimulating activity. *Clin Endocrinol (Oxford)*. 1993;38:345-350.
16. Tsuruta E, Tada H, Tamaki H, et al. Pathogenic role of asialo human chorionic gonadotropin in gestational thyrotoxicosis. *J Clin Endocrinol Metab*. 1995;80:350-355.
17. Yoshimura M, Pekary AK, Pang XP, Berg L, Goodwin TM, Hershman JM. Thyrotropic activity of basic isoelectric forms of human chorionic gonadotropin extracted from hydatidiform mole tissues. *J Clin Endocrinol Metab*. 1994;78:862-866.
18. Rodien P, Bremont C, Raffin Sanson ML, et al. Familial gestational hyperthyroidism caused by a mutant thyrotropin receptor hypersensitive to human chorionic gonadotropin. *N Eng J Med*. 1998;339(25):1823-1826.
19. Hamburger JI. Diagnosis and management of Graves' disease in pregnancy. *Thyroid*. 1992;2:219-224.
20. Mestman JH. Hyperthyroidism in pregnancy. *Best Pract Res Clin Endocrinol Metab*. 2004;18(2):267-288.
21. Anselmo J, Cao D, Karrison T, Weiss RE, Refetoff S. Fetal loss associated with excess thyroid hormone exposure. *JAMA*. 2004;292:691-695.
22. Casey BM, Dashe JS, Wells CE, McIntire DD, Leveno KJ, Cunningham FG. Subclinical hyperthyroidism and pregnancy outcomes. *Obstet Gynecol*. 2006;107:337-341.
23. Kung AWC, Jones BM. A change from stimulatory to blocking antibody activity in Graves' disease during pregnancy. *J Clin Endocrinol Metab*. 1998;83:514-518.
24. Higuchi R, Miyawaki M, Kumugai T, et al. Central hypothyroidism in infants who were born to mothers with thyrotoxicosis before 32 weeks gestation: 3 cases. *Pediatrics*. 2005;115: 623-625.
25. Klein RZ, Haddow JE, Faixt JD, et al. Prevalence of thyroid deficiency in pregnant women. *Clin Endocrinol (Oxford)*. 1991;35:41-46.
26. Casey BM, Dashe JS, Wells CE, et al. Subclinical hypothyroidism and pregnancy outcomes. *Obstet Gynecol*. 2005;105:239-245.
27. Morreale de Escobar G, Obregon MJ, Escobar del Rey. Is neuropsychological development related to maternal hypothyroidism or to maternal hypothyroxinemia. *J Clin Endocrinol Metab*. 2000;85:3975-3987.
28. Mandel SJ. Hypothyroidism and chronic autoimmune thyroiditis in the pregnant state: maternal aspects. *Best Pract Res Clin Endocrinol Metab*. 2004;18(2):213-224.
29. Alexander EK, Marqusee E, Lawrence J, Jarolim P, Fischer GA, Larsen PR. Timing and magnitude of increases in levothyroxine requirements during pregnancy in women with hypothyroidism. *N Engl J Med*. 2004;351:241-249.
30. Williams GR. Neurodevelopmental and neurophysiological actions of thyroid hormone. *J Neuroendocrinol*. 2008;20(6):784-794.
31. Bernal J. Action of thyroid hormone in brain. *J Endocrinol Invest*. 2002;25:268-288.
32. Haddow JE, Palomaki GE, Allan WC, et al. Maternal thyroid deficiency during pregnancy and subsequent neuropsychological development of the child. *N Engl J Med*. 341:549-555.
33. Pop VJ, Kuijpens JL, van Baar AL, et al. Low maternal free thyroxine concentrations during early pregnancy are associated with impaired psychomotor development in infancy. *Clin Endocrinol*. 1999;50:147-148.

34. Pop VJ, Brouwers EP, Vadert HL, Vulsma T, van Baar AL, de Vijlder JJ. Maternal hypothyroxinemia during early pregnancy and subsequent child development: a 3-year follow-up study. *Clin Endocrinol.* 2003;59:282-288.
35. Pop VJ, de Vries E, Van Baar Al, et al. Maternal thyroid peroxidase antibodies during pregnancy: a marker of impaired child development. *J Clin Endocrinol Metab.* 1995;80: 3561-3566.
36. Lazarus JH, Premawardhana LDKE. Postpartum thyroiditis. In: Weetman AP, ed. *Contemporary Endocrinology: Autoimmune Diseases in Endocrinology.* Totowa, NJ: Humana Press Inc; 2008:177-192.
37. Fantz CR, Dagogo-Jack S, Ladenson JH, Gronowski AM. Thyroid function during pregnancy. *Clin Chem.* 1999;45(12):2250-2258.
38. Glinoer D. What happens to the normal thyroid during pregnancy? *Thyroid.* 1999;9(7): 631-635.
39. Yoshimura M, Hershman JM, Pang XP, Berg L, Pekary AE. Activation of the thyrotropin (TSH) receptor by human chorionic gonadotropin and luteinizing hormone in Chinese hamster ovary cells expressing functional human TSH receptors. *J Clin Endocrinol Metab.* 1993;77(4):1009-1013.
40. Price A, Davies R, Heller SR, Milford-Ward A, Weetman AP. Asian women are at increased risk of gestational thyrotoxicosis. *J Clin Endocrinol Metab.* 1996;81(3):1160-1163.
41. Hegde UC. Immunomodulation of the mother during pregnancy. *Med Hypotheses.* 1991; 35(2):159-164.
42. Kung AW, Jones BM. A change from stimulatory to blocking antibody activity in Graves' disease during pregnancy. *J Clin Endocrinol Metab.* 1998;83(2):514-518.
43. Mandel SJ, Spencer CA, Hollowell JG. Are detection and treatment of thyroid insufficiency in pregnancy feasible? *Thyroid.* 2005;15(1):44-53.
44. Gu J, Soldin OP, Soldin SJ. Simultaneous quantification of free triiodothyronine and free thyroxine by isotope dilution tandem mass spectrometry. *Clin Biochem.* 2007;40(18): 1386-1391.
45. Soldin OP, Hilakivi-Clarke L, Weiderpass E, Soldin SJ. Trimester-specific reference intervals for thyroxine and triiodothyronine in pregnancy in iodine-sufficient women using isotope dilution tandem mass spectrometry and immunoassays. *Clin Chim Acta.* 2004;349(1-2): 181-189.
46. Fabian HM, Radestad IJ, Waldenstrom U. Characteristics of Swedish women who do not attend childbirth and parenthood education classes during pregnancy. *Midwifery.* 2004; 20(3):226-235.
47. Demers LM, Spencer CA. Laboratory medicine practice guidelines: laboratory support for the diagnosis and monitoring of thyroid disease. *Clin Endocrinol (Oxford).* 2003;58(2):138-140.
48. Fritz KS, Wilcox RB, Nelson JC. A direct free thyroxine (T4) immunoassay with the characteristics of a total T4 immunoassay. *Clin Chem.* 2007;53(5):911-915.
49. Wang R, Nelson JC, Weiss RM, Wilcox RB. Accuracy of free thyroxine measurements across natural ranges of thyroxine binding to serum proteins. *Thyroid.* 2000;10(1):31-39.
50. d'Herbomez M, Forzy G, Gasser F, Massart C, Beaudonnet A, Sapin R. Clinical evaluation of nine free thyroxine assays: persistent problems in particular populations. *Clin Chem Lab Med.* 2003;41(7):942-947.
51. Sapin R, d'Herbomez M. Free thyroxine measured by equilibrium dialysis and nine immunoassays in sera with various serum thyroxine-binding capacities. *Clin Chem.* 2003;49(9): 1531-1535.
52. Baloch Z, Carayon P, Conte-Devolx B, et al. Laboratory medicine practice guidelines. Laboratory support for the diagnosis and monitoring of thyroid disease. *Thyroid.* 2003;13(1): 3-126.
53. Abalovich M, Amino N, Barbour LA, et al. Management of thyroid dysfunction during pregnancy and postpartum: an Endocrine Society Clinical Practice Guideline. *J Clin Endocrinol Metab.* 2007;92(suppl 8):S1-S47.

54. Casey B. Maternal hypothyroidism and hyperthyroidism management. In: Queenan JT, Spong CY, Lockwood CJ, eds. *Management of High-Risk Pregnancy: An Evidence-Based Approach.* Massachusetts, MA: Wiley, John & Sons; 2007:187.

55. Gilbert RM, Hadlow NC, Walsh JP, et al. Assessment of thyroid function during pregnancy: first-trimester (weeks 9–13) reference intervals derived from Western Australian women. *Med J Aust.* 2008;189(5):250-253.

56. Gong Y, Hoffman BR. Free thyroxine reference interval in each trimester of pregnancy determined with the Roche Modular E-170 electrochemiluminescent immunoassay. *Clin Biochem.* 2008;41(10-11):902-906.

57. Panesar NS, Li CY, Rogers MS. Reference intervals for thyroid hormones in pregnant Chinese women. *Ann Clin Biochem.* 2001;38(pt 4):329-332.

58. Kung AW, Lao TT, Chau MT, Low LC. Goitrogenesis during pregnancy and neonatal hypothyroxinemia in a borderline iodine sufficient area. *Clin Endocrinol (Oxford).* 2000;53(6): 725-731.

59. Toldy E, Locsei Z, Rigo E, Kneffel P, Szabolcs I, Kovacs GL. Comparative analytical evaluation of thyroid hormone levels in pregnancy and in women taking oral contraceptives: a study from an iodine deficient area. *Gynecol Endocrinol.* 2004;18(4):219-226.

60. Marwaha RK, Chopra S, Gopalakrishnan S, et al. Establishment of reference range for thyroid hormones in normal pregnant Indian women. *BJOG.* 2008;115(5):602-606.

61. Antonangeli L, Maccherini D, Cavaliere R, et al. Comparison of two different doses of iodide in the prevention of gestational goiter in marginal iodine deficiency: a longitudinal study. *Eur J Endocrinol.* 2002;147(1):29-34.

62. Kurioka H, Takahashi K, Miyazaki K. Maternal thyroid function during pregnancy and puerperal period. *Endocr J.* 2005;52(5):587-591.

63. Goh KH, Ng ML, Roslan BA, Tan TT, Nasri BN, Khalid BA. Thyroid hormones and autoantibodies in pregnant patients with thyroid diseases. *Ann Acad Med Singapore.* 1993;22(4): 539-543.

64. Das SC, Isichei UP, Mohammed AZ, et al. Impact of iodine deficiency on thyroid function in pregnant African women—a possible factor in the genesis of 'small for dates' babies. *Afr J Med Med Sci.* 1994;23(3):239-247.

65. Yeo CP, Khoo DH, Eng PH, Tan HK, YO SL, Jacob E. Prevalence of gestational thyrotoxicosis in Asian women evaluated in the 8th to 14th weeks of pregnancy: correlations with total and free beta human chorionic gonadotrophin. *Clin Endocrinol (Oxford).* 2001;55(3): 391-398.

66. Eltom A, Elnagar B, Elbagir M, Gebre-Medhin M. Thyroglobulin in serum as an indicator of iodine status during pregnancy. *Scand J Clin Lab Invest.* 2000;60(1):1-7.

67. Soldin OP, Tractenberg RE, Hollowell JG, Jonklaas J, Janicic N, Soldin SJ. Trimester-specific changes in maternal thyroid hormone, thyrotropin, and thyroglobulin concentrations during gestation: trends and associations across trimesters in iodine sufficiency. *Thyroid.* 2004;14(12):1084-1090.

68. Stricker R, Echenard M, Eberhart R, et al. Evaluation of maternal thyroid function during pregnancy: the importance of using gestational age-specific reference intervals. *Eur J Endocrinol.* 2007;157(4):509-514.

69. Dhatt GS, Jayasundaram R, Wareth LA, et al. Thyrotrophin and free thyroxine trimester-specific reference intervals in a mixed ethnic pregnant population in the United Arab Emirates. *Clin Chim Acta.* 2006;370(1-2):147-151.

70. Price A, Obel O, Cresswell J, et al. Comparison of thyroid function in pregnant and non-pregnant Asian and western Caucasian women. *Clin Chim Acta.* 2001;308(1-2):91-98.

71. Pearce EN, Oken E, Gillman MW, et al. Association of first-trimester thyroid function test values with thyroperoxidase antibody status, smoking, and multivitamin use. *Endocr Pract.* 2008;14(1):33-39.

72. Lambert-Messerlian G, McClain M, Haddow JE, et al. First- and second-trimester thyroid hormone reference data in pregnant women: a FaSTER (First- and Second-Trimester Evaluation

of Risk for aneuploidy) Research Consortium study. *Am J Obstet Gynecol.* 2008;199(1):62. e1-e6.

73. Soldin OP, Soldin D, Sastogue M. Gestation-specific thyroxine and thyroid stimulating hormone levels in the United States and worldwide. *Ther Drug Monit.* 2007;29(5):553-559.

74. Kahric-Janicic N, Soldin SJ, Soldin OP, West T, Gu J, Jonklaas J. Tandem mass spectrometry improves the accuracy of free thyroxine measurements during pregnancy. *Thyroid.* 2007;17(4):303-311.

75. La'ulu SL, Roberts WL. Second-trimester reference intervals for thyroid tests: the role of ethnicity. *Clin Chem.* 2007;53(9):1658-1664.

76. Dashe JS, Casey BM, Wells CE, et al. Thyroid-stimulating hormone in singleton and twin pregnancy: importance of gestational age-specific reference ranges. *Obstet Gynecol.* 2005;106(4): 753-757.

77. Casey BM, Leveno KJ. Thyroid disease in pregnancy. *Obstet Gynecol.* 2006;108(5): 1283-1292.

78. Baloch Z, Carayon P, Conte-Devolx B, et al. Guidelines committee, national academy of clinical biochemistry. Laboratory medicine practice guidelines. Laboratory support for the diagnosis and monitoring of thyroid disease. *Thyroid.* 2003;13:3-126.

79. Soldin SJ, Soukhova N, Janicic N, Jonklaas J, Soldin OP. The measurement of free thyroxine by isotope dilution tandem mass spectrometry. *Clin Chim Acta.* 2005;358(1-2):113-118.

80. Feldt-Rasmussen U, Hyltoft PP, Blaabjerg O, Horder M. Long-term variability in serum thyroglobulin and thyroid related hormones in healthy subjects. *Acta Endocrinol (Copenhagen).* 1980;95(3):328-334.

81. Andersen S, Pedersen KM, Bruun NH, Laurberg P. Narrow individual variations in serum T(4) and T(3) in normal subjects: a clue to the understanding of subclinical thyroid disease. *J Clin Endocrinol Metab.* 2002;87(3):1068-1072.

82. Ankrah-Tetteh T, Wijeratne S, Swaminathan R. Intraindividual variation in serum thyroid hormones, parathyroid hormone and insulin-like growth factor-1. *Ann Clin Biochem.* 2008;45 (pt 2):167-169.

83. Biersack HJ, Hartmann F, Rodel R, Reinhardt M. Long term changes in serum T4, T3, and TSH in benign thyroid disease: proof of a narrow individual variation. *Nuklearmedizin.* 2004;43(5):158-160; quiz 162-163.

84. UK National Screening Committee. Criteria for appraising the viability, effectiveness and appropriateness of a screening programme. http://www.nsc.nhs.uk/pdfs/criteria.pdf. Accessed October 26, 2008.

85. Danese MD, Powe NR, Sawin CT, Ladenson PW. Screening formild thyroid failure at the periodic health examination: a decision and cost-effectiveness analysis. *JAMA.* 1996;276: 285-292.

86. Bona M, Santini F, Rivolta G, Grossi E, Grilli R. Cost effectiveness of screening for subclinical hypothyroidism in the elderly. A decision analyticalmodel. *Pharmacoeconomics.* 1998;14:209-216.

87. Baskin HJ, Cobin RH, Duick DS, et al. American Association of Clinical Endocrinologists medical guidelines for clinical practice for the evaluation and treatment of hyperthyroidism and hypothyroidism. *Endocr Pract.* 2002;8:457-469.

88. Surks MI, Ortiz E, Daniels GH, et al. Subclinical thyroid disease: scientific review and guidelines for diagnosis and management. *JAMA.* 2004;291:228-238.

89. Gharib H, Tuttle RM, Baskin HJ, Fish LH, Singer PA, McDermott MT. Subclinical thyroid dysfunction: a joint statement on management from the American Association of Clinical Endocrinologists, the American Thyroid Association, and the Endocrine Society. *J Clin Endocrinol Metab.* 2005;90:581-585.

90. British Thyroid Association. UK guidelines for the use of thyroid function tests. http://www. british-thyroid-association.org/Guidelines/ Published July 2006. Accessed October 28, 2008.

91. Committee on Patient Safety and Quality Improvement; Committee on Professional Liability. ACOG committee opinion No. 381: subclinical hypothyroidism in pregnancy. *Obstet Gynecol.* 2007;110:959-960.

92. Vaidya B. Universal screening for thyroid dysfunction in pregnancy? In: Lazarus JH, Pirags V, Butz S, eds. *Thyroid and Reproduction.* Thieme Verlag Stuttgart; 2009:153-159.
93. Dosiou C, Sanders GD, Araki SS, Crapo LM. Screening pregnant women for autoimmunethyroid disease: a cost-effectiveness analysis. *Eur J Endocrinol.* 2008;158(6):841-851.
94. Sonnenberg FA, Beck JR. Markov models in medical decision making: a practical guide. *Med Decis Making.* 1993;13:322-338.
95. Vaidya B, Anthony S, Bilous M, et al. Detection of thyroid dysfunction in early pregnancy: universal screening or targeted high-risk case finding? *J Clin Endocrinol Metab.* 2007;92(1): 203-207.

Chapter 12
Assessing Thyroid Function in the Elderly

Mary H. Samuels

12.1 Changes in Normal Thyroid Function with Aging

With aging, the normal thyroid gland has been reported to increase in size, although this is not consistent, and some studies show no changes in thyroid gland size or weight (reviewed in [1]). Other studies have reported increased rates of thyroid gland atrophy and fibrosis, although this may be due to underlying autoimmune thyroid disease in the population. Finally, thyroid nodules are much more common with aging, with nodules discovered by ultrasound in up to 50% of subjects over the age of 50 years [2].

A number of metabolic changes in thyroid hormone economy occur with aging (reviewed in [1]) (Table 12.1). Thyroid and renal clearance of iodine are decreased, and the daily production of throxine T4 is lower than in young subjects. This is balanced by decreased clearance of T4, and serum levels of T4 are maintained in the normal range. In contrast, triiodothyronine T3 levels may decrease by 10–20% with aging, while reverse T3 (rT3) levels may increase. These findings suggest that 5′-deiodinase activity decreases with aging. However, these changes are difficult to distinguish from those that occur with illness in many elderly subjects. Studies that carefully exclude elderly subjects with concurrent illnesses and medications tend to show fewer changes in thyroid hormone levels.

Serum TSH levels have been unchanged, lowered, or increased with aging in various reports. The normal diurnal variation in TSH levels, with higher levels at night, may be attenuated with aging. TSH responses to exogenous thyrotropin releasing hormone (TRH) have also been reported to be blunted in some studies, although others have reported normal or even enhanced responses. Again, is difficult to distinguish these changes from those that occur with illness, and healthier elderly subjects tend to have preserved TSH levels and TRH responses. This suggests that,

M. H. Samuels (✉)
Division of Endocrinology, Diabetes, and Clinical Nutrition, Oregon Health
& Science University, Portland, OR 97239, USA
e-mail: samuelsm@ohsu.edu

G. A. Brent (ed.), *Thyroid Function Testing*,
DOI 10.1007/978-1-4419-1485-9_12, © Springer Science+Business Media, LLC 2010

Table 12.1 Age-related changes in thyroid hormone economy (adapted from [1])

Parameter	Changes with aging
Thyroid iodine clearance	Decreased
Renal iodine clearance	Decreased
Daily T4 production	Decreased
Daily T4 clearance	Decreased
Serum T4 concentrations	Unchanged
Serum T3 concentrations	Unchanged to decreased
Serum reverse T3 concentrations	Unchanged to increased
Serum TSH concentrations	Usually unchanged
TSH responses to TRH	Unchanged to decreased
Diurnal variation in TSH levels	Unchanged to decreased

T4 thyroxine, *T3* triiodothyronine, *TSH* thyroid stimulating hormone, *TRH* thyrotropin releasing hormone

regardless of altered thyroid hormone economy with aging, the majority of healthy elderly subjects maintain normal thyroid function.

On the other hand, altered thyroid function is common in the elderly, and may have important clinical consequences. It can be challenging to accurately diagnose thyroid dysfunction in older patients, since presenting symptoms may be atypical, and other comorbid conditions may obscure the diagnosis. For these reasons, it is always important to consider the possibility of thyroid disease in elderly patients, and to accurately screen for it. The next two sections review the existent data on the prevalence, causes, clinical manifestations, diagnostic issues, and treatment of thyroid disease in older subjects.

12.2 Hypothyroidism in the Elderly

12.2.1 Prevalence

Hypothyroidism can be divided into overt hypothyroidism (elevated TSH, low free T4 [fT4] levels) and subclinical (or mild) hypothyroidism (elevated TSH, normal fT4 levels). The prevalence of hypothyroidism varies with age, gender, ethnicity, iodine content of the diet, and underlying prevalence of antithyroid antibodies in the population. In patients over the age of 60 years, the prevalence of overt hypothyroidism is between 2 and 10% [3]. Subclinical hypothyroidism is even more common, with three large population-based studies showing prevalence rates that increase with age, reaching 20% in subjects aged 80 years [4–6]. Most studies show that overt and subclinical hypothyroidism are more common in women, reflecting increased rates of autoimmune thyroid disease in women.

There is a high rate of progression from subclinical to overt hypothyroidism, especially in antibody-positive subjects. Long-term follow-up of subjects with elevated TSH levels and positive antithyroid peroxidase (anti-TPO) antibodies indicate that about 4% convert to overt hypothyroidism per year [7]. Higher TSH levels also predict higher rates of conversion to overt hypothyroidism. Thus, untreated subjects with subclinical hypothyroidism must be followed carefully for the development of overt hypothyroidism.

However, it should also be noted that there is a high rate of return to normal TSH levels in older subjects who have an elevated TSH. This rate of normalization depends on the initial TSH levels, with 50% of subjects who started with a TSH of 5–10 mU/L normalizing their TSH levels over time [8]. In contrast, in the same study, only 5% of subjects with initial TSH levels of 15–20 mU/L experienced normalization of their TSH levels. Normalization rates were also lower in subjects who had positive anti-TPO antibodies, as a marker for underlying autoimmune thyroid disease.

12.2.2 Etiology

In iodine-sufficient areas such as the United States, most overt and subclinical hypothyroidism is due to chronic autoimmune (Hashimoto's) thyroiditis. The prevalence of antithyroid antibodies increases with age, with frequencies as high as 30% in women older than 70 years [6]. The presence of these antibodies increases the risk of developing subclinical and overt hypothyroidism, and also the risk of progression from subclinical to overt hypothyroidism [7].

Less common causes of overt and subclinical hypothyroidism in the elderly include thyroid surgery, radiation therapy to the neck, radioactive iodine therapy of hyperthyroidism, or central hypothyroidism due to a pituitary or hypothalamic disorder. Finally, a number of medications can precipitate hypothyroidism in susceptible elderly patients; see Chap. 13 for a detailed discussion of these issues.

12.2.3 Clinical Manifestations

Many elderly hypothyroid patients manifest the classic symptoms and signs of overt hypothyroidism, including fatigue, cold intolerance, dry skin, and constipation. However, they may have lower rates of certain clinical findings such as weight gain, and many symptoms of hypothyroidism can be confused with other comorbid conditions that are common in this population [9] (Table 12.2). In addition, certain clinical manifestations may be accentuated in the elderly, including cardiac signs and mental status changes. Overt hypothyroidism may precipitate congestive heart failure or present as pseudo-dementia in this age range [10, 11]. For these reasons, an elderly patient who presents with any findings suggestive of hypothyroidism, or deterioration in cardiac status or mental function, should undergo testing for hypothyroidism.

Table 12.2 Comparison of clinical features of hypothyroidism in young versus old patients (from [9])

Clinical feature	Young patients (%)	Old patients (%)
Fatigue	83	68
Weakness	67	53
Mental slowness	48	45
Chilliness	65	35
Dry skin	45	35
Constipation	41	33
Depression	52	28
Anorexia	13	27
Slowed reflexes	31	24
Weight gain	59	23
Bradycardia	19	12
Hair loss	28	12

Clinical manifestations of subclinical hypothyroidism are controversial (reviewed in [12]). Some studies show increased rates of hypothyroid-type symptoms, decrements in quality of life, abnormal lipid levels, decreased left ventricular function, or neuropsychiatric dysfunction in subjects with subclinical hypothyroidism. Some treatment studies have shown improvements in these parameters when patients with subclinical hypothyroidism are given levothyroxine (L-T4), but this is inconsistent. Very few studies have singled out older subjects, and it is not clear whether the elderly have lower or higher rates of these effects. One recent study did report an increased risk of developing dementia in older women (but not men) with subclinical hypothyroidism, but this must be considered preliminary data which require confirmation in other studies [13]. There are no intervention studies that show the risk of dementia can be reduced with L-T4 therapy.

The most intensively studied area in subclinical hypothyroidism regards possible effects on the cardiovascular system, with outcomes including cardiac events and cardiovascular mortality [14]. There are a number of well-conducted, population-based epidemiology studies of this issue, with two recent metaanalyses of these studies [15, 16]. From these metaanalyses, an interesting age-related phenomenon has emerged. It appears that cardiovascular morbidity and mortality is only significantly increased in studies that included subjects younger than 65 years. In studies with older subjects, there was no increase in cardiovascular outcomes, and two studies in the "oldest old" (average age 78 and 85 years at study entry) showed a protective effect of subclinical hypothyroidism on physical function and mortality [17, 18]. These results can be interpreted to mean that the normal TSH range rises with age (further discussed below), and therefore elderly subjects with mild TSH elevations are in fact euthyroid, or that low thyroid function may protect the elderly in some way, perhaps by decreasing metabolic demands. However, there are no intervention studies of L-T4 treatment in subclinical hypothyroidism using cardiovascular endpoints, and these theories remain untested.

12.2.4   Diagnosis

The diagnosis of hypothyroidism is usually straightforward in the elderly, since TSH levels are almost always elevated. Exceptions include rare causes of central hypothyroidism, or supervening illnesses and medication use, which can lower TSH levels (discussed in Chaps. 4 and 13). There are other occasional causes of elevated TSH levels, including recovery from illness and medication effects, discussed in Chaps. 10 and 13. With these exceptions, serum TSH levels remain the best screening test for hypothyroidism in the elderly. Note that there has been recent controversy regarding the true upper limit of the normal range for TSH levels, especially in the elderly; this controversy is discussed below.

In a patient with an elevated TSH level, it is helpful to obtain a serum fT4 level, which will distinguish overt (low fT4) from subclinical (normal fT4) hypothyroidism. This distinction is important, since overt hypothyroidism should be treated, while there is controversy over whether to treat subclinical hypothyroidism (discussed below). Serum T3 levels are not helpful in diagnosing hypothyroidism, since they remain normal until the patient is severely hypothyroid, and may also be affected by nonthyroidal conditions and medications.

If the serum TSH is elevated but the fT4 is normal, it is advisable to wait a few months and repeat the TSH, prior to determining that the patient has sustained subclinical hypothyroidism. This is because a number of conditions can cause transient mild elevations in TSH levels, including recovery from illness, changes in medications, or various forms of temporary thyroiditis (subacute or silent). In addition, as described above, there are high rates of normalization of serum TSH levels in older subjects followed over time, particularly if the TSH is only minimally elevated [8].

Once overt hypothyroidism is diagnosed, it is not usually necessary to perform any further laboratory evaluation, since this would not change treatment decisions. In the case of subclinical hypothyroidism, the presence of serum anti-TPO antibodies may help predict the risk of developing overt hyperthyroidism, but measurement of these is optional. Thyroid ultrasounds or radionuclide scans should not be ordered in hypothyroid patients, unless there is a focal anatomic abnormality. These tests may show heterogeneous gland texture or uptake, which is common in Hashimoto's Disease. These can be confused with thyroid nodules, leading to unnecessary anxiety and testing.

12.2.5   Treatment

Once an elderly patient has been diagnosed with overt hypothyroidism, standard treatment is with synthetic L-T4. There is no role for other forms of thyroid hormone, including thyroid extract or T3 preparations, especially in the elderly, where they can precipitate angina and arrhythmias. L-T4 should be started at low doses (12.5–25 µg per day) in the elderly, to avoid acute adverse cardiac effects. Doses are adjusted every 6–8 weeks, following TSH levels, aiming for a mid-normal level. This can usually be achieved without adverse effects, unless the patient has severe coronary artery disease and cannot tolerate full replacement doses of L-T4 (reviewed in [1]).

Because of the controversy surrounding the normal TSH range and effects of subclinical hypothyroidism in the elderly, it is not clear whether elderly subjects with subclinical hypothyroidism should be treated, and what the target TSH level should be. With the absence of definitive data to answer those questions, this decision must be carefully individualized for a given patient. Many thyroid specialists recommend treating patients with serum TSH levels above 10 mU/L, but this may not be an optimal strategy in the elderly [12].

Average L-T4 replacement doses are lower in older patients, compared to young patients. This is due to the decreased clearance of T4 with age [19]. L-T4 absorption is decreased by food, conditions associated with impaired gastric acid production (such as atrophic gastritis, common in the elderly), and a number of medications discussed in Chap. 13. Other medications affect serum TBG levels, which can change L-T4 dose requirements. Patients receiving these medications may require significant adjustments of their L-T4 doses.

12.3 Hyperthyroidism in the Elderly

12.3.1 Prevalence

Hyperthyroidism can be divided into overt hyperthyroidism (low TSH, elevated fT4 and/or fT3 levels) and subclinical (or mild) hyperthyroidism (low TSH, normal fT4 and fT3 levels). The prevalence of hyperthyroidism depends on gender—the cutoff used to define a low TSH level—and the iodine intake of the population. Overall, the most common cause of hyperthyroidism in the population is overtreatment with thyroid hormone. If one excludes subjects treated with thyroid hormone, the prevalence of hyperthyroidism does not vary much with age. In the large US population-based National Health and Nutrition Examination Survey III (NHANES III), increased rates of hyperthyroidism were noted as the age range increased [5]. However, this increase was accounted for by subjects with known thyroid disease, most of whom were receiving L-T4. This indicated that these subjects had iatrogenic hyperthyroidism due to overtreatment with L-T4. When these subjects were excluded, there was a higher rate of hyperthyroidism in younger patients, probably indicating Graves' Disease, which is most common in young women. There was also a slight increase in the rate of hyperthyroidism in subjects over 80 years, which might indicate toxic multinodular goiter in this age range. Otherwise, rates of hyperthyroidism were fairly constant across age ranges at about 1–2% of the population. Women tend to have higher rates of hyperthyroidism than men, reflecting autoimmune disease, although this may become less apparent with aging, as toxic nodular goiter and medication use are more prevalent.

The prevalence of subclinical hyperthyroidism in older patients varies according to the population studied [3]. In the NHANES III study, half of the reported hyperthyroidism rate of 1–2% was overt, and half was subclinical, hyperthyroidism [5]. The natural history of subclinical to overt hyperthyroidism is quite variable, with some patients eventually progressing to overt hyperthyroidism, while others remain stable or revert to a normal TSH level (reviewed in [12]).

12.3.2   Etiology

In young patients, by far the most common cause of overt or subclinical hyperthyroidism is Graves' Disease, an autoimmune process that leads to stimulation of thyroid hormone synthesis and a diffuse toxic goiter. Graves' Disease remains a common cause of hyperthyroidism in older patients, but other etiologies become more frequent [20]. Toxic multinodular goiter is reported in about 50% of older patients with hyperthyroidism, especially in areas of low or borderline iodine intake. It occurs most often in patients with long-standing multinodular goiters, which gradually convert to toxic multinodular goiters over time. It can also be precipitated more abruptly by administration of a large iodine load, such as radiocontrast agents or amiodarone, to patients with nontoxic multinodular goiters. Less common causes of hyperthyroidism in older patients include subacute or silent thyroiditis, or rarely central hyperthyroidism due to a pituitary disorder with excess TSH secretion. Finally, a number of medications can cause hyperthyroidism; see Chap. 13 for further discussion. The most common medication to cause overt or subclinical hyperthyroidism in the elderly is thyroid hormone itself, since many patients who receive L-T4 (or other thyroid hormones) are inadvertently overtreated [4].

Amiodarone-induced thyrotoxicosis is a particular problem in the elderly, since amiodarone is most commonly prescribed to older subjects with significant cardiac disease or arrhythmias [21]. The onset of amiodarone-induced thyrotoxicosis can cause severe and abrupt deterioration in cardiac status in these patients. There are two types of amiodarone-induced thyrotoxicosis. Type 1 is due to the iodine load present in amiodarone, while Type 2 is a destructive thyroiditis. In theory, these two types of thyrotoxicosis can be distinguished by laboratory testing and thyroid ultrasound, and have different treatment options. However, in reality, an individual patient may have a mixed type, and the need for urgent treatment often precludes detailed laboratory testing. Patients receiving amiodarone should be monitored at 6 month intervals for thyroid hormone levels to screen for the onset of amiodarone-induced thyroid dysfunction.

12.3.3   Clinical Manifestations

Classic findings of overt hyperthyroidism in young patients include increased appetite, weight loss, heat intolerance, excessive sweating, diarrhea or loose stools, tremulousness, nervousness, tachycardia, and palpitations. Many of these findings are due to the hyperadrenergic state induced by hyperthyroidism. Older subjects may

Table 12.3 Comparison of clinical features of hyperthyroidism in young versus old patients (from [20, 22–25])

Clinical feature	Young patients (%)	Old patients (%)
Fatigue/weakness	61–84	27–56
Nervousness	42–99	20–38
Confusion	0	8–52
Sweating	39–95	0–38
Heat intolerance	49–92	0–63
Diarrhea	43	18
Palpitations	89	36–63
Increased appetite	38–61	0–36
Decreased appetite	4	32–36
Weight loss	29–85	35–83

also manifest hyperadrenergic and hypermetabolic symptoms and signs, but they are less common [20, 22–25] (Table 12.3). Instead, elderly patients often present with unexplained weight loss or cardiac decompensation, without the classic findings of hyperthyroidism. This phenomenon was first described in 1931 by Lahey as "apathetic hyperthyroidism" [26]. Fewer elderly patients with hyperthyroidism have a palpable goiter, further obscuring the diagnosis. If not recognized, apathetic hyperthyroidism can lead to an extensive and expensive evaluation for malignancy, gastrointestinal disorder, or cardiac disease.

Most of the data on clinical manifestations of subclinical hyperthyroidism have been in the areas of cardiac effects, bone loss, and neuropsychiatric effects (reviewed in [12]). However, few of these studies specifically evaluated older patients, and it is unclear whether these effects apply to the elderly. In addition, many of these studies involved patients receiving exogenous thyroid hormone, often in doses now considered excessive, and it is not clear whether the results apply to patients with endogenous hyperthyroidism.

A well-documented effect of either overt or subclinical hyperthyroidism in older patients is the risk of atrial fibrillation [27]. Many studies have shown that older patients with low TSH levels are at markedly increased risk of atrial fibrillation, compared to age-matched euthyroid subjects. Elderly patients with atrial fibrillation should always have TSH measured to rule out occult hyperthyroidism. The risk of atrial fibrillation is a major reason to consider treatment of even mild hyperthyroidism in the elderly, since older hyperthyroid patients with atrial fibrillation are at increased risk for cerebrovascular embolism and stroke.

Another recent area of concern is the possible link between subclinical hyperthyroidism and the development of dementia. A few recent epidemiologic studies have reported such a link, including the long-term Framingham study, which reported an increased risk in older women (but not men) [13]. However, the putative mechanisms are unclear, and the results require further confirmation with other population-based studies. There are no intervention studies that show the risk of developing dementia can be lowered by treating subclinical hyperthyroidism.

12.3.4 Diagnosis

The best screening test for hyperthyroidism in the elderly is a serum TSH level, which will be low in almost all cases of hyperthyroidism (rare exceptions include central hyperthyroidism due to pituitary tumors or other conditions). A normal TSH virtually rules out hyperthyroidism. However, many elderly subjects with low TSH levels do not have hyperthyroidism. A number of medications and acute or chronic illnesses can also cause low TSH levels in these patients (see Chaps. 10 and 13), although TSH levels are not usually undetectable. If an elderly patient has a low TSH level, a careful assessment and further laboratory testing are necessary to distinguish true hyperthyroidism from nonthyroidal illness or drug effects.

Older patients with low TSH levels require a serum fT4 level, which can help distinguish hyperthyroidism from nonthyroidal illness, and determine the extent of the hyperthyroidism. If the fT4 level is elevated, the patient has overt hyperthyroidism and requires treatment. If the fT4 level is normal, a serum T3 or fT3 level should be obtained. This is because many kinds of hyperthyroidism are characterized by relatively excessive T3 production, compared to T4 production. In some cases, this leads to pure "T3 toxicosis," which is treated as overt hyperthyroidism [28]. There are also cases of "T4 toxicosis," where the T4, but not the T3, is elevated. This is most commonly due to amiodarone or other iodine-induced hyperthyroid states, since iodine blocks T4 to T3 conversion [21]. It also appears to be more common in older subjects with hyperthyroidism of any cause, perhaps due to age-related decrease in T4 to T3 conversion. T4 toxicosis, like T3 toxicosis, is overt hyperthyroidism and needs to be treated.

If both the fT4 and T3 levels are normal in a patient with a low TSH, there are two possibilities: (1) The patient has subclinical hyperthyroidism. This is more likely if the TSH is undetectable, rather than low but detectable. (2) The patient has a nonthyroid cause of the low TSH, either an illness or a medication. It is important to distinguish these two etiologies, if possible, since treatment may be indicated for subclinical hyperthyroidism, but not for nonthyroidal illness.

Once a patient has been diagnosed with hyperthyroidism, a 24-hour radioactive iodine uptake is often obtained to determine the cause of the hyperthyroidism and determine the best treatment options. Graves' Disease presents as increased 24-hour radioiodine uptake, while toxic multinodular goiters may have normal or increased uptake. Hyperthyroidism due to excessive iodine intake, such as amiodarone-induced thyrotoxicosis, leads to little to no radioiodine uptake. A radioiodine scan may be added to the uptake test if there is concern about a toxic nodule or toxic multinodular goiter. A thyroid ultrasound may also be indicated if physical examination or the radioiodine scan indicates the presence of thyroid nodules.

12.3.5 Treatment

Treatment options for overt hyperthyroidism in the elderly depend to some extent on the severity of the hyperthyroidism, the medical condition of the patient, and the cause of the hyperthyroidism (reviewed in [1]). Radioactive iodine (I-131) is the definitive therapy for Graves' Disease or toxic multinodular goiter. Younger patients often proceed directly to radioactive iodine therapy without preceeding medical treatment, but this may not be advisable in an elderly patient or one with significant cardiac disease. This is because radioiodine causes temporary release of preformed thyroid hormone from the gland. In a young patient, this is well tolerated, but this can lead to cardiac decompensation in an older patient. For this reason, older patients are usually treated with a thionamide for a few weeks before proceeding to radioactive iodine treatment for Graves' Disease or toxic multinodular goiter. Methimazole is the preferred agent, since propylthiouracil has been associated with radioiodine resistance. The most common outcome of radioactive iodine therapy is long-term hypothyroidism (more common with Graves' Disease than with toxic multinodular goiter), so thyroid hormone levels in treated patients must be monitored for this development.

Therapy with thionamides is also appropriate for older patients with either Graves' Disease or toxic multinodular goiter, and is preferred in unstable patients, since the onset of action is much faster than with radioactive iodine. Propythiouracil and methimazole are both available, although methimazole is usually preferred, since it is more potent, can be given once a day, and is associated with fewer side effects. When given for Graves' Disease, the thionamide is usually discontinued after 12–18 months, to see if a remission has occurred. When given for toxic multinodular goiters, the agent must be given indefinitely.

Surgery is rarely indicated for hyperthyroidism, unless the patient has a very large goiter and obstructive symptoms, or a nodule that is suspicious for malignancy. The risks of surgery in an older hyperthyroid patient are considerable, and pretreatment with beta blockers and thionamides are advisable, if there are no contraindications.

Treatment of iodine-induced hyperthyroidism, such as hyperthyroidism associated with amiodarone, can be quite difficult [21]. Radioactive iodine is usually ineffective, given the large iodine load, and thionamides may have to be used in high doses, with variable efficacy. For Type 2 amiodarone-induced thyrotoxicosis, prednisone may be effective. Occasionally, these patients proceed to thyroidectomy, which is risky in a patient with decompensated cardiac disease.

There is controversy over whether subclinical hyperthyroidism should be treated in the elderly (reviewed in [12]). In a relatively healthy older patient with a mild decrease in serum TSH level, it may be sufficient to monitor the patient. However, as mentioned above, there is a significant risk of atrial fibrillation in older patients with subclinical hyperthyroidism [27]. In addition, at least in postmenopausal women, there may be accelerated loss of bone mass [29]. Finally, there is recent suggestive (although not conclusive) epidemiologic data on increased risks of dementia in subclinical hyperthyroidism in elderly women [13]. Given the variable risks, and the complexities of treatment, this decision should be carefully individualized for a given patient. In many cases, it is prudent to administer a trial of thionamide therapy to normalize serum TSH levels, rather than to proceed to radioactive iodine therapy.

12.4 Thyroid Nodules and Cancer

Thyroid nodules are very common in the population, and increase markedly in frequency with aging. By ultrasound or autopsy studies, almost 50% of subjects over the age of 50 years have thyroid nodules [2]. Most of these are small (less than 1 cm in diameter), and do not require further evaluation unless there are suspicious features. Patients with single palpable nodules often have multinodular goiters by ultrasound examination.

The recommended initial evaluation for a thyroid nodule is a serum TSH level, to rule out thyroid dysfunction [30]. Most patients with thyroid nodules have a normal TSH level, but occasional patients have suppressed TSH levels, consistent with a toxic nodular goiter, evaluated and treated as above. Patients with elevated TSH levels have hypothyroidism, which also needs to be evaluated and treated as above.

In addition to determination of thyroid function by TSH, patients with thyroid nodules should undergo a thyroid ultrasound [30]. This allows the number of nodules to be assessed, since many patients with single palpable nodules have additional nonpalpable nodules that need to be evaluated. It also allows the nodules to be characterized by size and ultrasound features, which help with the assessment for risk of malignancy. In general, nodules greater than 1–1.5 cm in diameter or those with suspicious ultrasound features should undergo fine needle aspiration biopsy to rule out thyroid cancer. The exception is "functioning" or "hot" nodules by radioiodine scan, which are virtually never malignant.

Thyroid cancer is most common in young patients, particularly young women. Although it is less common in older patients, it leads to increased morbidity and mortality with aging [31]. In fact, the single most important prognostic factor for thyroid cancer mortality is age, rising steeply after the age of 45 years. For this reason, thyroid nodules in the elderly should not be ignored, but should be evaluated aggressively, unless the patient is extremely old or medically frail, since early therapy may mitigate the detrimental effects of age on thyroid cancer mortality.

12.5 Challenges in Assessing Thyroid Function in the Elderly

12.5.1 What is the Normal TSH Range in the Elderly?

As TSH immunoassays have improved over the past 30 years, the upper limit of the TSH reference range has declined from about 10 mU/L to 4.0–4.5 mU/L with current assays. However, even with modern TSH assays, the TSH reference range does not follow a normal Gaussian distribution. It is skewed at the upper range, leading to an increased number of apparently healthy subjects with high-normal TSH levels. This is especially true with aging, as increasing numbers of older subjects have high-normal TSH levels compared to younger subjects [5].

Recent studies have attempted to discern why the TSH reference range is skewed at the upper end. The prevalence of anti-TPO antibodies increases as TSH levels increase within the normal range. In the NHANES III study, anti-TPO antibodies were present in 5.5% of subjects without any known thyroid disease who had TSH levels of 0.4–1.0 mU/L, but were present in 31% of subjects with TSH levels of 3.5–4.0 mU/L [5]. If subjects with positive anti-TPO antibodies were excluded, the upper limit of normal for TSH levels decreased from 4.5 to 4.12 mU/L. If the population was further constrained to younger subjects, ages 20–29 years, the upper limit of normal further decreased to 3.56 mU/L, illustrating the increased prevalence of high-normal TSH levels in aging.

These data have generated two opposing theories. The first argues that the skewed TSH distribution represents subjects with occult thyroid disease, as indicated at least partly by anti-TPO antibodies [32]. If this is the case, the argument concludes that the normal TSH range should be lowered to 3.5 mU/L. Other experts argue that the TSH normal range should be lowered even further, to 2.5 mU/L, which represents the upper 97.5th confidence interval for TSH levels with a Gaussian distribution [33]. This last suggestion has far-reaching public health implications, since millions of people in the United States would immediately be diagnosed with hypothyroidism. Since older subjects have higher TSH levels, many of these people would be elderly, with comorbidities that complicate decisions to treat with L-T4.

The second theory argues that the normal TSH range is skewed because TSH levels increase with aging, representing a normal resetting of the pituitary-thyroid axis with age [34]. A recent subanalysis of the NHANES data by age supports the latter hypothesis [35]. This study showed that TSH levels do follow a Gaussian distribution at each age range, with mean levels increasing slightly as one moves from younger to older populations. Ten percent of subjects over 80 years old without anti-TPO antibodies had TSH levels above 4.5 mU/L, and the upper 97.5th percentile for TSH levels in this age range was 7.5 mU/L. Another recent study excluded subjects with either anti-TPO antibodies or abnormal thyroid ultrasounds as markers for autoimmune thyroid disease, more rigorous exclusion criteria than in the NHANES III study [36]. The TSH distribution was still skewed in this reference population, further supporting the theory that the skewed TSH range is not merely an effect of autoimmune thyroid disease [36].

The most relevant point about this controversy is that very little is known regarding clinical effects of TSH levels in the upper-normal range, especially in the elderly (reviewed in [12]). There are a few studies that show correlations between TSH levels within the normal range and serum lipid levels, bone density, or progression to hypothyroidism. On the other hand, there is no apparent correlation between TSH levels within the normal range and symptoms or quality of life, and data on cardiovascular endpoints are mixed. Finally, in the "oldest old," lower thyroid function within the normal range appears to have a protective effect on functional status and mortality [17, 18]. Finally, it should be noted that there are no rigorous intervention trials in older subjects with high-normal or mildly elevated TSH levels and relevant clinical endpoints.

In the absence of consensus on this issue, one must use clinical judgment to decide what constitutes an abnormal TSH level in an older subject who may have nonspecific symptoms and other medical illnesses complicating the decision. It is prudent to err on the side of not treating older subjects with high-normal or mildly elevated TSH levels, given the recent NHANES III analysis and the absence of data showing beneficial clinical outcomes [35]. For example, one recent expert review concluded that treatment is not indicated in very elderly patients if serum TSH levels are lower than 10 mU/L [12]. Once a decision is made to treat an elderly patient, it is also prudent to choose conservative L-T4 doses, aim for a mid- to high-normal TSH level, and avoid overtreatment.

12.5.2   Altered Presentation of Thyroid Disease in the Elderly

As discussed above, hypothyroidism may present in an altered fashion in older patients. More importantly, most of the symptoms of hypothyroidism overlap those commonly seen with aging or with other medical conditions, including fatigue, weight gain, dry skin, cold intolerance, depression, cardiac symptoms, and cognitive decline. For this reason, the diagnosis of hypothyroidism can easily be overlooked in elderly patients with multiple comorbidities and symptoms. Although universal screening for hypothyroidism in the elderly is a controversial topic, there is no question that there should be a low threshold for obtaining a serum TSH in an elderly patient with any suggestion of hypothyroidism.

Older patients with hyperthyroidism often do not manifest the classic symptoms or signs of a hyperadrenergic and hypermetabolic state, as discussed above. Instead, many elderly hyperthyroid patients develop unexplained weight loss, anorexia, cardiac decompensation or arrhythmia, or neuropsychiatric symptoms. As in hypothyroidism, there should be a low threshold for suspecting hyperthyroidism in such patients and obtaining a serum TSH level.

12.5.3   The Effects of Comorbid Conditions and Drugs on Thyroid Function in the Elderly

A further challenge in diagnosing thyroid disease in the elderly is the confounding effect of other illnesses and medications on thyroid hormone levels in this population. These issues are discussed in detail in Chaps. 10 and 13. In a given patient with abnormal thyroid hormone levels, these issues must be factored into the decision regarding whether thyroid disease is present and should be treated.

12.5.4   Risks of Treatment in the Elderly

L-T4 treatment for hypothyroidism is generally considered to be safe, since L-T4 is identical to endogenous T4, and since serum TSH levels are a sensitive and accurate measure of L-T4 dose titration. However, inadvertent overtreatment remains a significant problem, with approximately 20% of L-T4 treated patients developing decreased serum TSH levels [4, 12]. This is a particularly relevant problem in the elderly, who could develop complications of excess L-T4, including weight loss, cardiac decompensation, arrhythmias, or bone loss. In addition, even physiologic L-T4 doses can precipitate angina in patients with significant underlying cardiac disease (reviewed in [1]). For these reasons, L-T4 therapy should be started in low doses in elderly patients, especially those with known cardiac disease, and dose adjustments should be made gradually. Target TSH levels should be conservative, given the recent data on normal TSH ranges in the elderly. Finally, since T4 clearance decreases with aging, lower doses of L-T4 are necessary in the elderly [19].

There are a number of treatment options for an elderly patient with hyperthyroidism, as discussed above. This decision depends on the severity and cause of the hyperthyroidism, the urgency for treatment, and other underlying medical conditions (especially cardiac disease). Radioactive iodine is an excellent choice for Graves' Disease and toxic nodular goiter in the elderly, but there is a risk of temporary exacerbation of the hyperthyroid state due to radiation-induced leakage of preformed hormone from the gland. While this is well tolerated in younger patients, it can lead to clinical deterioration in older patients. For this reason, it is prudent to treat the patient with a thionamide before proceeding to radioactive iodine, for a long enough time period to deplete the thyroid gland of excess hormone.

Thionamide therapy is an excellent alternative to radioactive iodine for Graves' Disease or toxic nodular goiter in older patients, but they must be informed of the risks, which include rash, bone marrow suppression, and hepatitis. These drugs should be used with caution in older subjects with underlying bone marrow or liver diseases. In almost all cases, methimazole is preferred over propylthiorucil, based on its longer half-life and better side-effect profile.

References

1. Hershman JM, Hassani S, Samuels MH. Thyroid diseases. In: Hazard WR, et al., eds. *Principles of Geriatric Medicine and Gerontology.* 6th ed. New York, NY: McGraw-Hill; 2008:1287-1304.
2. Mazzaferri EL. Management of a solitary thyroid nodule. *N Engl J Med.* 1993;328:553-559.
3. Samuels MH. Subclinical thyroid disease in the elderly. *Thyroid.* 1998;8:803-813.
4. Canaris GJ, Manowitz NR, Mayor G, Ridgway EC. The Colorado thyroid disease prevalence study. *Arch Intern Med.* 2000;160:526-534.
5. Hollowell JG, Staehling NW, Flanders WD, et al. Serum TSH, T(4), and thyroid antibodies in the United States population (1988 to 1994): National Health and Nutrition Examination Survey (NHANES III). *J Clin Endocrinol Metab.* 2002;87:489-499.
6. Tunbridge WM, Evered DC, Hall R, et al. The spectrum of thyroid disease in a community: the Whickham survey. *Clin Endocrinol (Oxford).* 1977;7:481-493.
7. Vanderpump MP, Tunbridge WM, French JM, et al. The incidence of thyroid disorders in the community: a twenty-year follow-up of the Whickham Survey. *Clin Endocrinol (Oxford).* 1995;43:55-68.

8. Díez JJ, Iglesias P. Spontaneous subclinical hypothyroidism in patients older than 55 years: an analysis of natural course and risk factors for the development of overt thyroid failure. *J Clin Endocrinol Metab.* 2004;89:4890-4897.

9. Doucet J, Trivalle C, Chassagne P, et al. Does age play a role in clinical presentation of hypothyroidism? *J Am Geriatr Soc.* 1994;42:984-986.

10. Davis JD, Tremont G. Neuropsychiatric aspects of hypothyroidism and treatment reversibility. *Minerva Endocrinol.* 2007;32:49-65.

11. Feldt-Rasmussen U. Treatment of hypothyroidism in elderly patients and in patients with cardiac disease. *Thyroid.* 2007;17:619-624.

12. Biondi B, Cooper DS. The clinical significance of subclinical thyroid dysfunction. *Endocr Rev.* 2008;29:76-131.

13. Tan ZS, Beiser A, Vasan RS, et al. Thyroid function and the risk of Alzheimer disease: the Framingham Study. *Arch Intern Med.* 2008;168:1514-1520.

14. Biondi B. Cardiovascular effects of mild hypothyroidism. *Thyroid.* 2007;17:625-630.

15. Ochs N, Auer R, Bauer DC, et al. Meta-analysis: subclinical thyroid dysfunction and the risk for coronary heart disease and mortality. *Ann Intern Med.* 2008;148:832-845.

16. Razvi S, Shakoor A, Vanderpump M, Weaver JU, Pearce SH. The influence of age on the relationship between subclinical hypothyroidism and ischemic heart disease: a metaanalysis. *J Clin Endocrinol Metab.* 2008;93:2998-3007.

17. Gussekloo J, van Exel E, de Craen AJ, Meinders AE, Frölich M, Westendorp RG. Thyroid status, disability and cognitive function, and survival in old age. *JAMA.* 2004;292:2591-2599.

18. van den Beld AW, Visser TJ, Feelders RA, Grobbee DE, Lamberts SW. Thyroid hormone concentrations, disease, physical function, and mortality in elderly men. *J Clin Endocrinol Metab.* 2005;90:6403-6409.

19. Sawin CT, Herman T, Molitch ME, London MH, Kramer SM. Aging and the thyroid. Decreased requirement for thyroid hormone in older hypothyroid patients. *Am J Med.* 1983;75:206-209.

20. Trivalle C, Doucet J, Chassagne P, et al. Differences in the signs and symptoms of hyperthyroidism in older and younger patients. *J Am Geriatr Soc.* 1996;44:50-53.

21. Basaria S, Cooper DS. Amiodarone and the thyroid. *Am J Med.* 2005;118:706-714.

22. Davis PJ, Davis FB. Hyperthyroidism in patients over the age of 60 years. Clinical features in 85 patients. *Medicine.* 1974;53:161-179.

23. Tibaldi JM, Barzel US, Albin J, Surks M. Thyrotoxicosis in the very old. *Am J Med.* 1986;81:619-622.

24. Nordyke RA, Gilbert FI, Harada ASM. Graves' Disease. Influence of age on clinical findings. *Arch Intern Med.* 1988;148:626-631.

25. Martin FIR, Deam DR. Hyperthyroidism in elderly hospitalized patients. Clinical features and treatment outcomes. *Med J Australia.* 1996;164:200-203.

26. Lahey FH. Apathetic thyroidism. *Ann Surg.* 1931;93:1026.

27. Sawin CT. Subclinical hyperthyroidism and atrial fibrillation. *Thyroid.* 2002;12:501-503.

28. Martino E, Pacchiarotti A, Aghini-Lombardi F, et al. Serum free thyroxine in patients with T3-toxicosis. *Acta Endocrinol (Copenhagen).* 1985;110:354-359.

29. Wexler JA, Sharretts J. Thyroid and bone. *Endocrinol Metab Clin North Am.* 2007;36: 673-705.

30. Cooper DS, Doherty GM, Haugen BR, et al. The American Thyroid Association Guidelines Taskforce. Management guidelines for patients with thyroid nodules and differentiated thyroid cancer. *Thyroid.* 2006;16:109-142.

31. Lin JD, Chao TC, Chen ST, Weng HF, Lin KD. Characteristics of thyroid carcinomas in aging patients. *Eur J Clin Invest.* 2000;30:147-153.

32. Spencer CA, Hollowell JG, Kazarosyan M, Braverman LE. National Health and Nutrition Examination Survey III thyroid-stimulating hormone (TSH)-thyroperoxidase antibody relationships demonstrate that TSH upper reference limits may be skewed by occult thyroid dysfunction. *J Clin Endocrinol Metab.* 2007;92:4236-4240.

33. Wartofsky L, Dickey RA. The evidence for a narrower thyrotropin reference range is compelling. *J Clin Endocrinol Metab.* 2005;90:5483-5488.

34. Surks MI, Goswami G, Daniels GH. The thyrotropin reference range should remain unchanged. *J Clin Endocrinol Metab.* 2005;90:5489-5496.
35. Surks MI, Hollowell JG. Age-specific distribution of serum thyrotropin and antithyroid antibodies in the US population: implications for the prevalence of subclinical hypothyroidism. *J Clin Endocrinol Metab.* 2007;92:4575-4582.
36. Hamilton TE, Davis S, Onstad L, Kopecky KJ. Thyrotropin levels in a population with no clinical, autoantibody, or ultrasonographic evidence of thyroid disease: implications for the diagnosis of subclinical hypothyroidism. *J Clin Endocrinol Metab.* 2008;93:1224-1230.

Chapter 13
Influence of Drugs on Thyroid Function Tests

Sonia Ananthakrishnan and Elizabeth N. Pearce

13.1 Introduction

Understanding and identifying medication-induced changes in thyroid function tests is crucial to avoid unnecessary investigations and treatment. This chapter discusses the effects of medications on the secretion, transport, metabolism, and absorption of thyroid hormones, both endogenous and exogenous (Fig. 13.1).

13.2 Alterations of Thyroid Hormone Secretion

Inhibition of thyroid hormone secretion can be induced with a variety of medications. Many of these medications are utilized to treat patients with hyperthyroidism, while decreased thyroid hormone levels are seen as a side effect of others.

13.2.1 Thionamides

Thionamides are compounds that are actively transported into the thyroid, where they inhibit both the organification of iodine and coupling of iodotyrosine residues, leading to a fall in serum throxine (T4) and triiodothyronine (T3) levels. Propylthiouracil (PTU) and methimazole (MMI) are the thionamides available in the United States. Carbimazole, which has an additional carboxy side chain that, when cleaved, converts it to MMI, is also available in Europe. The thionamides may also inhibit the process of thyroid hormone secretion, which can contribute to the decrease in serum T4 and T3 concentrations. Thyroid hormone levels are reduced within a few

S. Ananthakrishnan (✉)
Department of Medicine/Section of Endocrinology, Diabetes and Nutrition, Boston University School of Medicine, Boston, MA 02118, USA
e-mail: soniaa@bu.edu

G. A. Brent (ed.), *Thyroid Function Testing*,
DOI 10.1007/978-1-4419-1485-9_13, © Springer Science+Business Media, LLC 2010

Alterations of thyroid hormone secretion
Thionamides (decreased secretion)
Lithium (most commonly causes decreased secretion, also associated with thyroiditis and
rarely thyrotoxicosis)
Iodides (increased and decreased secretion, depending on baseline thyroid function)
Aminoglutethimide (decreased secretion)
Ethionamide (decreased secretion)

Changes in T4 and T3 Serum Transport Proteins
Increase TBG
Estrogen
SERMS
Narcotics
Mitotane
5-fluorouracil
Clofibrate
Decrease TBG
Androgens
Danazol
Nicotinic Acid
L-Asparaginase

Competition With T4 and T3 Binding Sites on Thyroid Hormone Binding Proteins
Aspirin
Salsalate
Furosemide (high dose)
Heparin

Induction of Metabolism
Phenytoin
Carbemazepine
Phenobarbitol
Oxcarbazepine
Rifampicin

Inhibition of 5'-Deiodination (activation from T4 to T3)
Amiodarone
Radiographic Contrast Agents (iopanoic acid)
Propylthiouracil
Beta Adrenergic Antagonists (high dose)
Glucocorticoids (dexamethasone)

Central TSH Suppression
Dopamine
Dobutamine
Octreotide
Glucocorticoids (dexamethasone)
Bexarotene
Metformin (though less well established)

Medications with Multiple Effects
Glucocorticoids (TSH suppression, reduced T4 to T3 conversion)
Amiodarone (See table 13.2)
Bexarotene (suppressed TSH, accelerated degradation)
Cytokines (thyroiditis)
Tyrosine kinase inhibitors (eg. sunitinib, sorafenib, and imatinib-impairs thyroid hormone synthesis,
associated with thyroiditis, influences thyroid hormone metabolism)

Fig. 13.1 Summary of medications that influence thyroid function arranged in categories based on
their likely mechanism of action. *T4* thyroxine, *T3* triiodothyronine, *TBG* thyroid binding globulin,
SERM selective estrogen receptor modifier, *TSH* thyrotropin

weeks in 90% of patients, making the thionamides effective treatment for patients with Graves' disease and other forms of hyperthyroidism [1].

In addition to decreasing thyroid hormone levels by direct effects on the thyroid, PTU inhibits the 5'-monodeiodinase that converts T4 to T3 in the periphery, which will be discussed elsewhere (Sect. 13.4.2.2).

13.2.2   Lithium

Lithium is commonly used to treat bipolar disorder and conduct disorder. Historically, patients on long-term therapy with lithium were noted to develop hypothyroidism and goiter. Lithium has multiple effects on thyroid function [2]. It causes inhibition of thyroid hormone secretion, hypothesized to be a result of decreased colloid droplet formation in the follicular cells of the thyroid [3–6]. Decreased serum levels of total T4 and T3 in turn lead to an increase in thyrotropin (TSH) concentration. Hypothyroidism occurs in up to 34% of patients. This typically occurs within the first 2 years of lithium use, but has been documented even after years of therapy [7–11]. Lithium-induced subclinical hypothyroidism, with an elevated serum TSH and normal free T4 and T3 values, is more common than overt hypothyroidism, and is more common in older women [12]. Changes in thyroid hormone secretion may also result in goiter, which can be found in up to 50% of patients within the first 2 years after starting lithium therapy [8, 9]. In addition to decreasing thyroid hormone secretion, animal studies have shown that lithium may also cause hypothyroidism by enhancing iodine trapping while inhibiting iodine release and coupling [4, 5, 13].

Lithium has also been associated with autoimmune thyroid disease. Patients who develop hypothyroidism while taking lithium have been noted to have a higher prevalence of pretreatment thyroid autoantibodies when compared to patients who remain euthyroid [10, 14, 15]. Lithium has also been reported to induce thyroid antibodies and histological features suggestive of autoimmune thyroiditis [9, 16–18].

Rarely, lithium use has been associated with thyrotoxicosis (decreased TSH and increased serum total T4 and T3 levels). Cases of Graves' disease, toxic nodular goiter, and thyroiditis have all been reported to be more frequent in lithium-treated patients than in the general population, with Graves' disease and thyroiditis being most common [18, 19].

Lithium effects on thyroid hormone secretion have led to its occasional therapeutic use in hyperthyroidism [20, 21] and for increasing radioiodine retention in the treatment of Graves' disease [22] or thyroid cancer [23].

13.2.3   Iodides

The effect of iodinated medications on the thyroid depends on baseline thyroid function (discussed in depth in Chap. 3). Overall, the thyroid follicular cell provides protection against wide variations in dietary intake of iodide via an autoregulatory mechanism, known as the acute Wolff–Chaikoff effect. In the setting of a large intake of iodine, escape from the acute Wolff-Chaikoff effect can occur and normal thyroid hormone synthesis and secretion resumes [24].

Iodine-induced hypothyroidism can occur in patients who ingest large quantities of inorganic iodide (typically greater than 1–2 mg/day), and fail to escape from the acute Wolff–Chaikoff effect. These patients usually have underlying thyroid disease, such as a history of autoimmune, subacute or postpartum thyroiditis, or Graves' disease that has been treated with partial thyroidectomy or radioactive iodine abla-tion [25, 26]. Also at risk are the elderly, newborns, and patients with other chronic illnesses such as cystic fibrosis or thalassemia major. In the setting of the large iodine load, these patients may experience a reduction in serum free T4 and T3 concentrations and a resultant increase in serum concentration of TSH [25, 27, 28]. Iodine-induced hypothyroidism typically resolves within 2–3 weeks of removing the source of excess iodine. If the iodine agent cannot be withdrawn, replacement levothyroxine therapy may be required. This overall effect of decreasing thyroid hormone levels is utilized in the therapy of hyperthyroidism, where administration of iodides causes transient suppression of T4 and T3 secretion [29].

Increased thyroid hormone levels due to iodine, known as iodine-induced hyper-thyroidism or the Jöd-Basedow phenomenon, can result when iodide-containing medications are administered to patients with autonomously functioning thyroid tissue in whom the acute Wolff–Chaikoff effect does not take place. This most com-monly occurs in regions of iodine deficiency, typically in patients with autonomous nodular goiter. In regions of iodine sufficiency, iodine-induced hyperthyroidism is less common overall, and may be seen in patients with latent Graves' disease or autonomous nodules [30, 31]. The risk of iodine-induced thyrotoxicosis is higher in patients with subclinical hyperthyroidism at baseline [32]. The elderly are at particular risk, given their increased prevalence of autonomous thyroid nodules and apathetic, or silent, Graves' disease [33, 34]. Excess iodide exposure from diet, drug therapy, or use of iodinated contrast agents in radiography leads to hyperthy-roidism, with increased free T4, normal-to-elevated free T3, and suppressed TSH concentrations [32, 35]. The hyperthyroidism typically occurs 4–8 weeks after the introduction of the iodine source. Clinical symptoms requiring therapy with antithy-roid agents may occur even after a single dose of iodide [35]. The thyroid hormone changes can last for several months following iodine discontinuation.

Many medications are sources of iodine. In addition to increased dietary iodine consumption, iodine-containing drugs that can produce these alterations in thyroid hormone levels are shown in Table 13.1 and include potassium iodine solutions, betadine vaginal douches, topical antiseptics, the antiamebic iodoquinol, and amio-darone, which is discussed separately below (Sect. 13.6.2) [36–39]. Radiographic contrast agents, for example, those used during coronary angiography or com-puted tomography, also contain significant amounts of iodine, and can lead to the changes in thyroid hormone levels discussed above. In addition, certain lipid-solu-ble radiocontrast agents can affect the deiodination of thyroid hormones, and will be

Table 13.1 Iodine-containing medications available in the United States

Antiarrhythmics	**Antiamebics**
Amiodarone (75 mg/200 mg tablet)	Iodoquinol (134 mg/tablet)
Iodides	**Topical antiseptics**
SSKI (38 mg/drop)	Povidone-Iodine (10 mg/mL)
Lugol's solution (5–6 mg/drop)	Clinoquinol cream (12 mg/gm)
Douches	**Ophthalmic solutions**
Povidone-Iodine (10 mg/mL)	Echothiophate iodide solution (5–41 ug/gtt)
Radiocontrast agents	**Anticellulite therapy**
Diatrizoate meglumine sodium (370 mg/mL)	Cellasene (720 µg/serving)
Iothalamate sodium (480 mg/mL)	

discussed elsewhere (Sect. 13.4.2.1). Radiocontrast agents deserve special attention due to their ubiquitous nature in clinical medicine [40].

13.2.4 Other Medications that Decrease Thyroid Hormone Secretion

Long-term use of aminoglutethimide, an aromatase inhibitor antineoplastic and antiadrenal agent, has been noted to cause decreases in serum total T4 and T3 concentrations. This may not be clinically significant, however, as patients in whom this has been described were being treated for postmenopausal breast cancer, and had thyroid hormone levels that remained in the normal range despite the small reduction [41, 42]. In addition, other medications such as tolbutamide (no longer used clinically) and sulfonamides have been reported to cause hypothyroidism in rare instances [43].

Ethionamide, used as a second-line agent for multi-drug resistant tuberculosis, is structurally similar to MMI, and causes decreases in serum total T4 and resultant increases in serum TSH concentrations by decreasing thyroid hormone synthesis and secretion. The resultant hypothyroidism is partially reversible following drug discontinuation [44, 45].

13.3 Changes in T4 and T3 Serum Transport Proteins

Thyroxine binding globulin (TBG), transthyretin, and albumin are the three major thyroid hormone binding proteins. Lipoproteins such as high-density lipoprotein (HDL) provide another transport vehicle for a much smaller amount of peripheral T4 and T3. Serum thyroid hormone kinetics are modified in the setting of changes in the concentrations of thyroid hormone binding proteins or in the affinity of thyroid hormones to the binding proteins.

13.3.1   Medications that Increase TBG

TBG binds over 70% of serum T4 and T3, and changes in TBG concentrations can thus affect total T4 and T3 levels [46].

13.3.1.1   Estrogens and Selective Estrogen Receptor Modulators

Oral estrogen therapy, used for estrogen replacement therapy or as an oral contraceptive, is known to increase hepatic production of TBG [47–51]. As estrogen increases, TBG sialyation increases, which reduces the rate of clearance of TBG and increases its half-life in a dose-dependent fashion [52]. This effect occurs after approximately 2 weeks of estrogen use, and a new thyroid hormone steady state is achieved after 4–8 weeks. Maintaining euthyroidism and a normal serum TSH level during this time depends on the ability of the thyroid to transiently increase T4 secretion. Women taking exogenous levothyroxine may need a dose increase in order to maintain euthyroidism. Commonly used doses of estrogen, such as ethinyl estradiol (20–30 µg daily) found in oral contraceptive pills, or conjugated estrogen (0.625 mg) cause up to a 50% increase in TBG concentration, which results in an increase in serum total T4 of up to 35%, and lesser increases of serum total T3. Transdermal estrogen, which bypasses the first pass effect on the liver, does not raise serum TBG or total T4 levels [48]. Progesterone therapy, used independently or in concert with estrogen therapy, has no independent effect on TBG concentrations.

SERMs, selective estrogen receptor modulators, including tamoxifene, droloxifene, and raloxifene, have been shown to reduce risks for breast cancer, postmenopausal osteoporosis, and serious cardiovascular disease. This class of medicines has a weak agonist effect on the liver, and thus increases TBG concentrations more modestly than oral estrogen therapy. Tamoxifen induces TBG and serum total T4 level increases, while raloxifene has been observed to cause less significant changes in both TBG and serum total T4 [53–55]. Droloxifene, a SERM structurally similar to tamoxifen, has been shown to increase serum TSH and TBG concentrations, but does not alter free T4 index values in postmenopausal women [56].

13.3.1.2   Narcotics

Long-term heroin and methadone use have been associated with increased TBG concentrations [57–59]. It is difficult to determine if the alteration of TBG is due to a specific effect of the narcotic, or from the coexistent liver dysfunction present in many of these patients. The free T4 index is normal in the majority of these patients [59]. Cocaine has not been shown to have a similar effect [60].

13.3.1.3 Other Medications that Increase TBG

Mitotane, used as long-term therapy in patients with adrenocortical carcinoma, has been shown to increase multiple hormone-binding globulins including TBG. This increase was reversed 1 year after mitotane was discontinued [61].

5-Fluorouracil, used weekly to treat breast cancer, has been noted to cause increased total serum T4 and T3 levels in the setting of unchanged serum free T4 levels and serum TSH levels. This change is hypothesized to occur due to TBG increases [62]. Clofibrate has similarly been noted to increase serum TBG concentrations [63].

13.3.2 Medications that Decrease TBG

13.3.2.1 Androgens

Contrary to the effects of estrogen, androgen therapy decreases levels of serum TBG concentrations. Total T4 and T3 hormone levels decrease, serum TSH is unchanged, and patients remain clinically euthyroid [64–66]. Hypothyroid women on levothyroxine who were treated with androgen therapy for breast cancer became hyperthyroid, requiring a reduction in levothyroxine dose [67]. The cause of the decrease in TBG concentration associated with androgen administration is not clear. It is believed that the effect is transcriptionally mediated, although cleavage of the protein may also play a role in increasing its clearance. Long-term use of glucocorticoids (discussed below) decreases serum TBG levels in a manner similar to androgen therapy (Sect. 13.6.1).

Danazol is a synthetic steroid with antigonadotropic properties used in young infertile women to treat endometriosis. It has been noted to cause changes in thyroid function tests. Total T4 levels were shown to decrease, with increased T3 uptakes, in eight patients receiving 800 mg of danazol daily for 1–5 months [67]. TSH and the free thyroid index (FTI) were normal, confirming that these patients were euthyroid during danazol therapy. This is thought to reflect danazol's androgen-like reduction in TBG rather than an actual decrease in thyroid function or interference with the pituitary-thyroid axis.

13.3.2.2 Other Medications that Decrease Serum TBG

Nicotinic acid, used for treatment of hypercholesterolemia, has been noted to decrease serum TBG concentrations by 25%. Decreases in serum total T4 are smaller, and no changes have been described in serum TSH or free thyroid hormone levels [68–70]. Patients studied were treated with nicotinic acid in doses of 3–6 g/day, used in combination with colestipol, for treating hypercholesterolemia. Colestipol has not been shown to have direct effects on the thyroid or to alter thyroid function tests [71].

L-asparaginase, an antineoplastic therapeutic, has also been associated with an acute deficiency of TBG [72].

13.3.3 Competition with T4 and T3 Binding Sites on Thyroid Hormone Binding Proteins

The binding sites for T4 and T3 on serum transport proteins can be inhibited by a variety of drugs, thus altering serum total T4 and T3 concentrations. Initially, free thyroid hormones increase due to drug displacement of T4, but after continued administration, free T4 and TSH levels normalize, and serum total T4 will decrease. Typically, this effect is seen when the offending medications are used in high dosages. These effects are well described *in vitro*, but are less well documented *in vivo*.

Salicylates, nonsteroidal antiinflammatory medicines (NSAIDs), inhibit T4 and T3 binding to both TBG and transthyretin when administered in doses greater than 2 g/day [73–75]. Similarly, the NSAID salsalate inhibits binding of these thyroid hormones to TBG alone, resulting in decreases of serum total T4 (up to 30%) and total T3 concentrations [76]. While the above studies have involved high dose, long-term NSAID use, effects on thyroid function tests have also been observed after shorter courses of therapy. Single-dose aspirin or salsalate decreases both total and free thyroid hormone measurements. One week of aspirin or salsalate decreased total T4, free T4 (salsalate only), total T3, free T3, and TSH [77]. Ibuprofen, naproxen, and indomethacin showed no effects on thyroid hormone levels after either a single dose or 1 week of therapy. Historically, fenclofenac was noted to displace T4 from its binding site as well, though this medication is no longer available [78].

Furosemide, a commonly used diuretic, has also been shown to inhibit T4 binding when used in doses higher than 80–100 mg daily [79–82]. This effect is seen more commonly with intravenous than with oral doses. The decrease in serum total T4 and increase in serum free T4 may be transient depending on a variety of factors, including the dosing frequency of furosemide, the rate of renal clearance, and the concentration of serum binding proteins, which can also bind this diuretic. It is important to note that both furosemide and aspirin (mentioned above) bind T4 sites on transport proteins with affinities several orders of magnitude less than that of T4.

Heparin similarly results in increased serum free T4 concentrations. Heparin activates endothelial lipoprotein lipase, which hydrolyzes triglycerides into free fatty acids. These free fatty acids then inhibit the protein binding of free T4 and free T3 [83–86]. Large doses of either subcutaneous or intravenous heparin, both fractionated and unfractionated, have been shown to increase plasma and decrease tissue concentrations of T4 *in vitro*, but have not been associated with clinical thyrotoxicosis. A similar effect has been noted when serum total and free T4 are measured shortly after an intravenous injection of 2,000 U of enoxaparin [87–89].

Flavons are naturally occurring substances similar in structure to thyroid hormone. In rats, a synthetic flavanoid has been noted to be a competitive inhibitor of thyroid hormone binding to transthyretin, but not of TBG. Naturally occurring flavanoids may have similar effects, but to a lesser degree [90, 91].

13.4 Metabolism of Thyroid Hormones

The hepatic metabolism and deiodination of T4 and T3 can be interrupted by many different medications.

13.4.1 Hepatic Metabolism

Induction of hepatic p450 enzyme pathways decreases serum T4 concentrations due to a decreased plasma half-life of thyroid hormones, and an increased metabolic clearance rate. These effects on thyroid hormone tests are pronounced in patients who have abnormalities in their baseline hypothalamic-pituitary-thyroid axis, and are unable to compensate appropriately for changes in thyroid hormone levels. Treated hypothyroid patients may need levothyroxine dose increases when concomitantly treated with drugs that induce p450 pathways.

13.4.1.1 Antiepileptics

Phenytoin and carbemazepine cause euthyroid hypothyroxinemia by augmenting the rate of thyroid hormone metabolism by induction of hepatic mixed-function oxygenases, the p450 complex. *In vitro* studies have shown that they also displace thyroid hormones from the serum binding proteins, principally TBG. Carbemazepine has a less potent effect on thyroid hormone levels when compared to phenytoin, but may potentiate the effects of other antiepileptic medications when used in combination. Phenytoin and carbemazepine decrease both total and free T4 and T3 concentrations. Total T4 levels can decrease as much as 40%, while less pronounced reductions are seen in total T3 [92–96].

Phenytoin may also decrease serum TSH levels and inhibit the TSH response to thyrotropin releasing hormone (TRH) [93, 97]. This suggests that phenytoin also interferes with cellular uptake of T3 and has stimulatory nuclear effects as a partial thyroid hormone agonist. In addition, the hypersensitivity syndrome associated with phenytoin has been associated with transient reversible hypothyroidism in five patients [43].

Similar to phenytoin and carbemazepine, phenobarbital activates hepatic microsomal enzymes that lead to increased T4 and T3 metabolism [98–100].

In patients who have a normal hypothalamic-pituitary-thyroid axis, serum total T4, total T3, and TSH concentrations remain within the normal range. However, patients who are hypothyroid and on levothyroxine therapy frequently require an increase in their levothyroxine dose when concomitantly treated with these antiepileptics.

Oxcarbazepine, an antiepileptic designed to reduce the side effects traditionally observed with antiepileptic drugs, has less of an effect on the hepatic p450 enzyme system. However, this medication is still associated with low serum total T4 concentrations and normal TSH levels, suggesting a possible central effect [101].

13.4.1.2 Rifampicin

Rifampicin, an antituberculosis drug, is another potent inducer of the hepatic p450 complex [102, 103]. Due to increased T4 clearance, significant decreases in serum total and free T4 are typically noted in patients treated with rifampicin. The changes in T4 are more profound than the changes in T3 levels, as glucuronidation of T4 is amplified, while T3 is metabolized by sulfation, which is not affected by changes in the hepatic mixed-function oxygenases. Normally, patients compensate for these changes by increasing thyroidal secretion of T4; this may result in an increase in thyroid size [104].

13.4.2 Deiodination

Deiodination, the sequential removal of iodine from T4, is discussed further in Chap. 1. It is the primary metabolic pathway of iodothyronine. Many drugs interfere with the activity of the deiodinase enzymes. T4 5′ deiodinase type 1 (D1) is the primary producer of T3 outside of the thyroid, and is the most common deiodinase targeted by drugs. Inhibition of this enzyme leads to decreased serum T3 concentrations. Reverse T3 (rT3) concentrations may be increased, as their metabolism depends on 5′-deiodinase type 1 (D1) activity. Iodinated medications are more potent inhibitors of deiodinase activity when compared to noniodinated medicines.

13.4.2.1 Iodinated Medications that Inhibit Deiodinases

One of the multiple effects of amiodarone on thyroid function tests is its inhibition of the T4 deiodinase type 1 (D1) enzyme. Amiodarone is further discussed below (Sect. 13.6.2).

Certain radiographic agents, in addition to causing iodine-induced hypo- or hyperthyroidism, are also inhibitors of T4 deiodination, and have been used in the treatment of hyperthyroidism [105–108]. These lipid-soluble radiocontrast agents (not currently available in the United States), such as iopanoic acid, sodium ipodate, and tyropanoate, cause decreased plasma clearance of T4, increased serum total and free T4, and decreased serum total and free T3. Like amiodarone, these radiographic agents likely inhibit 5'-deiodinase type 2 (D2) in addition to 5'-deiodinase type 1 (D1). The result is a transient initial increase in serum TSH that subsequently normalizes. These medications are slowly excreted and can cause prolonged hypothyroidism. These effects on thyroid function tests are in contrast to radiocontrast agents that are water-soluble, which do not inhibit deiodination.

13.4.2.2   Non-iodinated Medications that Inhibit Deiodinases

Propylthiouracil (PTU), in addition to its effects on decreasing thyroid hormone secretion, also inhibits the conversion of T4 to T3. PTU, but not MMI, inhibits the 5'-monodeiodinase that converts T4 to T3 in extrathyroidal tissue. This effect is achieved only with large doses of PTU (450–600 mg/day), and results in an approximate 25–30% reduction of serum T3 levels after 48 hours [109, 110]. Serum TSH concentrations may increase, and the TRH–stimulated TSH response is augmented. These thyroid hormone alterations are completely reversible when PTU is discontinued.

Beta-receptor antagonists in general can be useful in treating the symptoms of thyrotoxicosis, such as tachycardia, tremor, and anxiety, due to the suppression of sympathetic nervous system activity. However, propranolol, a nonselective beta-receptor antagonist, also has effects on the extrathyroidal metabolism of thyroid hormones via inhibition of the T4 5'-deiodinase (type 1) (D1). When given in doses greater than 160 mg/day, patients experience a modest decrease in serum T3 concentration, primarily from decreased conversion of T4, as well as less marked reductions in serum T4 [111, 112]. Reverse T3 levels increase from inhibited degredation. Patients typically remain euthyroid and have stable serum TSH values.

These effects on serum T4 and T3 concentrations are specific to propranolol, and are less applicable to the entire family of beta-receptor antagonists. Atenolol, metoprolol, and alprenolol (no longer used due to medication-induced esophagitis) have also been shown to decrease T3 levels in patients who are hyperthyroid, but not as consistently as and to a lesser degree than propranolol [113].

Dexamethasone similarly inhibits 5'deiodination and is discussed below (Sect. 13.6.1).

13.5   Central TSH Suppression

Several medications have been noted to inhibit pituitary TSH secretion, causing decreased serum TSH concentrations. Typically, this decrease is less pronounced than the TSH suppression that occurs in hyperthyroidism. These medication effects can be difficult to distinguish from the changes of non-thyroidal illness in the setting of severe illness, where many of these medications are frequently used.

Dopamine, when used in doses of at least 1 ug/kg per minute, has been shown to suppress serum TSH, the TRH-stimulated release of TSH, and the levels of TSH subunits alpha and beta [114–116]. Long-term use of a dopamine infusion may result in sustained reductions of TSH as well as reduced T4 and T3 secretion from the thyroid. It is important to note that these changes in thyroid function tests have not been definitively attributed to dopamine, as they may also be a result of underlying illness [117].

Similarly, one study showed that the use of high doses of dobutamine resulted in a significantly decreased TSH concentration in the acute setting, likely from central suppression [118]. TSH concentrations remained within the normal range in all subjects who started with a normal serum TSH, and remained above normal in the three dobutamine-treated subjects with elevated TSH at baseline.

Octreotide, a somatostatin analog, has been shown to decrease TSH secretion when used in doses higher than 100 ug/day, with subsequent reductions in T4 as well [119, 120]. This medication is occasionally used in the therapy of TSH-secreting adenomas in order to reduce TSH levels, restore euthyroidism, and shrink the adenoma. However, long-term use of octreotide does not result in sustained suppression of TSH concentrations, because resultant decreases in thyroid hormone secretion stimulate TSH secretion again.

Metformin has been associated with TSH suppression in both normal and hypothyroid individuals with and without levothyroxine therapy [121, 209]. Glucocorticoids and bexarotene have similar suppressive effects on TSH secretion and are discussed below (Sect. 13.6).

13.6   Medications with Multiple Effects

13.6.1   Glucocorticoids

Glucocorticoids are known to have a variety of effects on thyroid function. High doses of glucocorticoids, such as dexamethasone 0.5 mg or greater per day, or hydrocortisone 100 mg or greater per day, have been shown to reduce serum TSH levels due to central suppression of TSH secretion [122, 123]. The decrease in serum TSH is not as pronounced as the TSH reduction found in hyperthyroid patients. Within 48 hours of withdrawal of short-term glucocorticoids, TSH levels may transiently increase to above pretreatment levels. Long-term use of glucocorticoids does not result in sustained suppression of TSH concentrations, because a resultant decrease in thyroid hormone secretion stimulates TSH secretion again [124].

Higher doses of glucocorticoids, such as dexamethasone 4 mg/day, may cause a decrease in serum T3 concentrations within approximately 3 days. Nonthyroidal production of T3 decreases by up to 30% due to inhibition of the T4 5'deiodinase and increased rT3 production [125–129]. Long-term glucocorticoid therapy leads to a decrease in TBG concentration, probably due to decreased transcription, although cleavage of the protein also may play a role in increasing the clearance of TBG [130].

These effects on TBG and T3 are associated with insignificant reductions in serum T4 concentrations in normal patients. However, T4 secretion is decreased when high doses of dexamethasone are given to Graves' disease patients. It is unknown whether the decrease in T4 secretion is a direct result of thyroidal inhibition or because of decreased thyroid-stimulating immunoglobulin production.

Dexamethasone is the best-studied glucocorticoid, but the effects described above may apply to all glucocorticoids when given in comparable doses. These effects of reducing T3, and, to a lesser degree, T4, can be utilized clinically to decrease thyroid hormone concentrations in thyrotoxic patients.

13.6.2   Amiodarone

Amiodarone is an iodine-rich medication commonly used in the treatment of cardiac tachyarrythmias. The effects of amiodarone on thyroid function tests can be classified as either direct toxic effects from the medication, or effects related to iodine. Amiodarone is 37% iodine by weight. The average dose of 400 mg/day provides over 100 times the recommended daily allowance of iodine per day [131]. As a result, changes in thyroid function tests occur commonly in patients treated with amiodarone. These effects can be long lasting, as the half-life of amiodarone is 100 days. The risk of amiodarone-induced thyroid dysfunction ranges from 2 to 30%, and depends on two major factors: the individual's underlying thyroid status and regional dietary iodine intake [132].

Euthyroid patients with normal thyroid glands who are treated with amiodarone frequently experience changes in serum T4 and T3 concentrations, although approximately 90% remain euthyroid [133–135]. Typically, in the acute setting (less than 3 months) of amiodarone use, serum TSH and total and free T4 concentrations increase, while serum total and T3 concentrations decrease. This is due to direct inhibition of hepatic 5'-deiodinase type 1 (D1) and inhibition of entry of thyroid hormone into the peripheral tissue [136]. Serum TSH levels increase after the first day of therapy, while alterations of T3 and T4 concentrations occur 2–4 days later [137]. By 3–6 months after initiation of amiodarone TSH normalizes, with total and free T4 levels in the high-normal range and total T3 levels in the low-normal range in euthyroid individuals (Table 13.2).

Amiodarone-induced hypothyroidism can occur in patients with a variety of risk factors, including underlying Hashimoto's or autoimmune thyroiditis, positive antithyroid antibodies, previous radioactive iodine therapy history, or a partial thyroidectomy [138, 139]. Because these disorders are more common in women, amiodarone-induced hypothyroidism occurs more commonly in women than in men [134]. Overall, amiodarone-induced hypothyroidism is more common than hyperthyroidism in regions of iodine sufficiency, and may occur in up to 30% of patients

Table 13.2 Effects of amiodarone on thyroid function tests in euthyroid patients (adapted from [208])

Test	Duration of treatment	
	Subacute (up to 3 months)	Chronic (>3 months)
T4	Modest increase	Remains increased by up to 40% above baseline; may be in high reference range or modestly raised
T3	Decreased, usually to low reference range	Remains in low reference range or slightly low
TSH	Transient increase (up to 20 mU/L)	Normal, but may be periods of high or low values
rT3	Increased	Increased

taking amiodarone [132, 140, 141]. This hypothyroidism is a result of the inability of the thyroid to escape from the acute Wolff–Chaikoff effect, in the setting of the iodine load from amiodarone. This does not appear to be a dose-dependent effect. It may occur within 6–12 months after initiation of amiodarone therapy. Resolution, with normalization of serum TSH, can occur after 2–4 months of stopping the amiodarone, unless there is significant preexisting Hashimoto's thyroiditis.

Hyperthyroidism related to amiodarone administration, commonly referred to as amiodarone-induced thyrotoxicosis (AIT), is classified into two forms, either iodine-induced (Type I AIT) or an inflammatory thyroiditis (Type II AIT) [142]. The prevalence of these two types is thought to differ based on regional iodine dietary intake. In iodine-deficient regions, type I AIT predominates, while in iodine-sufficient areas such as the United States, AIT is less common overall, and AIT type II predominates [132, 134, 143]. Type I AIT, seen most commonly in individuals with autonomous thyroid glands who may have preexisting Graves' disease or multinodular goiter, results in augmented T4 and T3 production in the thyroid, and a suppressed TSH. This is a result of the excess iodine load provided by amiodarone and failure of the acute Wolff–Chaikoff effect [136]. Type II AIT is a destructive thyroiditis that results from the direct toxic effects of amiodarone on thyroid follicular cells, leading to increased total T4 and T3 concentrations. It lasts from weeks to months [144]. This can be followed by a hypothyroid phase and eventual recovery in most patients. Type I and type II AIT may coexist in a mixed form. Of special note is that the resultant thyrotoxicosis from amiodarone can potentiate the effects of other medications these arrhythmic patients may be taking, such as warfarin [145].

A lesser effect on thyroid function tests may result from amiodarone or its metabolite, desethylamiodarone, acting as a weak antagonist of thyroid hormone actions. The medication and/or its metabolite is a noncompetitive inhibitor of T3 binding to *E. coli*-expressed T3 receptor proteins *in vitro* [146, 147]. This effect has been hypothesized to provide a small contribution to the increase in serum TSH that is seen after initiation of amiodarone therapy. However, there is no *in vivo* data demonstrating that amiodarone creates selective target tissue resistance to T3, and it is likely that changes in TSH result primarily from decreased deiodination, as described above.

13.6.3 Bexarotene

Bexarotene, a retinoid X receptor-selective retinoid currently approved for use in the treatment of cutaneous T cell lymphoma and under investigation for treating other malignancies including thyroid carcinoma, has been observed to cause hypothyroidism with a variety of effects on thyroid function tests. Bexarotene suppresses TSH promoter activity, TSH mRNA synthesis, and subsequently TSH secretion, leading to central hypothyroidism with decreases in total T4 and T3 [148–150]. This medication has also been observed to cause changes in the peripheral metabolism of thyroid hormones, independent of effects on TSH secretion. Parallel decreases in serum T4, T3, and rT3 levels and a modest increase in the T3 to rT3 ratio observed in athyreotic patients suggest that accelerated degradation of these hormones occurs by pathways other than deiodination,such as hepatic conjugation [151].

13.6.4 Cytokines

Cytokine-based treatments have been associated with thyroid hormone abnormalities [152]. Both interferon-α and interleukin-2 have been associated with the novel development of anti-thyroperoxidase antibodies [153–155].

Up to 35% of patients treated with interferon-α may experience changes in thyroid hormone levels, although these changes do not consistently occur in the setting of the appearance of antibodies [156–159]. It is important to recognize that this therapy is used in individuals, including patients with hepatitis C and multiple sclerosis, who may be at a higher risk for autoimmune thyroid disease than the general population [160]. Interferon-α has been linked to both hypo- and hyperthyroidism, and although the mechanisms have not been fully elucidated, the changes are thought to be immune-mediated [161, 162]. Inflammatory thyroiditis with thyrotoxicosis followed by hypothyroidism has also been described [163–165]. Thyroid dysfunction of any type appears approximately 3 months after initiation of therapy, and persists for months after discontinuation [166]. Women and patients with preexisting thyroid auto-antibodies have been noted to be at an increased risk for thyroid dysfunction during treatment with interferon-α [157, 165]. Although there are case reports associating interferon-β with thyroid function changes, it is not clear that there is a true association [167].

Another cytokine, interleukin-2, has been associated with transient hypothyroidism in 15–40% of patients, as well as with autoimmune thyroiditis [165, 168, 169]. In these cases, alterations of thyroid function tests appear to resolve after cessation of the treatment [170]. Similar effects on thyroid function tests have been described with denileukin diftitox, a fusion toxin consisting of the enzymatic and translocating domain of diphtheria toxin and the ligand-binding domain of recombinant human interleukin-2 (IL-2) [171]. Interferon-γ may affect major histocompatibility complex class II expression that may increase thyroid autoimmunity [172, 173].

13.6.5 Other Medications with Effects on Thyroid Function Tests

The tyrosine kinase inhibitor, sunitinib, used for gastrointestinal stromal tumors (GIST) and metastatic renal cell carcinomas, may cause thyroid dysfunction and thyroid function test alterations. Up to 36% of patients on sunitinib have been noted to develop hypothyrodism, based on TSH elevation, at a mean of 50 weeks after the initiation of sunitinib therapy for GIST [174, 175]. The risk of hypothyroidism appears to increase with longer duration of sunitinib treatment, and may be reversible, although the time course of recovery is not certain. The hypothyroidism may be mediated by impaired thyroid hormone synthesis early after initiation of treatment, and followed later by thyroiditis [176]. The thyroiditis, which may include a period of thyrotoxicosis, can be followed by either transient or permanent hypothyroidism [177]. Alternatively, it has been suggested that sunitinib may inhibit thyroid hormone organification, or act as a noncompetitive inhibitor of thyroid peroxidase, similar in mechanism to MMI or PTU [178]. A recent study showed that sunitinib-induced hypothyroidism is not a result of inhibition of iodide uptake [179]. Sunitinib may also cause changes in thyroid function tests in thyroidectomized patients taking levothyroxine by accelerating the rate of thyroid hormone clearance [180].

Other tyrosine kinase inhibitors have similarly been linked to changes in thyroid hormone levels. Imatinib, also used to treat GIST, was noted to increase levothyroxine requirements in patients who had also undergone thyroidectomy, most likely to be related to increased hepatic metabolism of thyroid hormones [181]. Sorafenib, a vascular endothelial growth factor (VEGF) receptor tyrosine kinase inhibitor, has also been anecdotally noted to cause both hypo- and hyperthyroidism. Treatment has rarely been required. Motesanib, an oral inhibitor of the tyrosine kinases of VEGF receptors 1, 2, and 3, platelet-derived growth-factor receptor, and KIT, a tyrosine kinase receptor for mast/stem cell growth factor, recently studied in the treatment of advanced or metastatic radioiodine-resistant differentiated thyroid cancer, has been shown to increase serum TSH levels [182].

Thalidomide, originally marketed in 1956 as a sedative and withdrawn from the market due to teratogenicity, is now used as an immunomodulatory therapy for a variety of conditions including multiple myeloma. Thalidomide-induced hypothyroidism has been reported and up to 14% of patients on thalidomide treatment may become subclinically hypothyroid (TSH > 10 mu/L) by 3 months [183–185]. This thyroid dysfunction might contribute to some of the known side effects of thalidomide therapy, such as fatigue, constipation, and bradycardia [186]. The mechanism of hypothyroidism is thought to be the induction of autoimmune damage to the thyroid gland through the medication's immunomodulatory actions. It promotes the production of several cytokines and alters T cell populations, which may trigger an autoimmune response. An alternative hypothesis is that thalidomide inhibits secretion of thyroid hormones by a direct action on thyrocytes [187].

Quetiapine has been associated with changes in thyroid function tests [188, 189]. This medication, used as an antipsychotic treatment, causes decreases in both free and total T4 levels after approximately 6 weeks of therapy. No significant changes in TSH have been noted. The mechanism of thyroid hormone alteration has not been elucidated, and inhibition of thyroid hormone formation/secretion, alterations to hepatic metabolism, and changes to T4 and T3 deiodination have all been suggested.

13.7 Levothyroxine Absorption

The gastrointestinal tract plays a minor role in the metabolism of endogenous thyroid hormones, while exogenous levothyroxine requires an intact jejunum and ileum for adequate absorption. Eighty percent of orally ingested levothyroxine, used to treat hypothyroid and thyroid cancer patients, is absorbed within the first 3 hours following drug administration [190]. Because consistent and optimal absorption is essential, it is important to identify the prescription and over-the-counter medications that may interfere with the gastrointestinal (GI) absorption of levothyroxine, causing decreases in serum T4 concentrations, and resulting in increased TSH concentrations.

Aluminum hydroxide-containing antacids and sucralfate, used in the treatment of gastrointestinal ulcers have been shown to decrease levothyroxine absorption, though the latter less consistently so [191–194]. Newer medicines used to treat acid disorders in the GI tract, such as H2 blockers and proton pump inhibitors have not been shown to have similar inhibitory effects on levothyroxine absorption [195–198].

Ferrous sulfate and calcium carbonate independently cause decreased absorption of levothyroxine and increased serum TSH concentrations in levothyroxine treated patients [199–201]. Similarly, other elemental medications such as sevelamer hydrochloride and lanthanum carbonate, phosphate-binders used in the treatment of hyperphosphatemia in end-stage renal disease, and chromium picolinate (an over-the-counter nutritional supplement) have been recently shown to decrease levothyroxine absorption [202, 203]. Raloxifene, a SERM, also decreases levothyroxine absorption [204].

Cholestyramine, a bile acid sequestrant, decreases serum T4 and increases serum TSH concentrations in hypothyroid patients taking levothyroxine, but not in normal subjects [205, 206]. Similarly, colestipol and colesevelam, cholesterol-lowering bile acid sequestrants, cause parallel decreases in serum T4 concentrations. These medications are occasionally used to treat patients with both exogenous and endogenous hyperthyroidism [203, 207].

These changes in serum T4 and TSH can be minimized by instructing all patients to take levothyroxine and the above medications several hours apart.

13.8   Conclusions

There are drugs that may affect thyroid function in numerous ways. They can cause hypo- or hyperthyroidism, through effects on the thyroid axis at multiple levels. Understanding the effect of these medications on thyroid hormone concentrations, and the site of the drug interaction can aid clinicians in anticipating and adjusting for these changes, as well as utilizing these drugs in the therapy of thyroid disorders.

References

1. Cooper DS. Antithyroid drugs. *N Engl J Med.* 2005;352:905-917.
2. Bocchetta A, Loviselli A. Lithium treatment and thyroid abnormalities. *Clin Pract Epidemiol Ment Health.* 2006;2:23-27.
3. Williams JA, Berens SC, Wolff J. Thyroid secretion in vitro: inhibition of TSH and dibutyryl cyclic-AMP stimulated 131-I release by Li+1. *Endocrinology.* 1971;88:1385.
4. Berens SC, Bernstein RS, Robbins J, Wolff J. Antithyroid effects of lithium. *J Clin Invest.* 1970;49:1357.
5. Burrow GN, Burke WR, Himmelhoch JM, Spencer RP, Hershman JM. Effect of lithium on thyroid function. *J Clin Endocrinol Metab.* 1971;32:647.
6. Spaulding SW, Burrow GN, Bermudez F, Himmelhoch JM. The inhibitory effect of lithium on thyroid hormone release in both euthyroid and thyrotoxic patients. *J Clin Endocrinol Metab.* 1972;35:905.
7. Lazarus JH. The effect of lithium therapy on thyroid and thyrotropin-releasing hormone. *Thyroid.* 1998;8:909–913.
8. Perrild H, Hegedus L, Baastrup PC, Kayser L, Kastberg S. Thyroid function and ultrasonically determined thyroid size in patients receiving long-term lithium treatment. *Am J Psychiatry.* 1990;147:1518.
9. Bocchetta A, Bernardi F, Pedditzi M, et al. Thyroid abnormalities during lithium treatment. *Acta Psychiatr Scand.* 1991;83:193.
10. Emerson CH, Dysno WL, Utiger RD. Serum thyrotropin and thyroxine concentrations in patients recieving lithium carbonate. *J Clin Endocrinol Metab.* 1973;36:338.
11. Vincent A, Baruch P, Vincent P. Early onset of lithium-associated hypothyroidism. *J Psychiatry Neurosci.* 1993;18:74.
12. Kirov G, Tredget J, John R, Owen MJ, Lazarus JH. A cross-sectional and a prospective study of thyroid disorders in lithium-treated patients. *J Affect Disord.* 2005;87:313.
13. Bagchi N, Brown TR, Mack RE. Studies of the mechanism of inhibition of thyroid function by lithium. *Biochem Biophys Acta.* 1978;542:163.
14. Lindstedt G, Nilsson L-A, Walinder J, Skott A, Ohman R. On the prevalence, diagnosis and management of lithium-induced hypothyroidism in psychiatric patients. *Br J Psychiatry.* 1977;130:452-458.
15. Myers DH, Carter RA, Burns BH, Armond A, Hussain SB, Chengapa VK. A prospective study of the effects of lithium on thyroid function and on the prevalence of antithyroid antibodies. *Psychol Med.* 1985;15:55-61.

16. Wilson R, McKillop JH, Crocket GT, et al. The effect of lithium therapy on parameters thought to be involved in the development of autoimmune thyroid disease. *Clin Endocrinol.* 1991;34:357-361.

17. Mizukami Y, Michigishi T, Nonomura A, Nakamura S, Noguchi M, Takazakura E. Histoloigcial features of the thyroid gland in a patient with lithium induced thyrotoxicosis. *J Clin Pathol.* 1995;48:582-584.

18. Miller KK, Daniels GH. Association between lithium use and thyrotoxicosis caused by silent thyroiditis. *Clin Endocrinol (Oxford).* 2001;55:501-508.

19. Barclay ML, Brownlie BE, Turner J, Wells JE. Lithium associated thyrotoxicosis: a report of 14 cases, statistical analysis of incidence. *Clin Endocrinolo (Oxford).* 1994;40:759-764.

20. Lazarus JH, Addison GM, Richards AR, Owen GM. Treatment of thyrotoxicosis with lithium carbonate. *Lancet.* 1974;2:1160.

21. Boehm TM, Burman KD, Barnes S, Wartofsky L. Lithium and iodine combination therapy for thyrotoxicosis. *Acta Endocrinol (Copenhagen).* 1980;94:174.

22. Bogazzi F, Bertalena L, Brogioni S, et al. Comparison of radioiodine with radioiodine polus lithium in the treatment of Graves' hyperthyroidism. *J Clin Endocrinol Metab.* 1999;84:499-503.

23. Pons F, Carrio I, Estorch M, Ginjaume M, Pons J, Milian R. Lithium as an adjuvant of iodine-131 uptake when treating patients with well-differentiated thyroid carcinoma. *Clin Nucl Med.* August 1987;12(8):644-647.

24. Wolff J, Chaikoff IL. Plasma inorganic iodide as a homeostatic regulator of thyroid function. *J Biol Chem.* 1948;174:555.

25. Braverman LE. Iodine induced thyroid disease. *Acta Med Austriaca.* 1990;17(suppl 1):29-33.

26. Braverman LE. Iodine and the thyroid: 33 years of study. *Thyroid.* 1994;4:351.

27. Vagenakis AF, Braverman LE. Adverse effects of iodides on thyroid function. *Med Clin North Am.* 1975;59:1075.

28. Saberi M, Utiger RD. Augmentation of thyrotropin responses in thyrotropin-releasing hormone following small decreases in serum thyroid hormone concentrations. *J Clin Endocrinol Metab.* 1975;40:435.

29. Philippou G, Koutras DA, Piperingos G, Souvatzoglou A, Moulopoulos SD. The effect of iodide on serum thyroid hormone levels in normal persons, in hyperthyroid patients, and in hypothyroid patients on thyroxine replacement. *Clin Endocrinol (Oxford).* 1992;36:573-578.

30. Vagenakis AG, Wang CA, Burger A, Maloof F, Braverman LE, Ingbar SH. Iodide-induced thyrotoxicosis in Boston. *N Engl J Med.* 1972;287:523.

31. Fradkin JE, Wolff J. Iodide-induced thyrotoxicosis. *Medicine.* 1983;62:1.

32. Fricke E, Fricke H, Esdorn E, et al. Scintigraphy for risk stratification of iodine-induced thyrotoxicosis in patients receiving contrast agent for coronary angiography: a prospective study of patients with low thyrotropin. *J Clin Endocrinol Metab.* 2004;89:6092-6096.

33. Martin FI, Deam DR. Hyperthyroidism in elderly hospitalized patients. Clinical features and outcome. *Med J Aust.* 1996;164:200.

34. Tibaldi J, Barzel US, Albin J, Surks MI. Thyrotoxicosis in the very old. *Am J Med.* 1986;81:619.

35. Hintze G, Blombach O, Fink H, Burkhardt U, Kobberling J. Risk of iodine-induced thyrotoxicosis after coronary angiography: an investigation in 788 unselected subjects. *Eur J Endocrinol.* 1999;140:264-267.

36. l'Allemand D, Gruters A, Beyer P, Weber B. Iodine in contrast agents and skin disinfectants is the major cause for hypothyroidism in premature infants during intensive care. *Horm Res.* 1987;28:42.

37. Chanoine JP, Boulvain M, Bourdoux P, et al. Increased recall rate at screening for congenital hypothyroidism in breast fed infants born to iodine overloaded mothers. *Arch Dis Child.* 1988;63:1027.

38. Teng W, Shan Z, Teng X, et al. Effect of iodine intake on thyroid diseases in China. *N Engl J Med.* 2006;354:2783.

39. Pedersen IB, Laurberg P, Knudsen N, et al. An increased incidence of overt hypothyroidism after iodine fortification of salt in Denmark: a prospective population study. *J Clin Endocrinol Metab.* 2007;92:3122.

40. Conn JJ, Sebastian MJ, Deam D, Tam M, Martin FI. A prospective study of the effect of nonionic contrast media on thyroid function. *Thyroid.* 1996;6:107-110.

41. Dowsett M, Mehta A, Cantwell BMJ, Harris AL. Low-dose aminoglutethimide in postmenopausal breast cancer: effects on adrenal and thyroid hormone secretion. *Eur J Cancer.* 1991;27:846-849.

42. Figg WD, Thibault A, Sartor AO, et al. Hypothyroidism associated with aminoglutethimide in patients with prostate cancer. *Arch Intern Med.* 1994;154:1023-1025.

43. Gupta A, Eggo MC, Uetrecht JP, et al. Drug-induced hypothyroidism: the thyroid as a target organ in hypersensitivity reactions to anticonvulsants and sulfonamides. *Clin Pharmacol Ther.* 1992;51:56-67.

44. Drucker D, Eggo MC, Salit IE, Burrow GN. Ethionamide-induced goitrous hypothyroidism. *Ann Intern Med.* 1984;100:837-839.

45. McDonnell ME, Braverman LE, Bernardo J. Hypothyroidism due to ethionamide. *N Engl J Med.* 2005;352(26):2757-2759.

46. Bartalena L. Recent achievements in studies on thyroid hormone-binding proteins. *Endocr Rev.* 1990;11:47-64.

47. Knopp RH, Bergelin RO, Wahl PW, Walden CE, Chapman MB. Clinical chemistry alterations in pregnancy and oral contraceptive use. *Obstet Gynecol.* 1985;66:682-690.

48. Steingold KA, Matt DW, DeZiegler D, Sealey JE, Fratkin M, Reznikov S. Comparison of transdermal to oral estradiol administration on hormonal and hepatic parameters in women with premature ovarian failure. *J Clin Endocrinol Metab.* 1991;73:275-280.

49. Kuhl H, Jung-Hoffman C, Weber J, Boehm BO. The effect of a biphasic desogestrel-containing oral contraceptive on carbohydrate metabolism and various hormonal parameters. *Contraception.* 1993;47:55-68.

50. Geola FL, Frumar AM, Tataryn IV, et al. Biological effects of various doses of conjugated equine estrogens in postmenopausal women. *J Clin Endocrinol Metab.* 1980;51:620-625.

51. Ben-Rafael Z, Mastroianni L Jr, Struass JF III, Flickinger GL, Arendash-Durand B. Changes in thyroid function tests and sex hormone binding globulin associated with treatment by gonadotropin. *Fertil Steril.* 1987;48:318-320.

52. Bartalena L, Robbins J. Variations in thyroid hormone transport proteins and their clinical implications. *Thyroid.* 1992;2:237-245.

53. Mamby CC, Love RR, Lee KE. Thyroid function test changes with adjuvant tamoxifen therapy in postmenopausal women with breast cancer. *J Clin Oncol.* 1995;13:854-857.

54. Duntas LH, Mantzou E, Koutras DA. Lack of substantial effects of raloxifene on thyroxine-binding globulin in postmenopausal women: dependency on thyroid status. *Thyroid.* August 1, 2001;11(8):779-782.

55. Hsu SH, Cheng WC, Men-Wang J, Tsai KS. Effects of long-term use of Raloxifene, a selective estrogen receptor modulator, on thyroid function test profiles. *Clin Chem.* 2001;47:1865-1867.

56. Marqusee E, Braverman LE, Lawrence JE, Carroll JS, Seely EW. The effect of droloxifene and estrogen on thyroid function in postmenopausal women. *J Clin Endocrinol Metab.* 2000;85(11):4407-4410.

57. Azizi F, Vagenakis AG, Portnay GI, Braverman LE, Ingbar SH. Thyroxine transport and metabolism in methadone and heroin addicts. *Ann Intern Med.* 1974;80:194-199.

58. English TN, Ruxton D, Eastman CJ. Abnormalities in thyroid function associated with chronic therapy with methadone. *Clin Chem.* 1988;34:2202-2204.

59. Novick DM, Poretsky L, Kalin MF. Methadone and thyroid-function tests. *Clin Chem.* 1989;35:1807-1808.

60. Dhopesh VP, Burke WM, Maany I, Ravi NV. Effect of cocaine on thyroid functions. *Am J Drug Alcohol Abuse.* 1991;17:423-427.

61. van Seters AP, Moolenaar AJ. Mitotane increases the blood levels of hormone-binding proteins. *Acta Endocrinol Suppl (Copenhagen)*. 1991;124:526-533. [Erratum, Acta Endocrinol 1991;125:336].

62. Beex L, Ross A, Smals A, Klopenborg P. 5-Fluorouracil-induced increase of total serum thyroxine and triiodothyronine. *Cancer Treat Rep*. 1977;61:1291-1295.

63. McKerron CG, Scott RL, Asper SP, Levy RI. Effects of clofibrate (Atromid S) on the thyroxine-binding capacity of thyroxine-binding globulin and free thyroxine. *J Clin Endocrinol Metab*. 1969;29:957.

64. Deyssig R, Weissel M. Ingestion of androgenic-anabolic steroids induces mild thyroidal impairment in male body builders. *J Clin Endocrinol Metab*. 1993;76:1069-1071.

65. Malarkey WB, Strauss RH, Leizman DJ, Liggett M, Demers LM. Endocrine effects in female weight lifters who self-administer testosterone and anabolic steroids. *Am J Obstet Gynecol*. 1991;165:1385-1390.

66. Graham RL, Gambrell RD Jr. Changes in thyroid function tests during danazol therapy. *Obstet Gynecol*. 1980;55:395-397

67. Arafah BM. Decreased levothyroxine requirement in women with hypothyroidism during androgen therapy for breast cancer. *Ann Intern Med*. 1994;121:247-251.

68. Cashin-Hemphill L, Spencer CA, Nicoloff JT, et al. Alterations in serum thyroid hormonal indices with colestipol-niacin therapy. *Ann Intern Med*. 1987;107:324-329.

69. O'Brien T, Silverberg JD, Nguyen TT. Nicotinic acid-induced toxicity associated with cytopenia and decreased levels of thyroxine-binding globulin. *Mayo Clin Proc*. 1992;67:465-468.

70. Shakir KM, Kroll S, Aprill BS, Drake AJ III, Eisold JF. Nicotinic acid decreases serum thyroid hormone levels while maintaining a euthyroid state. *Mayo Clin Proc*. 1995;70:556-558.

71. Witztum JL, Jacobs LS, Schonfeld G. Thyroid hormone and thyrotropin levels in patients placed on colestipol hydrochloride. *J Clin Endocrinol Metab*. 1978;46:838-840.

72. Garnick MB, Larsen PR. Acute deficiency of thyroxine-binding globulin during L-asparaginase therapy. *N Engl J Med*. 1979;301:252.

73. Ratcliffe WA, Hazelton RA, Thompson JA. Effect of fenclofenac on thyroid-function tests. *Lancet*. 1980;1:432.

74. Baranetsky NG, Chertow BS, Webb MD, et al. Combined phenytoin and salicylate effects on thyroid function tests. *Arch Int Pharmacodyn Ther*. 1986;284:166-176.

75. Larsen PR. Salicylate-induced increases in free triiodothyronine in human serum: evidence of inhibition of triiodothyronine binding to thyroxine-binding globulin and thyroxine-binding prealbumin. *J Clin Invest*. 1972;51:1125-1134.

76. McConnell RJ. Abnormal thyroid function test results in patients taking salsalate. *JAMA*. 1992;267:1242-1243.

77. Samuels MH, Pillote K, Asher D, Nelson JC. Variable effects of nonsteroidal antiinflammatory agents on thyroid test results. *J Clin Endocrinol Metab*. December 2003;88(12):5710-5716.

78. Humphrey MJ, Capper SJ, Kurtz AB. Fenclofenac and thyroid hormone concentrations. *Lancet*. 1980;32:487-488.

79. Lim CF, Bai Y, Tpoliss DJ, Barlow JW, Stockgt JR. Drug and fatty acid effects on serum thyroid hormone binding. *J Clin Endocrinol Metab*. 1988;67:682-688.

80. Newnham HH, Hamblin PS, Long F, Lim CF, Topliss DJ, Stockigt JR. Effect of oral frusemide on diagnostic indices of thyroid function. *Clin Endocrinol (Oxford)*. 1987;26:423-431.

81. Stockigt JR, Lim CF, Barlow JW, et al. Interaction of furosemide with serum thyroxine binding sites: in vivo and in vitro studies and comparison with other inhibitors. *J Clin Endocrinol Metab*. 1985;60:1025-1031.

82. Stockigt JR, Topliss DJ. Assessment of thyroid function during high-dose furosemide therapy. *Arch Intern Med*. 1989;149:973-973.

83. Hershman JM, Jones CM, Bailey AL. Reciprocal changes in serum thyrotropin and free thyroxine produced by heparin. *J Clin Endocrinol Metab*. 1972;34:574-579.

84. Mendel CM, Frost PH, Kunitake ST, Cavalieri RR. Mechanism of the heparin-induced increase in the concentration of free thyroxine in plasma. *J Clin Endocrinol Metab*. 1987;65:1259-1264.

85. Mendel CM, Frost PH, Cavalieri RR. Effect of free fatty acids on the concentration of free thyroxine in human serum: the role of albumin. *J Clin Endocrinol Metab.* 1986;63:1394-1399.

86. Hollander CS, Scott RL, Burgess JA, Rabinowitz D, Merimee TJ, Oppenheimer JH. Free fatty acids: a possible regulator of free thyroid hormone levels in man. *J Clin Endocrinol Metab.* 1967;27:1219-1223.

87. Jain R, Uy HL. Increase in serum free thyroxine levels related to intravenous heparin treatment. *Ann Intern Med.* 1996;124:74-75.

88. Saeed-Uz-Zafar M, Miller JM, Breneman GM, Mansour J. Observations on the effect of heparin on free and total thyroxine. *J Clin Endocrinol Metab.* 1971;32:633-640.

89. Schwartz HL, Schadlow AR, Faierman D, Surk MI, Oppenheimer JH. Heparin administration appears to decrease cellular binding of thyroxine. *J Clin Endocrinol Metab.* 1973;36:598-600.

90. Abend SL, Fang SL, Alex S, et al. Rapid alteration in circulating free thyroxine modulates pituitary type II 5' deiodinase and basal thyrotropin secretion in the rat. *J Clin Invest.* 1991;88:899-903.

91. Chanoine JP, Alex S, Fang SL, et al. Role of transthyretin in the transport of thyroxine from the blood to the choroids plexus, the cerebrospinal fluid and the brain. *Endocrinology.* 1992;130:933-938.

92. Blackshear JL, Schultz AL, Napier JS, Stuart DD. Thyroxine replacement requirements in hypothyroid patients receiving phenytoin. *Ann Intern Med.* 1983;99:341-342.

93. Smith PJ, Surks MI. Multiple effects of 5,5'-diphenylhydantoin on the thyroid hormone system. *Endocr Rev.* 1984;5:514-524.

94. Liewendahl K, Tikanoja S, Helenius T, Majuri H. Free thyroxin and free triiodothyronine as measured by equilibrium dialysis and analog radioimmunoassay in serum of patients taking phenytoin and carbamazepine. *Clin Chem.* 1985;31:1993-1996.

95. Isojarvi JIT, Pakarinen AJ, Myllyla VV. Thyroid function in epileptic patients treated with carbamazepine. *Arch Neurol.* 1989;46:1175-1178.

96. Bentsen KD, Gram L, Veje A. Serum thyroid hormones and blood folic acid during monotherapy with carbamazepine or valproate: a controlled study. *Acta Neurol Scand.* 1983;67:235-241.

97. Surks MI, Ordene KW, Mann DN, Kumara-Siri MH. Diphenylhydantoin inhibits the thyrotropin response to thyrotropin-releasing hormone in man and rat. *J Clin Endocrinol Metab.* 1983;56:940-945.

98. Engler D, Burger AG. The deiodination of the iodothyronines and of their derivatives in man. *Endocr Rev.* 1984;5:151-184.

99. Oppenheimer JH, Bernstein G, Surks MI. Increased thyroxine turnover and thyroidal function after stimulation of hepatocellular binding of thyroxine by phenobarbital. *J Clin Invest.* 1968;47:1399-1406.

100. Cavalieri RR, Sung LC, Becker CE. Effects of phenobarbital on thyroxine and triiodothyronine kinetics in Graves' disease. *J Clin Endocrinol Metab.* 1973;37:308-316.

101. Miller J, Carney P. Central hypothyroidism with oxcarbazepine therapy. *Pediatr Neurol.* March 2006;34(3):242-244.

102. Isley WL. Effect of rifampin therapy on thyroid function tests in a hypothyroid patient on replacement L-thyroxine. *Ann Intern Med.* 1987;107:517-518.

103. Ohnahaus EE, Studer H. The effect of different doses of rifampicin on thyroid hormone metabolism. *Br J Clin Pharmacol.* 1980;9:285-286.

104. Christensen HR, Simonsen K, Hegedus L, et al. Influence of rifampicin on thyroid gland volume, thyroid hormones, and anti-pyrine metabolism. *Acta Endocrinol (Copenhagen).* 1989;121:406-410.

105. Burgi H, Wimpfheimer C, Burger A, et al. Changes of circulating thyroxine, triiodothyronine, and reverse triiodothyronine after radiocontrast agents. *J Clin Endocrinol Metab.* 1976;43:1203-1210.

106. Suzuki H, Kadena N, Takeuchi K, Nakagawa S. Effects of three-day oral cholecystography on serum iodothyronines and TSH concentrations:comparison of the effects among some

cholecystographic agents and the effects of iopanoic acid on the pituitary-thyroid axis. *Acta Endocrinol (Copenhagen)*. 1979;92:477-488.

107. Brown RS, Cohen JH, Braverman LE. Successul treatment of massive acute thyroid hormone poisoning with iopanoic acid. *J Pediatr.* 1998;132:902-905.

108. Meier CA, Burger AC. Effects of drugs and other substances on thyroid hormone synthesis and metabolism. In: Braverman LE, Utiger RD, eds. *The Thyroid: A Fundamental and Clinical Text.* Philadelphia, PA: Lippincott Williams and Wilkins; 2005:229-263.

109. Leonard JL, Rosenberg IN. Thyroxine 5'deiodinase activity of rat kidney: observations on activation by thiols and inhibition by propylthiouracil. *Endocrinology.* 1978;103:2137-2144.

110. Saberi M, Sterling FH, Utiger RD. Reduction in extrathyroidal triiodothyronine production by propylthiouracil in man. *J Clin Invest.* 1975;55:218-223.

111. Kristensen BO, Weeke J. Propranolol-induced increments in total and free serum thyroxine in patients with essential hypertension. *Clin Pharmacol Ther.* 1977;22:864-867.

112. Cooper DS, Daniels GH, Ladenson PW, Ridgway EC. Hyperthyroxinemia in patients treated with high-dose propranolol. *Am J Med.* 1982;73:867-871.

113. Perrild H, Hansen JM, Skovsted L, Christensen LK. Different effects of propranolol, alprenolol, sotalol, atenolol and metoprolol on serum T3 and serum rT3 in hyperthyroidism. *Clin Endocrinol (Oxford).* 1983;18:139-142.

114. Cooper, DS, Klibanski, A, Ridgway, EC. Dopaminergic modulation of TSH and its subunits: in vivo and in vitro studies. *Clin Endocrinol.* 1983;18:265.

115. Agner T, Hagen C, Andersen AN, Djursing H. Increased dopaminergic activity inhibits basal and metoclopramide-stimulated prolactin and thyrotropin secretion. *J Clin Endocrinol Metab.* 1986;62:778-782.

116. Kerr DJ, Singh VK, McConway MG, et al. Circadian variation of thyrotrophin, determined by ultrasensitive immunoradiometric assay, and the effect of low dose nocturnal dopamine infusion. *Clin Sci.* 1987;72:737-741.

117. Kaptein EM, Spencer CA, Kamiel MB, et al. Prolonged dopamine administration and thyroid hormone economy in normal and critically ill subjects. *J Clin Endocrinol Metab.*1980;51(2):387-393.

118. Lee E, Chen P, Rao H, Brumeister LA. Effect of acute high dose dobutamine administration on serum thyrotrophin (TSH). *Clin Endocrinol (Oxford).* 1999;50:487-492.

119. Chanson P, Weintraub BD, Harris AG. Octreotide therapy for thyroid-stimulating hormone-secreting pituitary adenomas: a follow-up of 52 patients. *Ann Intern Med.* 1993;119:236-240.

120. Bertherat J, Brue T, Enjalbert A, et al. Somatostatin receptors on thyrotropin-secreting pituitary adenomas: comparison with the inhibitory effects of octreotide upon in vivo and in vitro hormonal secretions. *J Clin Endocrinol Metab.* 1992;75:540-546.

121. Vigersky RA, Filmore-Nassar A, Glass AR. Thyrotropin suppression by metformin. *J Clin Endocrinol Metab.*2006;91(1):225-227.

122. Brabant A, Brabant G, Schuermeyer T, et al. The role of glucocorticoids in the regulation of thyrotropin. *Acta Endocrinol Suppl (Copenhagen).* 1989;121:95-100.

123. Samuels MH, Luther M, Henry P, Ridgway EC. Effects of hydrocortisone on pulsatile pituitary glycoprotein secretion. *J Clin Endocrinol Metab.* 1994;78:211-215.

124. Wilber JF, Utiger RD. The effect of glucocorticoids on thyrotropin secretion. *J Clin Invest.* 1969;48:2096-2103.

125. LoPresti JS, Eigen A, Kaptein E, Aderson KP, Spencer CA, Nicoloff JT. Alterations in 3,3'5'-triiodothyronine metabolism in response to propylthiouracil, dexamethasone, and thyroxine administration in man. *J Clin Invest.* 1989;84:1650-1656.

126. Degroot LJ, Hoye K. Dexamethasone suppression of serum T3 and T4. *J Clin Endocrinol Metab.* 1976;42:976-978.

127. Gamstedt A, Jarnerot G, Kagedal B. Dose related effects of betamethasone on iodothyronines and thyroid hormone-binding proteins in serum. *Acta Endocrinol Suppl (Copenhagen).* 1981;96:484-490.

128. Duick DS, Warren DW, Nicoloff JT, Otis CL, Croxson MS. Effect of single dose dexamethasone on the concentration of serum triiodothyronine in man. *J Clin Endocrinol Metab.* 1974;39:1151-1154.

129. Chopra IJ, Williams DE, Orgiazzi J, Solomon DH. Opposite effects of dexamethasone on serum concentrations of 3,3'5'-triiodothyronine (reverse T3) and 3,3'5-triiodothyronine (T3). *J Clin Endocrinol Metab.* 1975;41:911-920.

130. Emerson CH, Seiler CM, Alex S, Fang SL, Mori Y, DeVito WJ. Gene expression and serum thyroxine-binding globulin are regulated by adrenal status and corticosterone in the rat. *Endocrinology.* September 1993;133(3):1192-1196.

131. Basaria S, Cooper DS. Amiodarone and the thyroid. *Am J Med.* 2005;118:706.

132. Martino E. Environmental iodine intake and thyroid dysfunction during chronic amiodarone therapy. *Ann Intern Med.* 1984;101:28.

133. Figge HL, Figge J. The effects of amiodarone on thyroid hormone function: a review of the physiology and clinical manifestations. *J Clin Pharmacol.* 1990;30:588-595.

134. Trip MD, Wiersinga W, Plomp TA. Incidence, predictability, and pathogenesis of amiodarone-induced thyrotoxicosis and hypothyroidism. *Am J Med.* 1991;91:507-511.

135. Nademanee K. Amiodarone, thyroid hormone indices, and altered thyroid function: long-term serial effects in patients with cardiac arrhythmias. *Am J Cardiol.* 1986;58:981.

136. Martino E, Bartalena L, Bogazzi F, Braverman LE. The effects of amiodarone on the thyroid. *Endocr Rev.* 2001;22:240.

137. Iervasi G, Cleric A, Manfredi C, Sabatino L, Biagini A, Chopra IJ. Acute effects of intravenous amiodarone on sulphate metabolites of thyroid hormones in arrhythmic patients. *Clin Endocrinol (Oxford).* 1997;47:699-705.

138. Martino E, Aghini-Lombardi F, Mariotti S, Bartalena L, Braverman L, Pinchera A. Amiodarone: a common source of iodine-induced thyrotoxicosis. *Horm Res.* 1987;26:158.

139. Martino E. Amiodarone iodine-induced hypothyroidism: risk factors and follow-up in 28 cases. *Clin Endocrinol.* 1987;26:227.

140. Dunn JT. Guarding our nation's thyroid health. *J Clin Endocrinol Metab.* 2002;87:486.

141. Dayan CM, Daniels GH. Chronic autoimmune thyroiditis. *N Engl J Med.* 1996;335:99.

142. Bartalena L, Brogioni S, Grasso L, Bogazzi F, Burelli A, Martino E. Treatment of amiodarone-induced thyrotoxicosis, a difficult challenge: results of a prospective study. *J Clin Endocrinol Metab.* 1996;81:2930-2933.

143. Harjai KJ, Licata AA. Effects of amiodarone on thyroid function. *Ann Intern Med.* 1997;126:63.

144. Bartalena L, Grasso L, Brogioni S, Aghini-Lombardi F, Braverman LE, Martino E. Serum interleukin-6 in amiodarone-induced thyrotoxicosis. *J Clin Endocrinol Metab.* 1994;78:423-427.

145. Kurnik D, Loebstein R, Farfel Z, Ezra D, Halkin H, Olchovsky D. Complex drug-drug-disease interactions between amiodarone, warfarin, and the thyroid gland. *Medicine (Baltimore).* 2004;83:107.

146. Drvota V, Carlsson B, Haggblad J, Sylven C. Amiodarone is a dose dependent noncompetitive and competitive inhibitor of T3 binding to thyroid hormone receptor subtype beta 1, whereas disopyramide, lignocaine, propafenone, metoprolol, dl-sotalol, and verapamil have no inhibitory effect. *J Cardiovasc Pharmacol.* 1995;26:222-226.

147. van Beeren HC, Bakker O, Wiersinga WM. Desethylamiodarone interferes with the binding of co-activator GRIP-1 to the beta 1-thyroid hormone receptor. *FEBS Lett.* 2000;481:213-216.

148. Sherman SI, Gopal J, Haugen BR, et al. Central hypothyroidism associated with retinoid X receptor-selective ligands. *N Engl J Med.* 1999;340:1075-1079.

149. Sharma V, Hays WR, Wood WM, et al. Effects of rexinoids on thyrotrope function and the hypothalamic-pituitary-thyroid axis. *Endocrinology.* 2006;147:1438-1451.

150. Golden WM, Weber KB, Hernandez TL, Sherman SI, Woodmansee WW, Haugen BR. Single-dose rexinoid rapidly and specifically suppresses serum thyrotropin in normal subjects. *J Clin Endocrinol Metab.* 2007;92:124-130.

151. Smit JW, Stokkel MP, Pereira AM, Romijn JA, Visser TJ. Bexarotene-induced hypothyroidism: bexarotene stimulates the peripheral metabolism of thyroid hormones. *J Clin Endocrinol Metab.* 2007;92:2496.

152. Aijan RA, Watson PF, Weetman AP. Cytokines and thyroid function. *Adv Neuroimmunol.* 1996;6:359-386.

153. Surks M, Sievert R. Drugs and thyroid function. *N Engl J Med.* 1995;33:1688-1695.

154. Burman P, Totterman TH, Orgerbg K, Karlsson FA. Thyroid autoimmunity in patients on long term therapy with leukocyte derived interferon. *J Clin Endocrinol Metab.* 1986;63:1086-1090.

155. Baudin E, Marcellin P, Pouteau M, et al. Reversibility of thyroid dysfunction induced by recombinant alpha interferon in chronic hepatitis C. *Clin Endocrinol (Oxford).* 1993;39:657-661.

156. Russo MW, Fried MW. Side effects of therapy for chronic hepatitis C. *Gastroenterology.* 2003;124:1711-1719.

157. Deutsch M, Dourakis S, Manesis EK, et al. Thyroid abnormalities in chronic vital hepatitis and their relationship to interferon alfa therapy. *Hepatology.* 1997;26:206-210.

158. Villanueva RB, Brau N. Graves opthalmopathy associated with interferon-alfa therapy for hepatitis C. *Thyroid.* 2002;12:737-738.

159. Rotondi M, Mazziotti G, Biondi B, et al. Long-term treatment with interferon-beta therapy for multiple sclerosis and occurrence of Graves' disease. *J Endocrinol Invest.* 2000;23:321-324.

160. Antonelli A, Ferri C, Pampana A, et al. Thyroid disorders in chronic hepatitis C. *Am J Med.* 2004;117(1):60-61.

161. Primo J, Hinojosu J, Moles JR, et al. Development of thyroid dysfunction after α-interferon treatment for chronic hepatitis C. *Am J Gastroenterol.* 1993;88:1976-1977.

162. Schultz M, Muller R, von zur Muhlen A, Brabant G. Induction of hyperthyroidism by interferon-α-2b. *Lancet.* 1989;1:1452.

163. Schwartzentruber DJ, White DE, Zweig MH, Wientraub BD, Rosenberg SA. Thyroid dysfunction associated with immunotherapy for patients with cancer. *Cancer.* 1991;68:2384-2390.

164. Vialettes B, Guillaerand MA, Viens P, et al. Incidence rate and risk factors for thyroid dysfunction durgin recombinant interleukin-2 therapy in advanced malignancies. *Acta Endocrinol (Copenhagen).* 1993;129:31-38.

165. Vassilopoulou-Sellin R, Sella A, Dexeus FH, et al. Acute thyroid dysfunction (thyroiditis) after therapy with interleukin-2. *Horm Metab Res* 1992;24:434-438.

166. Carella C, mazziotti G, Morisco F, et al. Long-term outcome of interferon-alpha-induced thyroid autoimmunity and prognostic influence of thyroid autoantibody pattern at the end of treatment. *J Clin Endocrinol Metab.* 2001;86:1925-1929.

167. Durelli L, Ferrero B, Oggero A, et al. Thyroid function and autoimmunity during interferon ß-1b treatment: a multicenter prospective study. *J Clin Endocrinol Metab.* 2001;86:3525-3532.

168. Atkins MB, Mier JW, Parkinson DR, Gould JA, Berkman EM, Kaplan MM. Hypothyrodism after treatment with interleukin-2 and lymphokine-activated killer cells. *N Engl J Med.* 1988;318:1557-1563.

169. Kruit WHJ, Bolhuis RLH, Goey SH, et al. Interleukin-2-induced thyroid dysfunction is correlated with treatment duration but not with tumor response. *J Clin Oncol.* 1993;11:921-924.

170. Pearce EN, Farwell AP, Braverman LE. Thyroiditis. *N Engl J Med.* 2003;348:2646-2654.

171. Ghori F, Polder KD, Pinter-Brown LC, et al. Thyrotoxicosis after denileukin diftitox therapy in patients with mycosis fungoides. *J Clin Endocrinol Metab.* 2006;91:2205-2208.

172. Kraiem Z, Sobel E, Sadeh O, et al. Effects of gamma-interferon on DR antigen expression, growth, 3,5,3'-triiodothyronine sercretion, iodide uptake and cyclic adenosine 3',5'-monophosphate accumulation in cultured human thyroid cells. *J Clin Endocrinol Metab.* 1990;71:817-824.

173. Kasuga Y, Masubayashi S, Akasu F, Miller N, Jamieson C, Volpe R. Effects of recombinant human interleukin-2 and tumor necrosis factor-alpha with or without interferon-gamma on human thyroid tissues from patients with Graves' disease and from normal subjects xenografted into nude mice. *J Clin Endocrinolo Metab.* 1991;72:1296-1301.

174. Mannavola D, Coco P, Vannucchi G, et al. A novel tyrosine-kinase selective inhibitor, sunitinib, induces transient hypothyroidism by blocking iodine uptake. *J Clin Endocrinol Metab.* 2007;92:3531-3534.

175. Desai J, Yassa L, Marqusee E, et al. Hypothyroidism after sunitinib treatment for patients with gastrointestinal stromal tumors. *Ann Intern Med.* 2006;145:660-664.

176. Vetter Ml, Kaul S, Iqbal N. Tyrosine kinase inhibitors and the thyroid as both an unintended and an intended target. *Endocr Pract.* July-August 2008;14(5):618-624.

177. Faris JE, Moore AF, Daniels GH. Sunitinib (Sutent)-induced thyrotoxicosis due to destructive thyroiditis: a case report. *Thyroid.* 2007;17:1-3.

178. Wong E, Rosen LS, Mulay M, et al. Sunitinib induces hypothyroidism in advanced cancer patients and may inhibit thyroid peroxidase activity. *Thyroid.* 2007;17:351-355.

179. Salem AK, Fenton MS, Marion KM, Hershman JM. Effect of sunitinib on growth and function of FRTL-5 thyroid cells. *Thyroid.* 2008;18:631-635.

180. de Groot JW, Links TP, van Der Graaf WT. Tyrosine kinase inhibitors causing hypothyroidism in a patient on levothyroxine. *Ann Oncol.* 2006;17:1719-1720.

181. de Groot JW, Zonnenberg BA, Plukker JT, van Der Graaf WT, Links TP. Imatinib induces hypothyroidism in patients receiving levoythyroxine. *Clin Pharmacol Ther.* 2005;78:433-438.

182. Sherman SI, Wirth LJ, Droz JP, et al. Motesanib diphosphate in progressive differentiated thyroid cancer. *N Engl J Med.* 2008;359:31-42.

183. Alexander IRW. Acute myxoedema. *BMJ.* 1961;ii:1434.

184. Lillicrap DA. Myxoedema after thalidomide (Distaval). *BMJ.* 1962;i:477.

185. Badros AZ, Siegel E, Bodenner D, et al. Hypothyroidism in patients with multiple myeloma following treatment with thalidomide. *Am J Med.* 2002;112:412-413.

186. Calabrese L, Fleischer AL. Thalidomide: current and potential clinical applications. *Am J Med.* 2000;108:487-495.

187. Somers GF. Pharmacological properties of thalidomide, a new sedative hypnotic drug. *Br J Pharmacol.* 1960;15:111-116.

188. Kelly DL, Conley RR. Thyroid function in treatment-resistant schizophrenia patients treated with quetiapine, risperidone or fluphenazine. *J Clin Psychiatry.* 2005;66:1334-1335.

189. Dobbs RL. Thyroid function alterations following quetiapine initiation in a developmentally disabled adolescent. *Ann Pharmacother.* 2004;38:1541-1542.

190. Benvenga S, Bartolone L, Squadrito S, Lo Giudice F, Trimarchi F. Delayed intestinal absorption of levothyroxine. *Thyroid.* 1995;5:249-253.

191. Sperber AD, Liel Y. Evidence for interference with the intestinal absorption of levothyroxine by aluminum hydroxide. *Arch Intern Med.* 1992;152:183-184.

192. Liel Y, Sperber AD, Shany S. Nonspecific intestinal adsorption of levothyroxine by aluminum hydroxide. *Am J Med.* 1994;97:363-365.

193. Sherman SI, Tielens ET, Ladenson PW. Sucralfate causes malabsorption of L-thyroxine. *Am J Med.* 1994;96:531-535.

194. Campbell JA, Schmidt BA, Bantle JP. Sucralfate and the absorption of L- thyroxine. *Ann Intern Med.* 1994;121:152-152.

195. Ananthakrishnan S, Braverman LE, Levin R, Magnani B, Pearce EN. The effect of famotidine, esomeprazole, and ezetimibe on levothyroxine absorption. *Thyroid.* 2008;18:493-498.

196. Centanni M, Gargano L, Canettieri G, et al. Thyroxine in goiter, Helicobacter pylori infection, and chronic gastritis. *N Engl J Med.* 2006;354:1787-1795.

197. Dietrich JW, Gieselbrecht K, Holl RW, Boehm BO. Absorption kinetics of levothyroxine is not altered by proton-pump inhibitor therapy. *Horm Metab Res.* 2006;38:57-59.

198. Sachmechi I, Reich DM, Aninyei M, Wibowo F, Gupta G, Kim PJ. Effect of proton pump inhibitors on serum thyroid-stimulating hormone level in euthyroid patients treated with levothyroxine for hypothyroidism. *Endocr Pract.* 2007;13:345-349.

199. Campbell NRC, Hasinoff BB, Stalts H, Rao B, Wong NC. Ferrous sulfate reduces thyroxine efficacy in patients with hypothyroidism. *Ann Intern Med.* 1992;117:1010-1013.

200. Singh N, Singh PN, Hershman JM. Effect of calcium carbonate on the absorption of levothyroxine. *JAMA.* 2000;283:2822-2825.

201. Singh N, Weisler SL, Hershman JM. The acute effect of calcium carbonate on the intestinal absorption of levothyrxoine. *Thyroid.* 2001;11:967-971.

202. John-Kalarickal J, Pearlman G, Carlson HE. New medications which decrease levothyroxine absorption. *Thyroid.* 2007;17:763-765.

203. Weitzman SP, Ginsburg KC, Carlson HE. New medications which interfere with the absorption of levothyroxine. Paper presented at: 90th Annual Meeting of Endocrine Society; June 2008 Stony Brook University, San Francisco, CA.

204. Siraj ES, Gupta MK, Reddy SSK. Raloxifene causing malabsorption of levothyroxine. *Arch Intern Med.* 2003;163:1387-137.

205. Harmon SM, Seifert CF. Levothyroxine-cholestyramine interaction reemphasized. *Ann Intern Med.* 1991;115:658-659.

206. Witztum JL, Jacobs LS, Schonfeld G. Thyroid hormone and thyrotropin levels in patients placed on colestipol hydrochloride. *J Clin Endocrinol Metab.* 1978;46:838-840.

207. Shakir KMM, Michaels RD, Hays JH, Potter BB. The use of bile acid sequestrants to lower serum thyroid hormones in iatrogenic hyperthyroidism. *Ann Intern Med.* 1993;118:112-113.

208. Newman CM, Price A, Davies DW, Gray TW, Weetman AP. Amiodarone and the thyroid: a practical guide to the management of thyroid dysfunction induced by amiodarone therapy. *Heart.* 1998;79:121-127.

209. Cappelli C, Rotundi M, Pirola I, Agosit B, Gandossi E, Valentini U, DeMartino E, Cimino A, Chiovato L, Agabiti-Rosei E, Castellano M. TSH-lowering effect of metformin in type 2 diabetic patients: differences between euthyroid, untreated hypothyroid and euthyroid on L-T4 therapy patients. *Diabetes Care.* 2009 Sep;32(9):1589-1590.

Index

Lightning Source UK Ltd.
Milton Keynes UK
UKOW07f1459121214

243071UK00003B/15/P